McGraw-Hill's
EMT-Basic

Second Edition

Peter A. DiPrima, Jr., EMT-P
Instructor, Suffolk County Emergency Medical Services
Paramedic/Firefighter
Lakeland Fire Department
Suffolk County, New York

George P. Benedetto, Jr., DHA(c), EMT-P, MPA
Director, Simulation Laboratory
New York Hospital Queens
Flushing, New York

 Medical

New York   Chicago   San Francisco   Lisbon   London   Madrid   Mexico City   Milan   New Delhi
San Juan   Seoul   Singapore   Sydney   Toronto

McGraw-Hill's EMT-Basic, Second Edition

1 2 3 4 5 6 7 8 9 0   QDB/QDB   14 13 12 11

ISBN 978-0-07-175127-8
MHID 0-07-175127-0

Notice

Medicine is an ever-changing science. As new research and clinical experience broaden our knowledge, changes in treatment and drug therapy are required. The authors and the publisher of this work have checked with sources believed to be reliable in their efforts to provide information that is complete and generally in accord with the standards accepted at the time of publication. However, in view of the possibility of human error or changes in medical sciences, neither the authors nor the publisher nor any other party who has been involved in the preparation or publication of this work warrants that the information contained herein is in every respect accurate or complete, and they disclaim all responsibility for any errors or omissions or for the results obtained from use of the information contained in this work. Readers are encouraged to confirm the information contained herein with other sources. For example and in particular, readers are advised to check the product information sheet included in the package of each drug they plan to administer to be certain that the information contained in this work is accurate and that changes have not been made in the recommended dose or in the contraindications for administration. This recommendation is of particular importance in connection with new or infrequently used drugs.

This book was set in Minion by Glyph International.
The editors were Kirsten Funk and Robert Pancotti.
The production supervisor was Sherri Souffrance.
Project management was provided by Ranjit Kaur, Glyph International.
The text designer was Eve Siegel; the cover designer was Handel Low.
Quad/Graphics was printer and binder.

This book is printed on acid-free paper.

Library of Congress Cataloging-in-Publication Data

DiPrima, Peter A., Jr., author.
   McGraw-Hill's EMT-basic / Peter A. DiPrima Jr.,
George P. Benedetto Jr., —Second Edition.
      p. ; cm.
   EMT-basic
   Emergency medical technician-basic
   Includes bibliographical references and index.
   ISBN-13: 978-0-07-175127-8 (pbk. : alk. paper)
   ISBN-10: 0-07-175127-0 (pbk. : alk. paper)   1. Emergency medical technicians—Examinations, questions, etc.
  2. Emergency medicine—Examinations, questions, etc.   I. Benedetto, George P., Jr., author.   II. Title.   III. Title: EMT-basic.
IV Title: Emergency medical technician-basic.
   [DNLM: 1. Emergency Medical Services—United States—Examination Questions.   2. Emergencies—United States—
Examination Questions.   3. Emergency Medical Technicians—United States—Examination Questions.   4. Emergency Treatment—
United States—Examination Questions. WB 18.2]
   RC86.9.D56 2011
   616.02'5076—dc22

                                  2010050482

McGraw-Hill books are available at special quantity discounts to use as premiums and sales promotions, or for use in corporate training programs. To contact a representative, please e-mail us at bulksales@mcgraw-hill.com.

To my wife, Sue, and our children, Gabrielle and Jack, thank you for being there, with love.

PAD

To my daughter, Alessandra (Ale), you are the center of my universe and the reason I exist.
To my brothers and sisters, Nancy, George-Anne (Jan), Michael, Christopher, James, RoseMarie, and Paul, thank you for your loving support and encouragement; and to Angela, Anna, Christopher, and Peter, you four have made my life and career come full circle. I love and cherish you all so very much.
To Nayna Shah and Kenneth M. Rifkind, MD, FACS, my teachers, mentors, and friends for life. Thank you.

GPB

CONTENTS

*Online Practice Exam at **www.mcgrawhillemt.com***

PREFACE

The emergency medical technician performs a very unique service at the scene of an emergency, which cannot be rendered by any other emergency services profession. The concept of the team approach is important in responding to emergencies in the pre-hospital environment. Each health-care professional must not only perform the duties of his or her own role, but must understand the roles of other professionals involved. Everyone must work together in a coordinated and efficient manner to achieve optimal results for patient survival.

This review book is a complete resource for EMT-B training, which contains reader-friendly step-by-step explanations with comprehensive, stimulating, and challenging material that prepares and equips users for real on-the-job situations. With its use of the case study model, and the inclusion of areas above and beyond the DOT curriculum, this new, second edition of *McGraw-Hill's EMT-Basic* prepares users for success. Topics covered include an excellent introductory section that contains an overview of the human body, baseline vital signs, history taking, and ethical and legal issues. Subsequent chapters cover the airway; patient assessment; medical, behavioral, and obstetrics/gynecology; trauma; infants and children; operations; and advanced airway management. In addition, we have added a robust practice examination at the end of the book, which will assist the new or seasoned EMT in studying for their local state or national registry examination.

A free practice exam is also available online to help you prepare for exam day. Visit www.mcgrawhillemt.com to take the test and assess your results.

The review book also provides the theory adapted by the American Heart Association, Guidelines for Cardiopulmonary Resuscitation and Emergency Cardiovascular Care, the National Incident Management System, and updated hazardous materials information for the first responder.

We hope you enjoy utilizing this book as an adjunct learning tool. Be safe!

Peter A. DiPrima, Jr., EMT-P
George P. Benedetto, Jr., EMT-P

Exam Preparation Tips

Start studying now! Give yourself ample time to prepare by arranging your notes and making sure you have covered all the required course material. Organize all information that was given to you during your course—this includes textbooks, lecture notes, handouts, and the like.

ANATOMY OF A MULTIPLE-CHOICE QUESTION

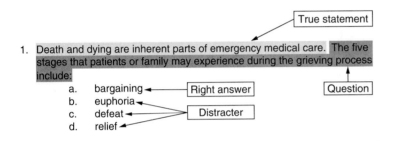

THE DO'S AND DON'TS OF ANSWERING MULTIPLE-CHOICE QUESTIONS

Do's

- If the question is "theoretical" carefully read and understand the stem of the question before looking at the alternatives. Circle or underline key words in the stem. Use your knowledge of headings to think about where in your text, lecture notes, etc. that question is drawn from. Recall a few relevant points about the information. This does not have to take much time but this recall is an essential step!

- Predict an answer, if possible.

- Uncover all of the alternatives and check the format of the question. Are one of the alternatives correct or can several or all of the alternatives be correct?

- Read each alternative carefully for understanding. Pay careful attention to qualifying words. Keeping the stem of the question in mind, respond to each alternative with a yes, no, or maybe/not sure.

- If you know the answer, carefully mark the correct answer on your answer sheet.

- If you do not know the answer, re-check the stem of the question. Narrow your choices, by eliminating any alternative that you know is incorrect. If two options still look equally tempting, compare each to the stem of the question, making sure that the one you eventually choose answers what is asked.

- If you are still not sure, make an educated guess.

- If you were unable to make a choice and need to spend more time with the question, or you answered the question but are not at all sure that you made the correct choice, put a big question mark beside that question, and move on to the next. Avoid getting bogged down on one question part of the way through the exam. It is much better to move on and finish all of those questions that you can answer and then to come back later to process the problematic questions. If necessary, when looking over the questions again, change an answer ONLY if you can logically justify the change.

Don'ts

- Don't select an alternative just because you remember learning the information in the course; it may be a "true" statement in its own right, but you have to make sure that it is the "correct" answer to the question.
- Don't pick an answer just because it seems to make sense.
- Don't dismiss an alternative answer because it seems too obvious and simple.
- Don't be wowed by fancy terms in the question.
- Don't pick "c" every time you are unsure of the answer.
- Don't pick your answer based on a pattern of responses.

PHYSICAL PREPARATION

It is crucial to know the material to pass the exam, but it is equally important to be prepared physically as well. Physical preparation includes staying healthy, getting adequate sleep, eating balanced meals, and exercising regularly. Reward yourself after a successful study session.

Finally, keep anxiety in check! Stretch, breathe deeply, breathe often, take frequent short breaks, and stay positive.

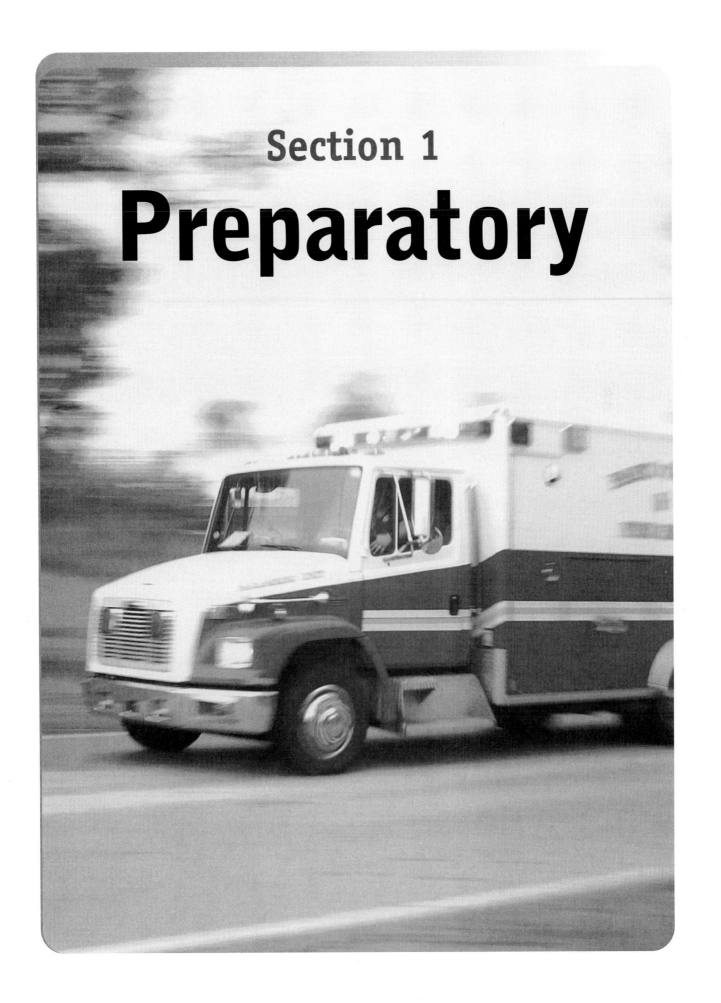

Section 1

Preparatory

Chapter 1
Introduction to Emergency Care

It is 5 AM on an already hot summer morning. An elderly woman wakes up to start her day. She rolls over to attempt to wake her husband who is due to go out for some early golf with his friends. She attempts to wake him, with no response. She nervously begins to shake him and yell his name, no response. She notices his face is cyanotic (blue) and he is not breathing, she yells for help and runs across the room to find the bedroom phone. She dials 911 frantically and begins giving the 911 operator her address and phone number. The emergency medical services (EMS) operator ascertains the medical complaint and prioritizes the assignment. A first-responder unit and a basic and advanced life support unit are dispatched for a priority assignment, "Elderly Male Unconscious, Not Breathing." The elderly woman is asked to stay on the phone and begin resuscitation efforts through the direction of the emergency medical dispatcher.

EARLY HISTORY OF EMERGENCY MEDICAL SERVICES

Throughout the evolution of paramedicine, there has been an ongoing association with military conflict. One of the first indications of a formal process for managing injured people dates from the Imperial Legions of Rome, where aging Centurions, no longer able to fight, were tasked with organizing the removal of the wounded from the battlefield and providing some form of care. Such individuals, although not physicians, were probably among the world's earliest surgeons, suturing wounds and completing amputations, not through training, but by default. This trend would continue throughout the Crusades, with the Knights Hospitallers of the Order of St. John of Jerusalem, known throughout the Commonwealth of Nations today as St. John Ambulance, filling a similar function.

The first vehicle that was specifically designed as an ambulance was created during the Napoleonic War, and called the *ambulance volante*. Created by Napoleon's Chief Surgeon, Baron Dominique Jean Larrey, this new horse-drawn contrivance was intended to transport the wounded rapidly to surgeons, waiting at the rear. Such vehicles were seen by the military as a general resource, and care of the wounded was not given much priority; it was not uncommon for such vehicles to be tasked with carrying fresh ammunition to the battlefront, before they transported the wounded back. The basic design of such vehicles remained unchanged for nearly 100 years.

Early Civilian Ambulance Services

While communities had organized to deal with the care and transportation of the sick and dying as far back as the plague in London, England (1598, 1665), such arrangements were typically temporary. In time, however, such arrangements began to formalize and become permanent. During the American Civil War, Jonathan Letterman had devised a system of forward first aid stations at the regimental level, where principles of triage were first instituted. Letterman, with the rank of major, served as the medical director of the Army of the Potomac. The United States Army had reeled from inefficient treatment of casualties, in part because of the adoption of new firearm technology such as breech-loading rifles and Minié ball systems. Letterman established mobile field hospitals to be located at division and corps headquarters. This was all connected by an efficient ambulance corps, established by him in August 1862, under the control of medical staff instead of the Quartermaster Department. He also arranged an efficient system for the distribution of medical supplies. His system was adopted by other Union armies and was eventually officially established as the medical procedure for the entirety of the United States' armies by an Act of Congress in March 1864.

Following the American Civil War, some veterans began to attempt to apply what they had seen on the battlefield to their own communities, through the creation of volunteer life-saving squads and ambulance corps. This translation to civilian use did not occur in the same way everywhere; in Britain, early civilian ambulances were often operated by the local hospital or police, while in some parts of Canada, it was common for the local undertaker (having the only transport in town in which one could lie down) to operate both the local furniture store (making coffins as a sideline) and the local ambulance service. In larger centers in various countries, such services might fall to the local Health Department, Police, Fire Department, or some combination of all of the above. Once again, the civilian model followed the lead of the military; although there were a handful of motorized ambulances just prior to the First World War (1914-1918), the concept of motorized ambulances was proven first on the battlefield, and spread rapidly to civilian systems immediately following the war.

There is some debate as to when the first formal training of "ambulance attendants" began. The generally accepted belief is that this occurred in the United States, at Roanoke, Virginia, with the Roanoke Life Saving and First Aid Crew, under Julian Stanley Wise, in 1928. While this may have been true of the United States, Canadian records indicate the members of the Toronto Police Ambulance Service received a mandatory 5 days of training, conducted by St. John, as early as 1889, and well-developed printed manuals, clearly beyond the scope of simple first aid, were present in England even earlier. In terms of advanced skills, it is known that, once again, the military led the way. During the Second World War (1939-1945) and the Korean Conflict, battlefield 'medics' were administering painkilling narcotics by injection, as emergency procedures, and 'pharmacists' mates on warships without physicians were permitted to do even more. Korea also marked the first widespread use of helicopters to evacuate the wounded from forward positions to medical units, coining the phrase 'medevac.' These innovations would not find their way into the civilian sphere for nearly 20 more years.

PRE-HOSPITAL MEDICINE

By the early 1960s, experiments in improving care had begun in some civilian centers. The first such experiment involved the provision of pre-hospital cardiac care by physicians in Belfast, Northern Ireland, in 1966. This was repeated in Toronto, Canada in 1968, using a single ambulance called Cardiac One, staffed by a regular ambulance crew, plus a hospital intern, who was tasked with performing the advanced procedures. While both of these experiments had certain levels of success, technology had not yet reached the required level (the Toronto 'portable' defibrillator/heart monitor was powered by lead-acid car batteries and weighed nearly 100 lb.). The required telemetry and miniaturization technologies already existed in the military, and particularly in the space program, but it would take several more years before they found their way to civilian applications. In North America, physicians were judged to be too expensive to be used in the pre-hospital setting, although such initiatives were implemented, and in some cases still operate, in the United Kingdom, Europe, and Latin America.

Around 1966, in a published report entitled "Accidental Death and Disability: The Neglected Disease of Modern Society," (known in EMS trade as the "White Paper") medical researchers began to reveal, to their astonishment, that soldiers who were seriously wounded on the battlefields of Vietnam had a better survival rate than those individuals who were seriously injured in motor vehicle accidents on California freeways. Early research attributed these differences in outcome to a number of factors, including comprehensive trauma care, rapid transport to designated trauma facilities, and a new type of medical corpsman, one who was trained to perform certain critical advanced medical procedures such as fluid replacement and airway management, which allowed the victim to survive the journey to definitive care. As a result, a series of grand experiments began in the United States. Almost simultaneously, and completely independent from one another, experimental programs began in a handful of US centers: Miami, Florida; Seattle, Washington; and Los Angeles, California. The first of these to go from being an experiment to being a working unit was in Los Angeles. With the passage of the Wedsworth-Townsend Act, other states would soon push their own paramedic bills through, and soon, every fire department in every major city in the country had their own paramedic squads. Each was aimed at determining the effectiveness of using firefighters to perform many of these same advanced medical skills in the pre-hospital setting in the civilian world. Many in the senior administration of the fire departments were initially quite opposed to this concept of 'firemen giving needles,' and actively resisted and attempted to cancel pilot programs more than once.

THE PUBLIC DISCOVERS "EMS AND PARAMEDICINE"

In a curious example of life imitating art, television producer Robert A. Cinader, working for producer Jack Webb of *Dragnet* and *Adam-12*, happened to be in Los Angeles' UCLA Harbor Medical Center, doing background research for a proposed new TV show about doctors, when he happened to encounter these 'firemen who spoke like doctors and worked with them.' This novel idea would eventually evolve into the *Emergency!* television series, which ran from 1972 to 1977, portraying the exploits of a new group called 'paramedics.' The show captured the imagination of emergency services personnel, the medical community, and the general public. When the show first aired in 1972, there were exactly six paramedic units operating in three pilot programs in the entire United States. No one had ever heard the term 'paramedic'; it is reported that one of the show's actors was initially concerned that the 'para' part of the term might involve jumping out of airplanes. By the time the program ended production in 1977, there were paramedics operating in every state. The show's technical advisor was a pioneer of paramedicine, James O. Page, then a Battalion Chief responsible for the paramedic program, but who would go on to help establish other paramedic programs in the United States, and to become the founding publisher of the *Journal of Emergency Medical Services* (JEMS).

Evolution and Growth

Throughout the 1970s and 1980s, the field continued to evolve, although in large measure on a local level. In the broader scheme of things the term *ambulance service* was replaced by *emergency medical service* in order to reflect the change from a transportation system to a system which provided actual medical care. The training, knowledge base, and skill sets of both paramedics and emergency medical technicians (both competed for the job title, and 'EMT-Paramedic' was a common compromise) were typically determined by what local medical directors were comfortable with, what it was felt that the community needed, and what could actually be afforded. There were also tremendous local differences in the amount and type of training required, and how it would be provided. This ranged from in-service training in local systems, through community colleges, and ultimately even to universities. In the United States, the community college training model remains the most common, although university-based paramedic education models continue to evolve. These variations in both educational approaches and standards led to tremendous differences from one location to another, and at its worst, created a situation in which a group of people with 120 hours of training, and another group (in another jurisdiction) with university degrees, were both calling themselves paramedics, there were some efforts made to resolve these discrepancies. The National Association of Emergency Medical Technicians (NAEMT) along with National Registry of Emergency Medical Technicians (NREMT) attempted to create a national standard by means of a common licensing examination, but to this day, this has never been universally accepted by all states, and issues of licensing reciprocity for paramedics continue. Nevertheless, if an EMT obtains certification through NREMT (NREMT-P, NREMT-I, NREMT-B), this is accepted by 40 of the 50 states in the United States. This confusion was further complicated by the introduction of complex systems of gradation of certification, reflecting levels of training and skill, but these too were for the most part purely local. The only truly common trend that would evolve was the relatively universal acceptance of the term Emergency Medical Technician being used to denote a lower level of training and skill than a Paramedic. In the UK, paramedics are being developed further, so a basic qualification of a paramedic is a foundation degree or diploma at university. Paramedics in the UK can now develop further to "Emergency Care Practitioner" and "Critical Care Practioner," providing extra clinical skills to their patients.

During the evolution of paramedicine, a great deal of both curriculum and skill set was in a state of constant flux. Permissible skills evolved in many cases at the local level, and were based upon the preferences of physician advisers and medical directors. Treatments would go in and out of fashion, and sometimes back in again. In some respects, the development seemed almost faddish. Technologies also evolved and changed, and as medical equipment manufacturers quickly learned, the pre-hospital environment was not the same as the hospital environment; equipment standards which worked fine in hospitals could not cope well with the less controlled pre-hospital environment. Physicians began to take more interest in paramedics from a research perspective as well. By about 1990, most of the trendiness in pre-hospital emergency care had begun to disappear, and was replaced by outcome-based research; the gold standard for the rest of medicine. This research began to drive the evolution of the practice of both paramedics and the emergency physicians who oversaw their work; changes to procedures and protocols began to occur only after significant outcome-based research demonstrated their need. Such changes affected everything from simple procedures, such as cardiopulmonary resuscitation (CPR), to changes in drug protocols. As the profession of paramedicine grew, some of its members actually went on to become not just research participants, but researchers in their own right, with their own projects and journal publications.

Changes in procedures also included the manner in which the work of paramedics was overseen and managed. In the earliest days of the field, medical control and oversight was direct and immediate, with paramedics calling into a local hospital and receiving orders for every individual procedure or drug. This still occurs in some jurisdictions, but is becoming very rare. As physicians began to build a bond of trust with paramedics, and experience in working with them, their confidence levels also rose. Increasingly, in many jurisdictions, day-to-day operations moved from direct and immediate medical control to pre-written protocols or 'standing orders,' with the paramedic typically only calling in for direction after the options in the standing orders had been exhausted. Medical oversight became driven more by chart review or rounds, than by step-by-step control during each call.

EMS SYSTEM

- EMS over the past 30 years has changed considerably.
- As an essential part of the EMS system, EMTs are usually one of the first medical professionals encountered by patients.

What Is an EMS System?

- EMS is a network of coordinated medical services that provide support and medical care to a given community.
- National Highway Traffic Safety Administration (NHTSA) Technical Assistance Program Standards for EMS include:
  1. Integration of health services
  2. EMS research
  3. Legislation and regulation
  4. System finance
  5. Human resources
  6. Medical direction
  7. Education systems
  8. Public education
  9. Prevention
  10. Public access
  11. Communication systems
  12. Clinical care
  13. Information systems
  14. Evaluation

Components of an EMS System

The "911" system emergency telephone number is utilized to gain access to emergency services such as fire, police, and EMS. Access to the EMS includes:

- Activation by citizens
- Dispatch of resources
- Out-of-hospital care (pre-hospital care)

- Transition of care (transfer of care between pre-hospital and in-hospital health-care providers)
- In-hospital care
- Rehabilitation

In some regions a nonemergent telephone number has been instituted, such as 311 in New York City.

There are four national recognized levels of pre-hospital care. They include:

1. First Responder (minimal training for emergencies)
2. EMT-Basic
3. EMT-Intermediate
4. EMT-Paramedic (highest level of pre-hospital care)

In various states other levels of training are available (ie, EMT-Cardiac Care).

KEY COMPONENTS OF A HEALTH-CARE SYSTEM

Emergency department (ED).

- Specialty facilities such as
  - Trauma centers
  - Burn centers
  - Pediatric centers
  - Poison centers
  - Other specialty centers—locally dependent (ie, venomous bite center, hyperbaric center, cardiac centers, stroke centers, etc.)
- Hospital personnel include:
  - Physicians
  - Nurses and other health professionals (physician assistant, respiratory therapist, nurse practitioners)

EMS personnel must be able to interact with other public safety workers; some examples include:

- Local law enforcement
- State and federal law enforcement
- Federal Emergency Management Agency (FEMA)—A division within the Department of Homeland Security
- Department of Homeland Security (DHS)

The roles and responsibilities of the EMT include:

- Personal safety (safety of crew, patient, and bystanders)
- Patient assessment
- Patient care based on assessment findings
- Lifting and moving patients safely
- Transport/transfer of care (transition of care)
- Record keeping/data collection
- Patient advocacy (protecting patient rights)

As an extension of the emergency department, EMTs are required to maintain professional attributes, such as:

- Neat and clean appearance
- A positive image

Clinical Significance

Review local and/or state emergency and nonemergency access phone numbers.

Clinical Significance

EMS is an extension of the emergency department.

- Up-to-date knowledge and skills, which includes continual medical education (CME), attending seminars, EMS regional updates
- Patient's needs prioritized without endangering self/crew
- Current knowledge of local, state, and national issues affecting EMS

QUALITY IMPROVEMENT

Quality improvement (QI) is a system of internal/external reviews and audits of all aspects of an EMS system. QI is important to an EMS system to identify aspects needing improvement; this ensures that the public receives the highest quality of pre-hospital care. Our role as EMTs in quality improvement includes:

- Neat, legible, and accurate documentation
- Attending CME that includes run review and call audits
- Gathering feedback from patients and hospital staff
- Conducting preventive maintenance
- Maintaining mastery skills performance

Clinical Significance

The goal of quality improvement is to *improve* patient care, not find fault.

ROLES OF THE SYSTEM MEDICAL DIRECTOR

The system medical director is a physician responsible for the clinical and patient care aspects of an EMS system or service.

- Every ambulance service/rescue squad must have physician medical direction. Types of medical direction include:
  - On-line (telephone, cell phone, satellite phone)
  - Radio (ultra high frequency [UHF], very high frequency [VHF] radio)
  - Off-line (standing orders, protocols)
- The relationship of the EMT and the systems medical director:
  - An EMT is the designated agent of the physician.
  - Care rendered is considered an extension of the medical director's authority (varies by state law). The EMT should review specific statutes and regulations regarding EMS in their state regarding specific health laws.

The system medical director is directly responsible for reviewing quality improvement.

? CHAPTER QUESTIONS

1. One important responsibility of the EMT is *patient advocacy*. This means the emergency provider is responsible for:

   a. providing emergency medical care

   b. gaining access to the patient

   c. ensuring scene safety by wearing body substance isolation

   d. protecting the patient's rights

2. A physician who is legally responsible for the clinical and patient care rendered by an EMS system is known as the systems:

   a. System medical director
   b. clinical manager
   c. chief medical officer (CMO)
   d. none of the above

3. The National Highway Traffic Safety Administration (NHTSA) provides suggested standards for EMS systems called the "Technical Assistance Program Assessment Standards." Which of the following is included as a standard of the NHTSA:

   a. system access
   b. EMS medical direction
   c. maintenance
   d. scheduling of personnel

4. Quality improvement includes finding fault of an EMT who is producing illegible ambulance run reports.

   a. True
   b. False

Chapter 2
Well-Being of the EMT

In the previous chapter, you and your partner responded to an elderly male in cardiac arrest. Upon arrival at the scene you evaluate scene safety, and determine the scene is safe to operate. You and your partner enter the apartment to find an elderly woman hysterically crying, screaming, "why me!" She is frantically attempting to perform cardiopulmonary resuscitation (CPR). You evaluate the elderly patient and determine whether he meets the criteria for obvious death. The elderly woman, distraught and angry, starts yelling and screaming at you and your partner. What should your next step be?

The myth of saving lives . . .

Somewhere along the way, the myth of saving lives found its way into the EMS profession. There are indeed times when EMS saves lives, but even in large EMS systems, this is by no means a daily occurrence. The vast majority of EMS providers are called upon simply to take care of people in need. Sometimes those needs are met with a combination of advanced invasive procedures, sophisticated pharmacology, and technical expertise. Other times, what a patient may need is a caring attitude, a few kind words, or safe transportation to an extended-care facility. Between these two extremes lie many shades of gray. One measure of an outstanding EMS professional is the ability to perceive a patient's real needs and to meet them.[1]

EMOTIONAL ASPECTS OF EMERGENCY CARE

Emergency medical technicians (EMTs) encounter death more frequently than the average person. As health-care professionals, we have very little training in dealing with people's emotions when they have lost a friend or family member. Dealing with a grieving family is quite difficult, and at times impossible. Therefore, understanding how to treat and react during these difficult times may allow us to better cope with survivors and their families.

The grieving process has five distinct or predictable stages. They are:

1. *Denial* ("Not me.")—Defense mechanism creating a buffer between shock of dying and dealing with the illness/injury.
2. *Anger* ("Why me?")—EMTs may be the target of the anger. Don't take anger or insults personally, be tolerant, and do not become defensive. Employ good listening and communication skills. Be empathetic.
3. *Bargaining* ("OK, but first let me . . .")—Agreement that, in the patient's mind, will postpone the death for a short time.

4. *Depression* ("OK, but I haven't . . .")—Characterized by sadness and despair. The patient is usually silent and retreats into his own world.

5. *Acceptance* ("OK, I am not afraid.")—Does not mean the patient will be happy about dying. The family will usually require more support during this stage than the patient.

Dealing with the needs of a dying patient and/or their family members includes performing the following:

- Show respect—Keep an open line of communication and allow the patient and family a means for privacy.
- Treat them with dignity by allowing them to feel in control.
- Family members may express rage, anger, and despair.
- Listen empathetically.
- Do not offer false reassurance.
- Use a gentle tone of voice.
- Let the patient know everything that can be done to help will be done.
- Use a reassuring touch, if appropriate.
- Comfort the family.
- Be respectful of religious beliefs and, when possible, honor requests of the family while adhering to regional or state protocols.

STRESS

In addition to responding to day-to-day assignments, EMTs encounter stressful situations while performing their duties. Examples of situations that may produce a stress response include:

- Mass casualty situations (ie, Oklahoma City bombing, September 11, Hurricane Katrina, Fort Hood Shooting, West Virginia mine explosion, etc.)
- Infant and child trauma (ie, child struck by a car)
- Amputations
- Infant/child/elder/spouse abuse
- Death/injury of coworker or other public safety personnel

The EMT will experience personal stress as well as encounter patients and bystanders in severe distress. Therefore, understanding how to manage stress and stressful situations is paramount. Remember, what constitutes an emergency to others may not necessarily be an emergency to you; be respectful!

Stress Management

EMTs should recognize warning signs of stress:

- Irritability to coworkers, family, friends
- Inability to concentrate
- Difficulty sleeping/nightmares
- Anxiety
- Indecisiveness
- Guilt
- Loss of appetite
- Loss of interest in sexual activity
- Isolation
- Loss of interest in work

Keeping Stress Under Control

Reducing stress by making lifestyle changes is helpful for "burnout." Lifestyle changes include:

- Changing your diet
- Reducing sugar, caffeine, and alcohol intake
- Avoiding fatty foods
- Increasing carbohydrates
- Exercising regularly
- Practicing relaxation techniques, meditation, and visual imagery
- Balancing work, recreation, family, health, and the like

Work environment changes can reduce stress.

- Request work shifts allowing for more time to relax with family and friends.
- Request a rotation of duty assignment to a less busy area.
- Seek/refer professional help (employee assistance program [EAP]).

CRITICAL INCIDENT RESPONSE

Critical incident stress debriefing (CISD) or critical incident stress management (CISM) is a team of peer counselors and mental health professionals who help emergency care workers deal with critical incident stress.

A meeting is held within 24 to 72 hours of a major incident.

- Open discussion of feelings, fears, and reactions.
- Not an investigation or interrogation.
- All information is confidential.
- CISD leaders and mental health personnel evaluate the information and offer suggestions on overcoming the stress.

CISD/CISM is designed to accelerate the normal recovery process after experiencing a critical incident.

- Works well because feelings are ventilated quickly.
- Debriefing environment is nonthreatening.
- The EMT should review how to access their local CISD system.

Comprehensive critical incident stress management includes:

- Preincident stress education
- On-scene peer support
- One-on-one support
- Disaster support services
- Defusing
- CISD
- Follow-up services
- Spouse/family support
- Community outreach programs
- Other health and welfare programs such as the employee assistance program (EAP)

Clinical Significance

Universal precautions involve the use of protective barriers such as gloves, gowns, aprons, masks, or protective eyewear, which can reduce the risk of exposure of the health-care worker's skin or mucous membranes to potentially infective materials. In addition, under universal precautions, it is recommended that all health-care workers take precautions to prevent injuries caused by needles, scalpels, and other sharp instruments or devices.

SCENE SAFETY

Body Substance Isolation (Bio-Hazard)

EMT and Patient Safety Takes Priority!

- Hand washing before and after an assignment is the number-one way to prevent transmission of infection or disease.
- Any infectious waste should be disposed of in a bio-hazard container (Fig. 2-1a)
- Eye protection (Fig. 2-1b)
  - Eye protection must be worn when there is a chance for an eye injury to occur (ie, broken glass in a motor vehicle collision).
  - If prescription eyeglasses are worn, removable side shields can be applied to them.
  - Goggles are *not* required, but should be worn when bodily fluids are present.
- Gloves (Fig. 2-1c)
  - Gloves (vinyl or latex) should be worn on every assignment to reduce the risk of exposure.
  - Gloves must be worn when there is any contact with blood or body fluids.
  - Gloves should be changed in between contact with different patients.
  - Gloves (utility).
- Gowns (Fig. 2-1d) are needed for large splash situations such as with field delivery and major trauma.
- Masks (Fig. 2-1e)
  - Surgical type for possible blood splatter (worn by care provider)
  - High efficiency particulate air (HEPA) respirator if patient suspected for or diagnosed with tuberculosis (worn by care provider)
  - Airborne disease—surgical type mask (worn by patient)

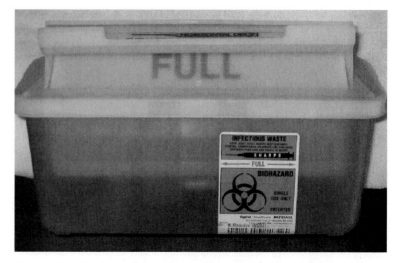

Figure 2-1a   Sharps container. *(Used with permission from Peter DiPrima.)*

Figure 2-1b Eye protection. *(Used with permission from Peter DiPrima.)*

- Requirements and availability of specialty training:
  - Hazardous Waste Operations and Emergency Response standard (HAZWOPER) training.
  - Review Occupational Safety and Health Administration (OSHA)/state regulations regarding body substance isolation (BSI).
  - Review local notification and testing in an exposure incident.

Clinical Significance

Vinyl gloves/nitrile gloves should be utilized if the EMT has a latex allergy. Latex precautions should also be observed when confronted with a patient with latex allergies.

Figure 2-1c Gloves. *(Used with permission from Peter DiPrima.)*

Figure 2-1d   Gown. *(Used with permission from Peter DiPrima.)*

Figure 2-1e   Mask. *(Used with permission from Peter DiPrima.)*

PERSONAL PROTECTION AT HAZARDOUS MATERIALS INCIDENTS

- Identify possible hazards from a distance.
- Carrying binoculars on the ambulance is good for assessing a scene at a distance.
- Placards located on buildings or trucks aid in the identification of substances (Fig. 2-2).
- Carry the most updated version of the *Emergency Response Guidebook*, published by the United States Department of Transportation (Fig. 2-3).[2]

PROTECTIVE CLOTHING FOR HAZ-MAT INCIDENTS

- Haz-mat incidents require specialized hazardous material (haz-mat) suits.
- Haz-mat incidents require special training in the use of Self Contained Breathing Apparatus (SCBA).
- Haz-mat scenes are controlled by specialized haz-mat teams.

EMTs provide emergency care only after the scene is safe and patient contamination has been eliminated. EMS personnel not operating in the capacity of a haz-mat response team should operate in the "cold zone." Review Chapter 41 for an in-depth review of haz-mat operating zones.

RESPONSIBILITY AT RESCUE INCIDENTS

Identify and reduce potential life threats, such as:

- Downed electrical lines
- Fire
- Explosion
- Haz-mat

Figure 2-2 Placard example. *(Used with permission from Peter DiPrima.)*

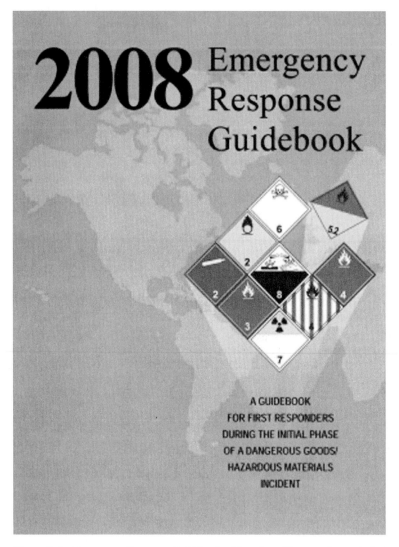

Figure 2-3   Emergency Response Guidebook. *(From http://hazmat.dot.gov/pubs/ erg/gydebook.htm.)*

EMTs should request assistance from trained personnel early in an incident. EMTs should wear proper protective clothing such as:

- Turnout gear
- Puncture-proof gloves
- Helmet
- Eyewear

OPERATIONS AT THE SCENE OF A VICTIM OF VIOLENCE ASSIGNMENT

Scene security should always be controlled by law enforcement before the EMT provides patient care. Violence toward EMS personnel can occur when:

- Perpetrator of the crime is still on the scene
- Bystanders interfere with patient care
- Family members interfere with patient care

Behavior at a crime scene:

- Do not disturb the scene unless required for medical care.
- Maintain the chain of evidence.
- When in doubt, request assistance from law enforcement.

PROTECTION FROM COMMUNICABLE DISEASES

Routes of transmission for communicable diseases:

- Direct contact
- Indirect contact—spread by inanimate objects
- Vectorborne—carried by insects

Diseases of Concern for Pre-hospital Personnel

- Herpes simplex
- Syphilis
- Human immunodeficiency virus (HIV)
- Hepatitis B and C virus
- Meningitis
- Tuberculosis

Potentially Infectious Bodily Fluids

- Blood, semen, vaginal secretions
- Cerebrospinal fluids
- Pleural, synovial fluids
- Peritoneal and amniotic fluids
- Saliva
- Fixed tissue or organ
- All other body fluids that may be contaminated such as:
  - Urine
  - Vomitus
  - Saliva
  - Sweat
  - Feces
  - Sputum
  - Tears
  - Nasal secretions

Prevention

- OSHA establishes guidelines in reducing risk in the workplace.
- OSHA requires all EMTs to be trained to handle bloodborne pathogens.
- Hand washing and washing body areas exposed to blood or body fluids immediately after contact is an important means of preventing infection.
- Gloves should be worn when it is likely there will be contact with blood or other fluids.

Suggested immunizations EMTs should have are:

1. Tetanus prophylaxis
2. Hepatitis B vaccine
3. Verification of immune status with respect to commonly transmitted contagious diseases such as varicella, mumps, measles, rubella
4. Access or availability of immunizations in the community (influenza)
5. Annual tuberculin purified protein derivative (PPD) testing

? CHAPTER QUESTIONS

1. One of the five stages of death and dying is:

   a. relief
   b. bargaining
   c. elation
   d. overcoming

2. An EMT should wear specific body substance isolation (BSI) clothing to avoid being exposed to infectious diseases. An example of BSI would be:

   a. leather gloves
   b. a helmet
   c. turnout gear
   d. latex/nitrile gloves

3. What stage of death or dying is characterized by sadness and despair? The patient is usually silent and retreats into his own world ("OK, but I haven't . . .").

   a. Depression
   b. Anger
   c. Despair
   d. Denial

4. The number-one way an EMT can prevent infection is to vigorously wash their hands after every assignment:

   a. True
   b. False

References

1. American College of Emergency Physicians. In: Peter T, Pons MC, Cason D, eds. *Paramedic Field Care*. 1st ed. St. Louis: Mosby-Year Book; 1997.

2. US Department of Transportation, Transport Canada, and the Secretariat of Communications and Transportation of Mexico (SCT). *Emergency Response Guidebook*. Washington, DC: US Department of Transportation; 2004.

Chapter 3
Medical, Legal, and Ethical Issues

You respond to an unconscious patient at an adult community within your response area. Upon arrival, the patient's wife meets you at the door and briefs you on the patient's extensive cancer medical history and provides you and your partner with a valid out-of-hospital do not resuscitate (DNR) order. You assess the patient and determine he meets the criteria for death. A few moments later, the patient's children show up and begin questioning why resuscitative efforts have not started. Your partner explains to the family the patient's wishes, and they begin to get very upset about the decision not to resuscitate. What should you and your partner do?

MEDICAL ETHICS

Eth-ics\ `e-thiks`\ *n:* the principles of conduct governing an individual or a group.[1] In 1978, the National Association of Emergency Medical Technicians (NAEMTs) adopted the EMT Code of Ethics.[2] Professional status as an EMT and EMT-Paramedic is maintained and enriched by the willingness of the individual practitioner to accept and fulfill obligations to society, other medical professionals, and the profession of Emergency Medical Technician. As an Emergency Medical Technician-Paramedic, I solemnly pledge myself to the following code of professional ethics: A fundamental responsibility of the Emergency Medical Technician is to conserve life, to alleviate suffering, to promote health, to do no harm, and to encourage the quality and equal availability of emergency medical care.

The emergency medical technician provides services based on human need, respect for human dignity, and is unrestricted by consideration of nationality, race, creed, color, or status. The emergency medical technician does not use professional knowledge and skills in any enterprise detrimental to the public well-being.

LEGAL DUTIES TO THE PATIENT, MEDICAL DIRECTOR, AND PUBLIC

- Providing for the well-being of the patient by rendering necessary interventions outlined in the scope of practice.
- Legal duties are defined by state legislation and are enhanced by medical direction through the use of protocols and standing orders.
- Legal right to function as an EMT may be contingent upon the following:
  - Medical direction
  - Telephone/radio communications
  - Approved standing orders/protocols
  - Responsibility to medical direction

MEDICAL ETHICS AND ETHICAL RESPONSIBILITIES

- Always make the physical/emotional needs of the patient a priority.
- Practice/maintain skills to the point of mastery.
- Attend continuing education/refresher programs.
- Critically review performances, seeking ways to improve response time, patient outcome, and communication.
- Honesty in reporting.

ADVANCE DIRECTIVES

Honoring patient preferences is a critical element in providing quality end-of-life care. To enable physicians and other health-care providers to discuss and convey a patient's wishes regarding cardiopulmonary resuscitation (CPR) and life-sustaining treatment.

Out-of-hospital DNR orders (Fig. 3-1):

- Patient has the right to refuse resuscitative efforts.
- Requires written order from a physician.
- The EMT should review state and local legislation/protocols relative to DNR orders and advance directives.

**State of New York
Department of Health**

**Nonhospital Order Not to Resuscitate
(DNR Order)**

Person's name_____
Date of Birth__ / __ / __

Do not resuscitate the person named above.

Physician's Signature_____
Print Name_____
License Number_____
Date__ / __ / __

It is the responsibility of the physician to determine, at least every 90 days, whether this order continues to be appropriate, and to indicate this by a note in the person's medical chart. The issuance of a new form is NOT required, and under the law this order should be considered valid unless it is known that it has been revoked. This order remains valid and must be followed, even if it has not been reviewed within the 90-days period.

Figure 3-1   DNR order. (*From http://www.health.state.ny.us/publications/4182/index.htm.*)

- When in doubt or when written orders are not present, the EMT should begin resuscitation efforts.
- In New York State the Medical Orders for Life Sustaining Treatment form (MOLST) was created by the Community-wide End of Life Palliative Care Initiative to provide a single document that would function as an actionable medical order and could transition with a patient through all health-care settings. It is intended that the form will be transported with the patient between different health-care settings in order that their wishes for life-sustaining treatment and CPR will be clearly indicated.

If the EMT is unsure about the next course of action, the EMT should begin resuscitation and contact medical control for definitive direction.

FORMS OF CONSENT

Expressed Consent

- Patient must be of legal age and able to make a rational decision.
- Patient must be informed of the steps of the procedures and all related risks.
- Consent must be obtained from every conscious, mentally competent adult before rendering any treatment.

Implied Consent

- Consent assumed from the unconscious patient requiring emergency intervention.
- Based on the assumption that the unconscious patient would consent to life-saving interventions.

Children and Mentally Incompetent Adults

- Consent for treatment must be obtained from the parent or legal guardian.
- When life-threatening situations exist and the parent or legal guardian is not available for consent, emergency treatment should be rendered based on implied consent.

Emancipation Issues

A patient legally underage but is recognized by the state as having the legal capacity to consent. Criteria for being emancipated vary among states.

ASSAULT/BATTERY

- An EMT can be charged with assault/battery when proper consent is not elicited. This includes the following instances:
- Unlawfully touching a patient without his/her consent.
- Providing emergency care when the patient does not consent to the treatment.

Refusals of Treatment and/or Transport

- The patient has the right to refuse treatment.
- The patient may withdraw from treatment at any time. Example: an unconscious patient regains consciousness and refuses transport to the hospital.

REFUSAL OF MEDICAL ASSISTANCE

You have been advised that you require medical assistance and that this pre-hospital care provider is prepared to render pre-hospital care and to transport you to a hospital. You have further been advised that your refusal to accept such medical assistance may imperil your health, or result in death.

You have nonetheless refused to accept pre-hospital care and/or transportation to a hospital, as documented on Page 2 of the Pre-hospital Care Report. You have agreed to assume all risks, consequences and costs of your decision not to accept pre-hospital care and/or transportation to a hospital, and you release the provider of pre-hospital care service, and its employees, agents and independent contractors, from any liability arising from your decision.

Figure 3-2 Patient privacy practices from the electronic patient care reporting (ePCR). HealthEMS ePCR form.

- Refusals must be made by mentally competent adults following the rules of expressed consent.
- The patient must be informed of and fully understand all the risks and consequences associated with refusal of treatment/transport, and must sign a "release from liability" form (Fig. 3-2).
- When in doubt, err in favor of providing care.
- Documentation is a key factor in protecting the EMT legally during, and after a patient refuses treatment and transportation.
  - Competent adult patients have the right to refuse treatment.
  - Before the EMT leaves the scene, he/she should:
    - Try again to persuade the patient to go to a hospital.
    - Ensure the patient is able to make a rational, informed decision, that is, ensure the patient is not under the influence of alcohol or drugs, or illness/injury affecting rational decision making.
    - Inform the patient why he should go and what may happen to him if he does not.
    - Consult medical direction as directed by local protocol.
    - Consider assistance of law enforcement.
    - Document any assessment findings and emergency medical care given, and if the patient still refuses, then have the patient sign a refusal form.
    - The EMT should never make an independent decision not to transport.

ABANDONMENT

Termination of care without assuring the continuation of care at the same level or higher.

NEGLIGENCE

Deviation from the accepted standard of care resulting in further injury to the patient. Components needed to prove negligence include:

- Duty to act
- Breach of the duty
- Injury/damages were inflicted (physical/psychological)
- The actions of the EMT caused the injury/damage

DUTY TO ACT

A contractual or legal obligation must exist.

- *Implied*
  - Patient calls for an ambulance and the dispatcher confirms that an ambulance will be sent.
  - Treatment has begun.
- *Formal*
  - Ambulance service has a written contract with a municipality. Specific clauses within the contract should indicate when service can be refused to a patient.
- Legal duty to act may not exist. May be a moral/ethical consideration.
- In some states, while off duty, if the EMT comes upon an accident while driving, they must stop and help.
- When driving the ambulance not in the company's service area and EMT observes an accident.
  - Moral/ethical duty to act
  - Risk management
  - Documentation
- "- - - how a reasonably prudent person with similar training & experience would act under similar circumstances, with similar equipment, and in the same place."

PATIENT CONFIDENTIALITY/CONFIDENTIAL INFORMATION

- Patient history gained through interview
- Assessment findings
- Treatment rendered

HEALTH INSURANCE PORTABILITY AND ACCOUNTABILITY ACT

These are the requirements that are most relevant to ambulance service providers. For more detail, see the HHS Fact Sheet or the complete Privacy Rule.

- A covered provider must provide patients with notice of their privacy rights and its privacy practices, but need not obtain prior consent that would inhibit patient access to health care.
- Patients must grant permission in advance for each type of nonroutine use or disclosure, but providers may use one form for all of them.
- A covered entity must obtain prior written authorization to use protected health information for marketing purposes.
- Only the minimum necessary protected health information may be disclosed without authorization.
- A covered entity must account for disclosures of protected health information in the 6 years prior to the individual's request, with some exceptions, such as individual authorization.
- An individual may request restriction of use and disclosure of protected health information.
- Administratively, a covered entity must implement administrative, technical, and physical safeguards:

- It must implement policies and procedures to comply with HIPAA, document all policies and procedures, written communications, required actions, and personnel designations, and maintain them for 6 years.
- It must train its workforce, provide a complaint process, apply workforce sanctions for violations, mitigate harmful effects of improper use and disclosure, not retaliate, not require rights waived, designate a privacy official and contact person, and establish permitted uses and disclosures for its business associates.

- Releasing confidential information:
  - Requires a written release form signed by the patient. Do not release on request, written or verbal, unless legal guardianship has been established.
  - When a release is not required, other health-care providers need to know information to continue care. State law requires reporting incidents such as rape, abuse, or gunshot wounds.

SPECIAL SITUATIONS

Donor/Organ Harvesting

Donor/organ harvesting requires a signed legal permission document. The EMT's role in organ harvesting includes:

- Identifying the patient as a potential organ donor.
- Establishing communication with medical direction.
- Providing care to maintain viable organs.

Medical Identification Insignia (Medical Alert Tag)

- Bracelet, necklace, card (Fig. 3-3)
- Indicates a serious medical condition of the patient, such as:
  - Allergies to food, medication, and the like
  - Serious medical conditions (epilepsy, diabetes, stroke, etc.)
  - Others (DNR bracelet)

Potential Crime Scene/Evidence Preservation

- Dispatch should notify police personnel.
- Responsibility of the EMT:
  - Emergency care of the patient is the EMTs *first* priority.

Figure 3-3   Medical alert tag. *(From http://dhfs.wisconsin.gov/ ems/ images/MedAlert_front.jpg.)*

- ○ Every attempt should be made *not* to disturb any item at the scene unless emergency care requires it. Observe and document anything unusual at the scene using an Unusual Occurrence document.
- ○ Documentation on the Pre-Hospital Care Report should include patient assessment and treatment only. Any other documentation related to the incident or assignment should be included on a report of Unusual Occurrence document.

SPECIAL REPORTING SITUATIONS

Established by state legislation and may vary from state to state. Common reporting situations for EMS providers include instances of abuse, such as:

- Child abuse (Fig. 3-4)
- Elderly abuse
- Spousal abuse

Figure 3-4 Report of suspected child abuse. *(From http://www.health.state.ny.us/publications/4182/index.htm.)*

Incidents Involving a Crime

- Wounds obtained by violent crime, sexual assault, animal bites
- Infectious disease exposure
- Patient restraint laws (forcing someone to be transported against their will)
- Mental incompetence (ie, intoxication with injuries)

? CHAPTER QUESTIONS

1. Refusals must be made by a mentally competent adult following the rules of expressed consent.

   a. True
   b. False

2. All of the following are components of establishing negligence, except when:

   a. the EMT's action or lack of action incurs injury to the patient
   b. the EMT has violated the standard of care
   c. there was a duty to act
   d. the EMT was being paid at the time of the incident

3. When a patient is unable to make a rational decision regarding consent to emergency care, the EMT will care for the patient based on what form of consent:

   a. expressed
   b. minor
   c. informed
   d. implied

4. An EMT performed his initial assessment on a patient who was experiencing chest pain and shortness of breath. After initiating care, the EMT transported the patient to the hospital and did not provide a proper transition of care between the hospital staff and the EMS crew. In addition, the EMT did not wait to get a proper signature from the receiving hospital nurse or physician. This EMT could be legally liable for:

   a. negligence
   b. gross negligence
   c. abandonment
   d. violating the standard of care

5. By law, the EMT is authorized to release confidential information without the patient's permission in all of the following situations except when:

   a. information is requested by a member of the press
   b. another health-care provider needs information for the continuity of care
   c. the EMT is legally subpoenaed
   d. the third-party billing form requires the information

References

1. Merriam Webster's Medical Dictionary. Massachusetts, MA: Merriam Webster Mass Market; 1995.
2. Charles Gillespie. EMT Code of Ethics, adopted by NAEMT.

Chapter 4
The Human Body

You arrive on-scene and ensure the scene is safe to operate. In the apartment you find an 89-year-old woman semi-Fowler's on a couch. She is complaining of crushing substernal chest pain radiating to her mid-scapular region, left shoulder, and mandible. She also complains of associated shortness of breath, nausea, and vomiting. You begin performing the initial assessment and determine any life threats. You and your partner form a general impression of the patient. You then move on to assessing mental status and note the patient is alert to person, place, and time. As you determine if the patient's airway is patent, you ask the patient to open her mouth and inspect her oropharynx. As you move on in the assessment, you establish the patient is breathing at a rate of 20, shallow and labored. Upon auscultation, you listen to the right and left midaxillary line and note equal lung sounds bilateral, equal chest rise, and no signs of trauma. Oxygen is administered via nonrebreather at 15 L/min. Circulation is assessed by taking a radial pulse located on the distal end of the arm just proximal to the thumb in the ridge located where the radius bone meets the hand. You establish that her heart rate is 88 and irregular. The patient is kept in a position of comfort and your assessment continues.

ANATOMICAL TERMINOLOGY

Normal *anatomical position* is defined as a person standing, facing forward, palms facing forward (Fig. 4-1).

- An anatomical plane is a surface in which if any two points are taken, a straight line that is drawn to join these two points lies wholly within that plane or surface.
- Midline—Imaginary line drawn vertically through the middle of the body: Nose through the umbilicus (belly button).
  ○ Divides the body into right and left halves.
- Midaxillary—Imaginary line drawn vertically from the middle of the armpit to the ankle.
  ○ Divides the body into anterior and posterior.

Clinical Significance

Anatomical terms are used in medicine to describe location, comparison, or position. These terms are vital in proper communication/documentation.

Descriptive Anatomical Terms/Definitions

- *Torso*—Trunk of the body
- *Medial*—Toward the middle
- *Lateral*—A point that is more distant from the midsagittal or median plane
- *Proximal*—Closer to any point of reference

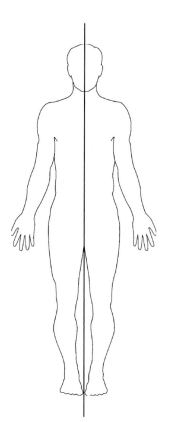

Figure 4-1 Anatomical position.

- *Distal*—Farther from any point
- *Superior*—Toward the head
- *Inferior*—Toward the feet
- *Anterior*—Toward the front
- *Posterior*—Toward the back
- *Right and left*—Toward the right or left
- *Midclavicular*—Imaginary line in the center of the clavicle
- *Bilateral*—Both sides
- *Dorsal*—Toward the back
- *Ventral*—Toward the front
- *Plantar*—Pertaining to the sole of the foot
- *Palmar*—Pertaining to the palm
- *Prone*—Face down
- *Supine*—Face up
- *Fowler's*—Sitting in a 90-degree angle
- *Trendelenburg*—Supine, lower body elevated above head
- *Shock position*—Body supine, legs elevated 8 to 12 in

COMPONENTS OF THE SKELETAL SYSTEM

The function of the skeletal system is to provide the body shape, protect vital internal organs, and assist in body movement. The skeletal system consists of 206 bones (Fig. 4-2).

Skull

Houses and protects the brain

Facial Bones

- Orbit
- Nasal bone
- Maxilla
- Mandible (jaw)
- Zygomatic bones (cheeks)

Spinal Column

- Cervical (neck)—7 vertebrae
- Thoracic—12 vertebrae
- Lumbar—5 vertebrae
- Sacral (sacrum)—5 vertebrae
- Coccyx—4 vertebrae

Thorax

Ribs

- 12 pair
- Attached posterior to the thoracic vertebrae
- Pairs 1 to 10 attached anterior to the sternum
- Pairs 11 and 12 floating

Figure 4-2 Skeletal system.

Sternum (Breastbone)

- Manubrium (superior portion of sternum)
- Body (middle)
- Xiphoid process (inferior portion of sternum)

Pelvis

- Iliac crest (wings of pelvis)
- Pubis (anterior portion of pelvis)
- Ischium (inferior portion of pelvis)

Lower Extremities

- Greater trochanter (ball) and acetabulum (socket of the hip bone)
- Femur
- Patella (knee cap)
- Tibia
- Fibula
- Medial and lateral malleolus
- Tarsals and metatarsals
- Calcaneus
- Phalanges

Upper Extremities

- Clavicle
- Scapula
- Acromion (tip of shoulder)
- Humerous
- Olecranon (elbow)
- Radius
- Ulna
- Carpals
- Metacarpals
- Phalanges

Joints—Where Bones Connect to Other Bones

Types of joints include:

- Ball and socket (eg, hip and shoulder)
- Hinged (eg, elbow and knee)

RESPIRATORY SYSTEM

Brings oxygen into the body and eliminates carbon dioxide (CO_2) from the body.

- Nose and mouth
- Pharynx
- Oropharynx
- Nasopharynx

Clinical Significance

Sellick maneuver—The application of digital pressure to the cricoid cartilage to reduce gastric distention

Clinical Significance

Initial Assessment
- *Airway*
  - Suction the oropharynx/nasopharynx as needed.
  - Insert an oropharyngeal or nasopharyngeal airway; if the patient gags, remove the airway and prepare for suction.
- *Breathing*
  - *Inspect* the chest.
  - *Palpate* the chest for symmetry, paradoxical movement, and crepitus.
  - *Auscultate* lung sounds.
  - *Seal/stabilize* any punctures or flail segments.
  - *Administer oxygen* nonrebreather mask, bag-valve-mask with reservoir, or nasal cannula.

Clinical Significance

Although these ranges are considered normal for the adult, child, and infant, it is important to remember, that abnormal findings, such as perioral cyanosis, tripoding, tachypnea, and altered mental status, in conjunction with these ranges, are clinical findings of respiratory distress/failure.

- Epiglottis—A leaf-shaped structure that prevents food and liquid from entering the trachea during swallowing
- Trachea (windpipe)
- Cricoid cartilage—Firm cartilage ring forming the lower portion of the larynx
- Larynx (voice box)
- Bronchi—Two major branches of the trachea to the lungs (bronchus subdivides into smaller air passages ending at the alveoli)
- Lungs
- Diaphragm

Inhalation (Active)

- Diaphragm and intercostal muscles contract, increasing the size of the thoracic cavity
- Diaphragm moves slightly downward, flares lower portion of rib cage
- Ribs move upward/outward
- Air flows into the lungs

Exhalation (Passive)

- Diaphragm and intercostal muscles relax, decreasing the size of the thoracic cavity
- Diaphragm moves upward
- Ribs move downward/inward
- Air flows out of the lungs

Respiratory Physiology

How does the respiratory system work?

Alveolar/Capillary Exchange

- Oxygen-rich air enters the alveoli during each inspiration.
- Oxygen-poor blood in the capillaries passes into the alveoli.
- Oxygen enters the capillaries as carbon dioxide enters the alveoli.

Capillary/Cellular Exchange

- Cells give up carbon dioxide to the capillaries.
- Capillaries give up oxygen to the cells.

Adequate Breathing—Normal Rate/Ranges

- Adult—12 to 20/min
- Child—15 to 30/min
- Infant—25 to 50/min

Respiratory Assessment

Rhythm

- Regular/irregular

Quality

- Breath sounds—Present and equal
- Chest expansion—Adequate and equal
- Effort of breathing—Use of accessory muscles predominantly in infants and children

Depth (Tidal Volume)

- Adequate/inadequate breathing.
- Rate—Outside of normal ranges.
- Rhythm—Regular/irregular.
- Quality:
  ◦ Breath sounds—Diminished or absent
  ◦ Chest expansion—Unequal or inadequate
  ◦ Increased effort of breathing—Use of accessory muscles, predominantly in infants and children
- Inadequate/shallow.
- The skin may be pale or cyanotic (blue) and cool and clammy. **Hypoxia** is a pathological condition in which the body as a whole (**generalized hypoxia**) or a region of the body (**tissue hypoxia**) is deprived of adequate oxygen supply.
- There may be retractions above the clavicles, between the ribs, and below the rib cage, especially in children.
- Nasal flaring may be present, especially in children.
- In infants, there may be "see-saw" breathing where the abdomen and chest move in opposite directions.
- Agonal respirations (occasional gasping breaths) may be seen just before death.

PEDIATRIC ANATOMY CONSIDERATIONS

- Mouth and nose—All structures are smaller and more easily obstructed than in adults.
- Pharynx—Infants' and children's tongues take up proportionally more space in the mouth than adults.
- Trachea (windpipe):
  ◦ Infants and children have narrower tracheas that are obstructed more easily by swelling.
  ◦ The trachea is softer and more flexible in infants and children.
- Cricoid cartilage—Like other cartilage in the infant and child, the cricoid cartilage is less developed and less rigid.
- Diaphragm—The chest wall is softer, so infants and children tend to depend more heavily on the diaphragm for breathing.

CIRCULATORY (CARDIOVASCULAR) SYSTEM

Heart (Size, Shape, and Position)

- Muscular pump
- Size of the patient's fist
- Weighs 10 oz

Clinical Significance

Signs of accessory muscle use in infants and children include intercostal/supraclavicular retractions.

Clinical Significance

A swollen throat from the streptococcus infection (strep throat) can cause significant narrowing of the pediatric airway.

- Located in *mediastinum,* area between the lungs
- *Base*—Broad superior portion of heart
- *Apex*—Inferior end, tilts to the left, tapers to point

Heart Muscle

- Epicardium (visceral pericardium)
  - Serous membrane that covers the heart
- Myocardium
  - Thick muscular layer
  - Fibrous skeleton—Network of collagenous and elastic fibers
    — Provides structural support
    — Attachment for cardiac muscle
    — Nonconductor important in coordinating contractile activity
- Endocardium
  - Smooth inner lining

Heart Chambers

- Four chambers (two atria, two ventricles)
- Right and left atria
  - Two superior chambers
  - Receive blood returning to heart from veins; veins carry blood back to the heart
- Right and left ventricles
  - Two inferior chambers
  - Pump blood into arteries; arteries carry blood away from the heart

Atrium

- Right atrium—Receives blood from the veins of the body; pumps oxygen-poor blood to the right ventricle
- Left atrium—Receives oxygenated blood from the pulmonary veins (lungs); pumps oxygen-rich blood to the left ventricle

Ventricle

- Right ventricle—Pumps oxygen-poor blood to the lungs
- Left ventricle—Pumps oxygen-rich blood to the body

► **Note:**

Valves prevent backflow of blood.

Follow a Drop of Blood Through the Heart

Deoxygenated blood enters the right atrium through the superior and inferior vena cava, and the coronary sinus. Deoxygenated blood is then pumped from the right atrium to the right ventricle through the tricuspid valve. Once deoxygenated blood fills the right ventricle, it is then pumped through the pulmonic semilunar valve into the pulmonary artery (still deoxygenated blood). Blood flows through the pulmonary artery to the lungs for gas exchange through the alveolar/capillary membrane. Once gas exchange occurs (oxygen/carbon dioxide), blood flows into the left atrium through the pulmonary vein (oxygenated blood). As it fills the left atrium, oxygenated

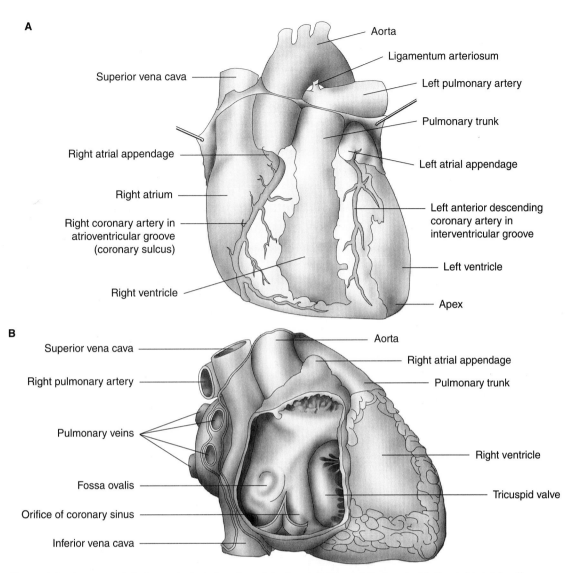

Figure 4-3 Anatomy of the heart. A. Anterior view of the heart. B. View of the heart with the right atrial wall reflected to show the right atrium. *(Reprinted with permission from Cheitlin MD, Sokolow M, McIllroy MB. Clinical Cardiology. 6th ed. Originally published by Appleton & Lange. Copyright 1993 by The McGraw-Hill Companies, Inc.)*

blood is then pumped to the left ventricle passing through the mitral valve. Once the left ventricle is filled, oxygenated blood is pumped through the aortic semilunar valve into the aorta to the entire body (Fig. 4-3).

CARDIAC CONDUCTIVE SYSTEM

- The heart is more than just a muscle.
- The heart has specialized contractile and conductive tissue.
  - *Automaticity*—Ability to generate an electrical impulse without stimulation from another source
  - *Excitability*—Ability to respond to an electrical stimulus (This is a property of all myocardial cells.)
  - *Conductivity*—Ability to propagate an impulse from cell to cell

Electrical Impulses

- *SA node*—Primary pacemaker, initiates heartbeat, sets heart rate
- *Fibrous skeleton insulates atria from ventricles*
- *AV node*—Electrical gateway to ventricles
- *AV bundle*—Pathway for signals from AV node
- *Right and left bundle branches*—Divisions of AV bundle that enter interventricular septum and descend to apex
- *Purkinje fibers*—Upward from apex spread throughout ventricular myocardium

Sinoatrial (SA) Node (Dominant Pacemaker of the Heart)

- Located in the right atrium near the entrance of the superior vena cava
- Intrinsic rate *60 to 100* beats per min

Atrioventricular (AV) Node

- Responsible for creating a slight delay in conduction before sending the impulse to the ventricles
- Impulse travel time 0.08 to 0.16 second
- No pace-making properties in the node itself
- AV junction tissue has intrinsic rate of *40 to 60* beats per min

Bundle of His

- Bundle of fibers coming from the AV node, located at the top of the interventricular septum
- Considered part of the AV junction
- Makes the electrical connection between the atria and ventricles

Bundle Branches

- Created by the bifurcation of the Bundle of His into left and right bundle branches
- Carry electrical impulse at high velocity to the interventricular septum and each ventricle simultaneously
- Rate of *20 to 40* per min

Purkinje Fibers

- Terminal ends of the bundle branches
- Network of fibers helping to spread the impulse throughout the ventricular walls
- Rapid impulse 0.08 to 0.09 s
- Rate of *20 to 40* per min

Blood Vessels

Arteries—Carry blood away from the heart to the rest of the body

Major Arteries of the Body

- Coronary arteries—Vessels that supply the heart with oxygen-rich blood.
- Aorta (oxygen-rich blood)—Major artery originating from the heart, lying in front of the spine in the thoracic and abdominal cavities.
  - Divides at the level of the navel into the iliac arteries.

- Pulmonary (oxygen-poor blood) artery—Originating at the right ventricle, carries oxygen-poor blood to the lungs.
- Carotid (oxygen-rich blood)—Major arteries of the neck.
  - Supplies the head with blood.
  - Pulsations can be palpated on either side of the neck.
- Femoral (oxygen-rich blood)—Major artery of the thigh.
  - Supplies the lower extremities with blood.
  - Pulsations can be palpated in the groin area (the crease between the abdomen and thigh).
- Radial (oxygen-rich blood)—Major artery of the lower arm.
  - Pulsations can be palpated at the wrist thumb side.
- Brachial (oxygen-rich blood)—An artery of the upper arm.
  - Pulsations can be palpated on the inside of the arm between the elbow and the shoulder.
  - Used when determining blood pressure (BP) using a BP cuff (sphygmomanometer) and a stethoscope.
- Posterior tibial—Pulsations can be palpated on the posterior surface of the medial malleolus.
- Dorsalis pedis—An artery in the foot.
  - Pulsations can be palpated on the anterior surface of the foot.
- Arteriole—The smallest branch of an artery leading to the capillaries.
- Capillaries—Tiny blood vessels that connect arterioles to venules.
  - Found in all parts of the body.
  - Allow for the exchange of nutrients and waste at the cellular level.

Major Veins

- Venule—The smallest branch of a vein leading to the capillaries
- Veins—Vessels that carry blood back to the heart
- Pulmonary vein (only vein that carries oxygen-rich blood in the adult body)—Carries *oxygen-rich* blood from the lungs to the left atrium
- Venae cavae—Carries oxygen-poor blood back to the right atrium
- Superior vena cava
- Inferior vena cava

Blood Composition

- Red blood cells
  - Carry oxygen to organs utilizing hemoglobin found in the cytoplasm.
  - Carries carbon dioxide away from organs.
  - Hemoglobin is what gives the blood its distinctive red color.
- White blood cells—Part of the body's defense against infections.
- Plasma—Fluid that carries the blood cells and nutrients.
- Platelets—Essential for the formation of blood clots.

Cardiovascular Physiology

- How is a pulse generated?
- Left ventricle contracts sending a wave of blood through the arteries. Can be palpated anywhere an artery simultaneously passes near the skin surface and over a bone.

Clinical Significance

In the initial assessment it is important to assess circulation. While assessing the "C" in ABC (airway, breathing, circulation), we will:

- Correct any life-threatening bleeding.
- Assess skin color, temperature, and moisture.
- Assess pulse rate and quality.

Peripheral Circulation

- Radial
- Brachial
- Posterior tibial
- Dorsalis pedis

Where are these pulses palpated?

Central Circulation

- Carotid artery
- Femoral artery

Where are these pulses palpated?

Blood Pressure

- Systolic—The pressure exerted against the walls of the artery when the left ventricle contracts
- Diastolic—The pressure exerted against the walls of the artery when the left ventricle is at rest

MUSCULOSKELETAL SYSTEM

Function of the musculoskeletal system:

- Gives the body shape
- Protects internal organs
- Provides for movement

Types of Muscle

Voluntary (Skeletal)

- Attached to the bones
- Form the major muscle mass of the body
- Controlled by the nervous system and brain; voluntary muscles can be contracted and relaxed by the will of the individual
- Responsible for movement

Involuntary (Smooth)

- Found in the walls of the tubular structures of the gastrointestinal tract and urinary system, as well as the blood vessels and bronchi.
- Control the flow through these structures.
- Carry out the automatic muscular functions of the body.
- Individuals have no direct control over these muscles.
- Respond to stimuli such as stretching, heat, and cold.

Cardiac

- Found only in the heart
- Involuntary muscle—Has its own supply of blood through the coronary artery system
- Can tolerate interruption of blood supply for only very short periods
- Automaticity—The ability of the muscle to contract on its own

NERVOUS SYSTEM

Function—Controls the voluntary and involuntary activity of the body

- Central nervous system (consists of the brain and spinal cord)
  - Brain—Located within the cranium
  - Spinal cord—Located within the spinal column from the brain through the lumbar vertebrae
- Peripheral nervous system
  - Sensory—Carry information from the body to the brain and spinal cord
  - Motor—Carry information from the brain and spinal cord to the body

INTEGUMENTARY SYSTEM

Function of the Skin

- Protects the body from the environment, bacteria, and other organisms
- Helps regulate the temperature of the body
- Senses heat, cold, touch, pressure and pain; transmits this information to the brain and spinal cord via the sensory portion of the peripheral nervous system

Layers of the Skin

(Fig. 4-4)

- Epidermis—Outermost layer of skin
- Dermis—Deeper layer of skin containing sweat and sebaceous glands, hair follicles, blood vessels, and nerve endings
- Subcutaneous layer—Fatty tissue

Figure 4-4 Layers of the skin. *(Reprinted with permission from Brunicardi FC, Andersen DK, Billiar TR, et al (eds). Schwartz's Principles of Surgery, 8th ed. New York: McGraw-Hill, 2005, p. 430.)*

ENDOCRINE SYSTEM

- Function—Secretes chemicals, such as insulin and adrenalin, responsible for regulating body activities and functions. The endocrine system is a vital system that aids in maintaining homeostasis in the body.
- Homeostasis—The ability or tendency of an organism or a cell to maintain internal equilibrium by adjusting its physiological processes.

? CHAPTER QUESTIONS

1. The functions of the body are called its:

   a. physiology
   b. kinesiology
   c. pathology
   d. microbiology

2. The term that refers to a position closer to the midline is:

   a. medial
   b. lateral
   c. posterior
   d. anterior

3. The structure that carries air downward from the larynx to the lungs is the:

   a. bronchus
   b. pharynx
   c. epiglottis
   d. trachea

4. The chamber that pumps oxygen-rich blood out of the heart for distribution to the rest of the body is the:

   a. right atrium
   b. right ventricle
   c. left atrium
   d. left ventricle

5. The pulse that is located in the foot is the:

   a. carotid
   b. femoral
   c. brachial
   d. dorsalis pedis

Chapter 5
Baseline Vital Signs and History Taking

You respond to an adult female having difficulty breathing. Upon arrival you find a 23-year-old woman in obvious respiratory distress secondary to asthma. You perform an initial assessment and begin treatment with an albuterol nebulizer at 6 L/min. As treatment is being rendered, your partner begins eliciting the past medical history. What questions should you ask?

GENERAL INFORMATION

- Chief complaint—Why emergency medical services (EMS) was notified (ie, "My chest hurts.")
- Age—Years, months, days
- Gender—Male or female
- Race
- Estimated weight of patient

BASELINE VITAL SIGNS

Breathing

- Assessed by observing the patient's chest rise and fall.
- Rate is determined by counting the number of breaths in a 30 second period and multiplying by 2. Care should be taken not to inform the patient, to avoid influencing the rate.
- Quality of breathing can be determined while assessing the rate. Quality can be placed in one of the following categories:
  - Normal—average chest wall motion, not using accessory muscles
  - Shallow—slight chest or abdominal wall motion
  - Labored
    - An increase in the effort of breathing
    - Grunting and stridor
    - Use of accessory muscles
    - Nasal flaring, supraclavicular, and intercostal retractions in infants and children
    - Sometimes gasping
    - Noisy—An increase in the audible sound of breathing; may include snoring, wheezing, gurgling, crowing

Pulse

- Initially a radial pulse should be assessed in all patients 1 year or older. In patients less than 1 year of age, a brachial pulse should be assessed.
- If the pulse is present, assess rate and quality.
- Rate is the number of beats felt in 30 second multiplied by 2.
- Quality of the pulse can be characterized as:
  - Strong
  - Weak
  - Regular
  - Irregular
  - Absent (If absent, begin cardiopulmonary resuscitation [CPR] at a compression to ventilation rate of 30:2.)
- If peripheral pulse is not palpable, assess carotid pulse.
- Use caution. Avoid excess pressure on geriatrics. Never attempt to assess carotid pulse on both sides at one time.

Clinical Significance

An emergency medical technician (EMT) can estimate a systolic blood pressure by palpating specific pulses.
- Radial pulse: 80 systolic
- Femoral pulse: 70 systolic
- Carotid pulse: 60 systolic

Skin

Assess skin to determine perfusion

- The patient's color should be assessed in the nail beds, oral mucosa, and conjunctiva.
- In infants and children, palms of hands and soles of feet should be assessed.
- Normal skin appearance—Pink.
- Abnormal skin colors:
  - Pale—Indicating poor perfusion (impaired blood flow)
  - Cyanotic (blue-gray)—Indicating inadequate oxygenation or hypoperfusion
  - Flushed (red)—Indicating exposure to heat or carbon monoxide poisoning (late sign)
  - Jaundice (yellow)—Indicating liver abnormalities such as hepatitis, liver failure, liver cancer
- The patient's temperature should be assessed by placing the back of your hand on the patient's skin.
  - Normal—Warm
  - Abnormal skin temperatures
    — Hot—Indicating fever or an exposure to heat
    — Cool—Indicating poor perfusion or exposure to cold
    — Cold—Indicating extreme exposure to cold
- Assess the condition of the patient's skin.
  - Normal—Dry
  - Abnormal—Skin is wet (diaphoretic), moist, or dry
- Assess capillary refill in infants and children less than 6 years of age
  - Capillary refill in infants and children is assessed by pressing on the patient's skin or nail beds and determining the time for return to initial color.
  - Normal capillary refill in infants and children is less than 2 second.
  - Abnormal capillary refill in infants and children is greater than 2 second.

Clinical Significance

Skin temperature is best assessed by using a thermometer (ie, tympanic thermometer or oral thermometer).

Pupils

Pupils are assessed by briefly shining a light into the patient's eyes, and determining size and reactivity.

- Dilated (very big), normal, or constricted (small)
- Equal or unequal
- Reactivity—Whether or not the pupils change in response to the light
  - Reactive—Change when exposed to light
  - Nonreactive—Do not change when exposed to light
  - Equally or unequally reactive

Blood Pressure

- Assess systolic and diastolic pressures.
- Systolic blood pressure is the first distinct sound of blood flowing through the artery as the pressure in the blood pressure cuff is released. This is a measurement of the pressure exerted against the walls of the arteries during contraction of the heart.
- Diastolic blood pressure is the point during deflation of the blood pressure cuff at which sounds of the pulse beat disappear. It represents the pressure exerted against the walls of the arteries while the left ventricle is at rest.
- There are two methods of obtaining blood pressure:
  - Auscultation—The EMT will listen for the systolic and diastolic sounds.
  - Palpation—In certain situations, the systolic blood pressure may be measured by feeling for return of pulse with deflation of the cuff.
- Blood pressure should be measured in all patients older than 3 years of age.
- The general assessment of the infant or child patient, such as appearing sick, in respiratory distress, or unresponsive, is more valuable than vital sign numbers.
- Reassessment of vital signs:
  - Vital signs should be assessed and recorded every 15 minutes at a minimum in a stable patient.
  - Vital signs should be assessed and recorded every 5 minutes in an unstable patient.
  - Vital signs should be assessed following all medical interventions.

OBTAIN A SAMPLE HISTORY

Use the mnemonic *SAMPLE*:

Signs/Symptoms

- Sign—Any medical or trauma condition displayed by the patient and identifiable by the EMT, that is, hearing = respiratory distress, seeing = bleeding, feeling = skin temperature
- Symptom—Any condition described by the patient, that is, shortness of breath, nausea, chest pain

Allergies

- Medications
- Food
- Environmental allergies
- Consider medical identification tag

Medications (Prescription)

- Nonprescription
- Current
- Recent
- Consider medical identification tag

Pertinent Past History

- Medical (prior intubations in an asthmatic)
- Surgical (recent surgery)
- Trauma
- Consider medical identification tag

Last Oral Intake—Solid or Liquid

- Time
- Quantity

Events

Leading to the injury or illness (ie, chest pain with exertion, or chest pain while at rest)

Clinical Significance

Patient compliance with taking medication in accordance with his/her physician.

? CHAPTER QUESTIONS

1. In a blood pressure reading of 120/80, the 120 refers to the diastolic pressure and the 80 refers to the systolic pressure.

   a. True
   b. False

2. The "L" in SAMPLE stands for:

   a. length of illness
   b. last doctor's visit
   c. length of chief complaint
   d. last oral intake

3. The term used to describe a weak, rapid pulse is:

   a. mottled
   b. reedy
   c. thready
   d. bounding

4. The skin color that indicates inadequate breathing or heart attack is:

   a. flushed
   b. blue-gray
   c. jaundice
   d. yellow

Chapter 6
Preparing to Lift and Move Patients

Your ambulance is dispatched to an 18-story multiple dwelling. Dispatch data states you are responding for a person with abdominal pain in the hallway of the 17th floor. Upon arrival at the scene, you enter the lobby of the building and summon an elevator. The elevator arrives and you and your partner realize the stretcher will not fit in the elevator. Your partner runs out and gets the stair chair from the ambulance while you hold the elevator. When you arrive on the 17th floor, you find a patient in his 20s complaining of abdominal pain. You open the stair chair and have the patient sit down while you elicit a medical history. You begin to move the patient downstairs to the ambulance using a stair chair for patient transport.

BODY MECHANICS

- Proper body mechanics while lifting include:
  - Using your legs, not your back, to lift.
  - Keeping weight as close to your body as possible.
- Guidelines for lifting:
  - Consider weight of patient and need for additional help.
  - Know physical ability and limitations.
  - Lift without twisting.
  - Have feet positioned properly.
  - Communicate clearly and frequently with partner.
- Safe lifting of cots and stretchers. When possible use stretchers that have a mechanical lift. (Fig. 6-1)
  - When possible, use a stair chair instead of a stretcher if medically appropriate.
  - Know or find out the weight to be lifted.
  - Use at least two people.
  - Ensure enough help is available. Use an even number of people to lift so that balance is maintained.
  - Know or find out the weight limitations of equipment being used. (Average new-style stretchers have a 700 lb maximum weight limit.)
  - Know what to do with patients who exceed weight limitations of equipment.
  - Using power-lift or squat-lift position (best defense against injury), keep back locked into normal curvature. The power-lift position is useful for individuals with weak knees or thighs. The feet are a comfortable

Figure 6-1   Mechanical lift stretcher (Stryker). *(Used with permission from Peter DiPrima.)*

distance apart. The back is tight and the abdominal muscles lock the back in a slight inward curve. Straddle the object. Keep feet flat. Distribute weight to balls of feet or just behind them. Stand by making sure the back is locked in and the upper body comes up before the hips.

- Use power grip to get maximum force from hands. The palm and fingers come into complete contact with the object and all fingers are bent at the same angles. The power grip should always be used in lifting. This allows for maximum force to be developed. Hands should be at least 10 in apart.
- Lift while keeping back in locked-in position.
- When lowering cot or stretcher, reverse steps.
- Avoid bending at the waist.

• Carrying precautions
- Transport on devices that can be rolled.
- Know or find out the weight to be lifted.
- Know limitations of the crew's abilities.
- Work in a coordinated manner and communicate with partners.
- Keep the weight as close to the body as possible.
- Keep back in a locked-in position and refrain from twisting.
- Flex at the hips, not the waist; bend at the knees.
- Do not hyperextend the back (do not lean back from the waist).

• One-handed carrying technique
- Pick up and carry with the back in the locked-in position.
- Avoid leaning to either side to compensate for the imbalance.

- Correct carrying procedure on stairs
  - When possible, use a stair chair instead of a stretcher.
  - Keep back in locked-in position.
  - Flex at the hips, not the waist; bend at the knees.
  - Keep weight and arms as close to the body as possible.
- Reaching
  - Keep back in locked-in position.
  - When reaching overhead, avoid hyperextended position.
  - Avoid twisting the back while reaching.
  - Avoid reaching in front of the body for long periods.
  - Avoid situations where prolonged (more than a minute) strenuous effort is needed in order to avoid injury.
- Log rolling a patient
  - Keep back straight while leaning over patient.
  - Lean from the hips.
  - Use shoulder muscles to help with roll.
- Pushing and pulling guidelines
  - Push, rather than pull, whenever possible.
  - Keep back locked-in position.
  - Keep line of pull through center of the body by bending knees.
  - Keep weight close to the body.
  - Push from the area between the waist and shoulder.
  - If weight is below waist level, use kneeling position.
  - Avoid pushing or pulling from an overhead position, if possible.
  - Keep elbows bent with arms close to the sides.

PRINCIPLES OF MOVING PATIENTS

- As a general rule, a patient should be moved immediately (emergency move) only when there is a/an:
  - Immediate danger to the patient if not moved.
  - Fire or danger of fire.
  - Explosives or other hazardous materials.
  - Inability to protect the patient from other hazards at the scene.
  - Inability to gain access to other patients in a vehicle who need life-saving care.
  - Life-saving care cannot be given because of the patient's location or position.
- A patient should be moved quickly (urgent move) when there is immediate threat to life.
  - Altered mental status
  - Inadequate breathing
  - Shock (hypoperfusion)
- If there is no threat to life, the patient should be moved when ready for transportation (nonurgent move).

Using Emergency Moves

- The greatest danger in moving a trauma patient quickly is the possibility of aggravating a spine injury.

- In an emergency, every effort should be made to pull the patient in the direction of the long axis of the body to provide as much protection to the spine as possible.
- It is impossible to remove a patient from a vehicle quickly and at the same time provide as much protection to the spine as can be accomplished with an interim immobilization device.
- If the patient is on the floor or ground, they can be moved by:
  ○ Pulling on the patient's clothing in the neck and shoulder area.
  ○ Putting the patient on a blanket and dragging the blanket.
  ○ Putting the emergency medical technician's (EMT's) hands under the patient's armpits (from the back), grasping the patient's forearms, and dragging the patient.
- Rapid extrication of a patient sitting in vehicle involves the following processes:
  ○ One EMT gets behind the patient and brings the cervical spine into a neutral in-line position and provides manual immobilization.
  ○ A second EMT applies a cervical immobilization device as the third EMT first places the long backboard near the door and then moves to the passenger seat.
  ○ The second EMT supports the thorax as the third EMT frees the patient's legs from the pedals.
  ○ At the direction of the second EMT, he and the third EMT rotate the patient in several short, coordinated moves until the patient's back is in the open doorway and his feet are on the passenger seat.
  ○ Since the first EMT usually cannot support the patient's head any longer, another available EMT or a bystander supports the patient's head as the first EMT gets out of the vehicle and takes support of the head outside of the vehicle.
  ○ The end of the long backboard is placed on the seat next to the patient's buttocks. Assistants support the other end of the board as the first EMT and the second EMT lower the patient onto it.
  ○ The second EMT and the third EMT slide the patient into the proper position on the board in short, coordinated moves.
  ○ Several variations of the technique are possible, including assistance from bystanders. This must be accomplished without compromise to the spine.

Using Nonemergent Moves

Direct Ground Lift (No Suspected Spine Injury)

- Two or three rescuers line up on one side of the patient.
- Rescuers kneel on one knee (preferably the same for all rescuers).
- The patient's arms are placed on his chest if possible.
- The rescuer at the head places one arm under the patient's neck and shoulder and cradles the patient's head. He places his other arm under the patient's lower back.
- The second rescuer places one arm under the patient's knees and one arm above the buttocks.
- If a third rescuer is available, he should place both arms under the waist and the other two rescuers slide their arms either up to the midback or down to the buttocks, as appropriate.

- On signal, the rescuers lift the patient to their knees and roll the patient in toward their chests.
- On signal, the rescuers stand and move the patient to the stretcher.
- To lower the patient, the steps are reversed.

Extremity Lift (No Suspected Extremity Injuries)

- One rescuer kneels at the patient's head and one kneels at the patient's side by his knees.
- The rescuer at the head places one hand under each of the patient's shoulders while the rescuer at the foot grasps the patient's wrists.
- The rescuer at the head slips his hands under the patient's arms and grasps the patient's wrists.
- The rescuer at the patient's foot slips his hands under the patient's knees.
- Both rescuers move up to a crouching position.
- The rescuers stand up simultaneously and move with the patient to a stretcher.

Transfer of Supine Patient from Bed to Stretcher Direct Carry

- Position cot perpendicular to bed with head end of cot at foot of bed.
- Unbuckle straps.
- Both rescuers stand between bed and stretcher, facing patient.
- First rescuer slides arm under patient's neck and cups patient's shoulder.
- Second rescuer slides hand under hip and lifts slightly.
- First rescuer slides other arm under patient's back.
- Second rescuer places arms underneath hips and calves.
- Rescuers slide patient to edge of bed.
- Patient is lifted/curled toward the rescuers' chests.
- Rescuers rotate and place patient gently onto cot.

Draw Sheet Method

- Loosen bottom sheet of bed.
- Position cot next to bed.
- Prepare cot-adjust height, lower rails, unbuckle straps.
- Reach across cot and grasp sheet firmly at patient's head, chest, hips, and knees.
- Slide patient gently onto cot.

Proper Patient Positioning During Transport

- An unresponsive patient without suspected spine injury should be moved into the recovery position by rolling the patient onto his side (preferably the left) without twisting the body.
- A patient with chest pain or discomfort or difficulty in breathing should sit in a position of comfort as long as hypotension is not present.
- A patient with suspected spine injury should be immobilized on a long backboard.
- A patient in shock (hypoperfusion) should have his legs elevated 8 to 12 in.
- For the pregnant patient with hypotension, an early intervention is to position the patient on her left side.
- A patient who is nauseated or vomiting should be transported in a position of comfort; however, the EMT should be positioned appropriately to manage the airway.

? CHAPTER QUESTIONS

1. When lifting a heavy object, avoid using the muscles of your:

   a. back
   b. arms
   c. shoulders
   d. legs

2. When performing a log roll, an EMT should:

   a. bend over the patient
   b. lean from the hips
   c. twist and pull simultaneously
   d. lean from the waist

3. The preferred device for carrying a conscious medical patient down a flight of stairs is the:

   a. stair chair
   b. reeves sleeve
   c. ambulance stretcher
   d. backboard

4. All of the following techniques will help prevent injuries when lifting or moving patients except the:

   a. power lift
   b. back lift
   c. power grip
   d. squat lift

CROSSWORD

Across

1. Listening with a stethoscope.
4. Away from the attached limb or origin.
5. The pneumonic for stress debriefing.
8. _____ substance isolation.
10. The middle layer of the skin.
12. An agency that coordinates emergency care as part of the continuum of care.

Down

1. The patient may project feelings of _____ at family of EMS.
2. The top number of the blood pressure.
3. Permission obtained from a parent or legal guardian for emergency treatment of a patient who is not of legal age or is unconscious.
6. When lifting use the _____ _____ to maintain control of the device.
7. Towards the middle.
9. EMS should be a patient _____.
11. An abnormal sign found when evaluating the skin (diaphoresis).

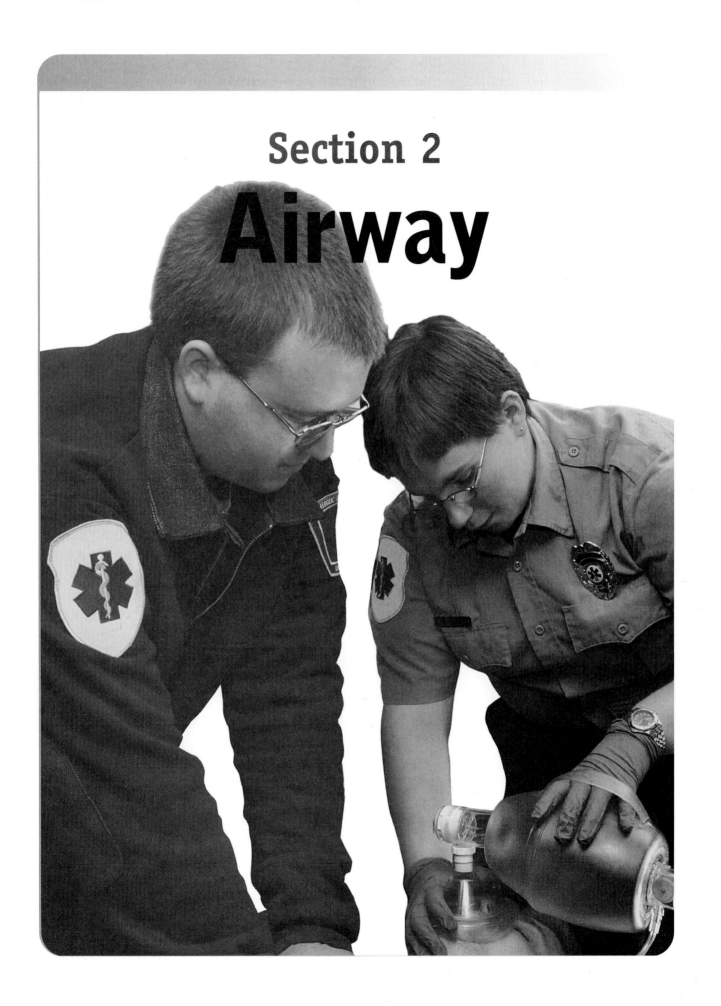

Section 2
Airway

Chapter 7

Airway Management, Ventilation, and Oxygen Therapy

It is 11:30 p.m. in a suburban town. A 40-year-old woman has just gone to bed when she begins to complain of difficulty in breathing. The patient's husband summons EMS. A few moments later, you are dispatched to this location for a person having respiratory difficulty from asthma. When you arrive you find a woman 40 years old sitting in her kitchen, obviously breathing heavy (in severe distress), sitting tripod with accessory muscle use, trying to speak but is unable because she is only able to speak in one-word sentences. She says, "I......can't.......breathe, my.........asthma." Your next action should be to?

RESPIRATORY ANATOMY REVIEW

Upper Airway

- Nose and mouth (Fig. 7-1)
- Pharynx—U-shaped muscular structure located between the oral and nasal cavity, posterior to the larynx
  - Oropharynx—Encompassed by the soft palate above and the epiglottis below
  - Nasopharynx—Situated behind the nasal cavity, above the soft palate
- Epiglottis—A leaf-shaped structure that prevents food and liquid from entering the trachea during swallowing
- Trachea (windpipe)
- Cricoid cartilage—Firm cartilage ring forming the lower portion of the larynx
- Larynx (voice box)

Lower Airway

- Bronchi—Two major branches of the trachea to the lungs. Bronchus subdivides into smaller air passages ending at the alveoli
- Lungs
- Diaphragm

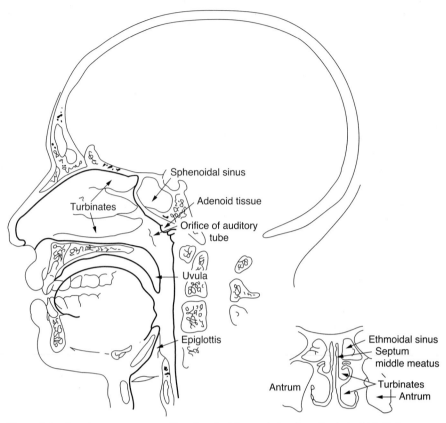

Figure 7-1   Respiratory anatomy. *(Reprinted with permission from Levitzky MG. Pulmonary Physiology. 7th ed. New York: McGraw-Hill.)*

- Inhalation (active)
  - Diaphragm and intercostal muscles contract, increasing the size of the thoracic cavity.
  - Diaphragm moves slightly downward.
  - Ribs move upward/outward.
  - Air flows into the lungs.
- Exhalation (passive)
  - Diaphragm and intercostal muscles relax, decreasing the size of the thoracic cavity.
  - Diaphragm moves upward.
  - Ribs move downward/inward.
  - Air flows out of the lungs.

RESPIRATORY PHYSIOLOGY

(Fig. 7-2)

- Alveolar/capillary exchange (site of gas exchange).
- Oxygen-rich air enters the alveoli during each inspiration.
- Oxygen-poor blood in the capillaries passes into the alveoli.
- Oxygen enters the capillaries as carbon dioxide enters the alveoli.
- Capillary/cellular exchange:
  - Cells give up carbon dioxide to the capillaries.
  - Capillaries give up oxygen to the cells.

Clinical Significance

Although these ranges are considered normal for the adult, child, and infant, it is important to remember that abnormal findings, such as perioral cyanosis, tripodding, tachypnea, and altered mental status, in conjunction with these ranges, are clinical findings of respiratory distress/failure.

Figure 7-2 A. Respiratory physiology. B. Respiratory anatomy. *(Reprinted with permission from Fishman AP et al., eds. Fishman's Pulmonary Diseases and Disorders. 3rd ed. New York: McGraw-Hill, 1998.)*

ADEQUATE BREATHING

Normal Rate

- Adult—12 to 20/min
- Child—15 to 30/min
- Infant—25 to 50/min

Rhythm

- Is the rhythm regular or irregular?

Quality

- Breath sounds—Present and equal
- Chest expansion—Adequate and equal
- Minimum effort of breathing—Use of accessory muscles (predominantly in infants and children)

Depth (Tidal Volume)

- Adequate tidal volume for the adult patient is approximately 500 cc.

EVALUATION OF INADEQUATE BREATHING

- Rate—Outside of normal ranges
- Rhythm—Irregular?
- Quality:
  - Breath sounds—Diminished or absent
  - Chest expansion—Unequal or inadequate
  - Increased effort of breathing—Use of accessory muscles (predominantly in infants and children)
- Depth (tidal volume)—Inadequate/shallow
- The skin may be pale or cyanotic (blue) and cool and clammy
- There may be retractions above the clavicles, between the ribs, and below the rib cage, especially in children
- Nasal flaring may be present, especially in children
- In infants, there may be "see-saw" breathing where the abdomen and chest move in opposite directions
- Agonal respirations (occasional gasping breaths) may be seen just before death

PEDIATRIC ANATOMY CONSIDERATIONS

- Mouth and nose—In general, all structures are smaller and more easily obstructed than in adults.
- Pharynx—Infants' and children's tongues take up proportionally more space in the mouth than adults.
- Trachea (windpipe).
  - Infants and children have narrower tracheas that are obstructed more easily by swelling.
  - The trachea is softer and more flexible in infants and children.

- Cricoid cartilage—Like other cartilage in the infant and child, the cricoid cartilage is less developed and less rigid.
- Diaphragm—Chest wall is softer; infants and children tend to depend more heavily on the diaphragm for breathing.

ADEQUATE AND INADEQUATE ARTIFICIAL VENTILATION

- An emergency medical technician (EMT) is artificially ventilating a patient adequately when:
  - The chest rises and falls with each artificial ventilation.
  - The rate is sufficient, approximately 10 to 12 per minute for adults and 12 to 20 times per min for children and infants.
  - Heart rate returns to normal with successful artificial ventilation.
- Artificial ventilation is inadequate when:
  - The chest does not rise and fall with artificial ventilation.
  - The rate is too slow or too fast.
  - In pediatric patients heart rate does not return to normal with artificial ventilation.
  - Skin color does not improve.

OPENING THE AIRWAY

- Head-tilt-chin-lift when no neck injury suspected (Fig. 7-3)
- Jaw thrust when EMT suspects spinal injury (Fig. 7-4)
- Assess need for suctioning

TECHNIQUES OF SUCTIONING

- Utilize proper body substance isolation
- Purpose of suctioning:
  - Remove blood, other liquids, and food particles from the airway.
  - Some suction units are inadequate for removing solid objects like teeth, foreign bodies, and food.
  - A patient needs to be suctioned immediately when a gurgling sound is heard with artificial ventilation.

TYPES OF SUCTION UNITS

- Mounted (Fig. 7-5A)
- Portable suction units (Fig. 7-5B)
- Hand operated (Fig. 7-5C)

Suction Catheters

- Hard or rigid ("tonsil sucker," "tonsil tip") Yankauer.
  - Used to suction the mouth and oropharynx of an unresponsive patient.
  - Should be inserted only as far as you can see.
  - Use rigid catheter for infants and children, but take caution not to touch back of airway.

Figure 7-3 Head-tilt-chin-lift. *(Reprinted with permission from Stone CK, Humphries RL. Current Diagnosis and Treatment: Emergency Medicine. 6th ed. New York: McGraw-Hill.)*

- Soft (French)
  - Useful for suctioning the nasopharynx and in other situations where a rigid catheter cannot be used.
  - Should be measured so that it is inserted only as far as the base of the tongue.

Techniques of Use

- Suction device should be inspected on a regular basis before it is needed. A properly functioning unit with a gauge should generate 300 mm Hg vacuum. A battery-operated unit should have a charged battery.
- Turn on the suction unit.
- If there is no measuring gauge, allow suction tubing to begin suctioning on your finger. Turn the suction unit off; if tubing stays attached, there is adequate suction.
- Attach a catheter.
- Use rigid catheter when suctioning mouth of an infant or child.
- Often will need to suction nasal passages; should use a bulb suction or French catheter with low to medium suction.

Figure 7-4A Modified jaw thrust. *(Reprinted with permission from Stone CK, Humphries RL. Current Diagnosis and Treatment: Emergency Medicine. 6th ed. McGraw-Hill.)*

- Insert the catheter into the oral cavity without suction. Insert only to the base of the tongue (as far as you can see).
- Apply suction. Move the catheter tip side to side.
- Suction for no more than 15 second at a time.

Figure 7-4B Modified jaw thrust. *(Used with permission from Peter DiPrima.)*

Figure 7-5A   Onboard suction unit. *(Used with permission from Peter DiPrima.)*

Figure 7-5B   Portable suction unit. *(Used with permission from Peter DiPrima.)*

Figure 7-5C   Manual suction device. *(Used with permission from Peter DiPrima.)*

- ○ In infants and children, shorter suction time should be used.
- ○ If the patient has secretions or emesis that cannot be removed quickly and easily by suctioning, the patient should be log rolled and the oropharynx should be cleared.
- ○ If patient produces frothy secretions as rapidly as suctioning can remove, suction for 15 seconds, artificially ventilate for 2 minutes, then suction for 15 seconds, and continue in that manner. Consult medical direction for this situation.
- ○ If necessary, rinse the catheter and tubing with water to prevent obstruction of the tubing from dried material.

TECHNIQUES OF ARTIFICIAL VENTILATION

- Methods for ventilating a patient by the EMT are as follows:
  - ○ Two-person bag-valve-mask (Fig. 7-6A)
  - ○ Flow-restricted, oxygen-powered ventilation device
  - ○ One-person bag-valve-mask (Fig. 7-6B)
- Use of body substance isolation
- Mouth-to-mouth—Review technique learned in BCLS course
- Mouth-to-mask (Fig. 7-6C)
- Bag-valve-mask—The mask should be connected to high flow oxygen = 15 L/min. (Fig. 7-7)
- The bag-valve-mask consists of a self-inflating bag, one-way valve, face mask, and oxygen reservoir. It needs to be connected to oxygen to perform effectively.
- Bag-valve-mask pros/cons:
  - ○ Maximum volume is approximately 1600 mL
  - ○ Provides less volume than mouth-to-mask
  - ○ Bag-valve-mask ventilation is challenging for a single EMT because maintaining an airtight seal requires considerable practice for competency.
  - ○ Two EMTs using the device will be more effective.
  - ○ Position self at top of patient's head for optimal performance.
  - ○ Adjunctive airways (oral or nasal) may be necessary in conjunction with bag-valve-mask.
  - ○ May produce gastric inflation with positive pressure ventilation.
- The bag-valve-mask should have:
  - ○ A self-refilling bag.
  - ○ A nonjam valve that allows a maximum oxygen inlet flow of 15 L/min.
  - ○ No pop-off valve or the pop-off valve must be disabled. Failure to do so may result in inadequate artificial ventilations.
  - ○ Standardized 15/22 mm fittings.
  - ○ An oxygen inlet and reservoir to allow for high concentration of oxygen.
  - ○ A true valve for nonrebreather.
  - ○ Ability to perform in all environmental conditions and temperature extremes.
  - ○ Availability in infant, child, and adult sizes.

Clinical Significance

During cardiopulmonary resuscitation (CPR), tidal volumes of approximately 500-600 cc are sufficient. Equivalent to 6-7 mL/kg.

Figure 7-6A   BVM with modified jaw thrust maneuver (two rescuers). *(Used with permission from Peter DiPrima.)*

Figure 7-6B   BVM with the head-tilt-chin-lift (one rescuer). *(Used with permission from Peter DiPrima.)*

Figure 7-6C   Adult BVM. *(Reprinted with permission from Tintinalli JE, Kelen GD, Stapczynski JS. Tintinalli's Emergency Medicine: A Comprehensive Study Guide, 6th ed. New York: McGraw-Hill.)*

Figure 7-7A   Adult bag-valve-mask. *(Used with permission from Peter DiPrima.)*

Figure 7-7B   Pediatric bag-valve-mask. *(Used with permission from Peter DiPrima.)*

Figure 7-7C   Infant bag-valve-mask. *(Used with permission from Peter DiPrima.)*

Using the Bag-Valve-Mask and the Head-Tilt-Chin-Lift

- Use when trauma is not suspected; after opening airway, select correct mask size (adult, infant, or child).
  - Position thumbs over top half of mask, and index and middle fingers over bottom half.
  - Place apex of mask over bridge of nose, then lower mask over mouth and upper chin.
  - If mask has large round cuff surrounding a ventilation port, center port over mouth.
  - Use ring and little fingers to bring jaw up to mask.
  - Connect bag to mask if not already done.
  - Have assistant squeeze bag with two hands until chest rises.
  - If alone, form a "C" around the ventilation port with thumb and index finger; use middle, ring, and little fingers under jaw to maintain chin lift and complete the seal.
  - Key is to observe adequate chest rise. Repeat a minimum of every 5 to 6 seconds for adults and every 3 seconds for children and infants.
  - If chest does not rise and fall, reevaluate.
    — If chest does not rise, reposition head.
    — If air is escaping from under the mask, reposition fingers and mask.
    — Check for obstruction.
    — If chest still does not rise and fall, use alternative method of artificial ventilation, for example, pocket mask or manually triggered device.
  - If necessary, consider use of adjuncts, such as an oropharyngeal or nasopharyngeal airway.

Using the Bag-Valve-Mask and Modified Jaw Thrust

- Use with suspected trauma
  - After opening airway, select the correct mask size (adult, infant, or child).
  - Immobilize head and neck, that is, have an assistant hold head manually or use your knees to prevent movement.
  - Position thumbs over top half of mask, and index and middle fingers over bottom half.
  - Place apex of mask over bridge of nose, then lower mask over mouth and upper chin. If mask has large round cuff surrounding a ventilation port, center port over mouth.
  - Use ring and little fingers to bring jaw up to mask *without* tilting head or neck.
  - Connect bag to mask if not already done.
  - Have assistant squeeze bag with two hands until chest rises.
  - Repeat every 5 to 6 seconds for adults and every 3 to 5 seconds for children and infants, continuing to hold jaw up without moving head or neck.
  - If chest does not rise, reevaluate.
    — If abdomen rises, reposition jaw.
    — If air is escaping from under the mask, reposition fingers and mask.

— Check for obstruction.

— If chest still does not rise, use alternative method of artificial ventilation, such as a pocket face mask.

Flow-Restricted, Oxygen-Powered Ventilation Devices

- Flow-restricted, oxygen-powered ventilation devices (for use in adults only) should provide:
  - A peak flow rate of 100% oxygen at up to 40 L/min
  - An inspiratory pressure relief valve that opens at approximately 60 cm water and vents any remaining volume to the atmosphere or ceases gas flow
  - An audible alarm that sounds whenever the relief valve pressure is exceeded
  - Satisfactory operation under ordinary environmental conditions and extremes of temperature
  - A trigger positioned so that both hands of the EMT can remain on the mask to hold it in position
- *Use when no neck injury is suspected.*
  - After opening airway, insert correct size oral/nasal airway and attach adult bag-valve-mask.
  - Position thumbs over top half of mask, and index and middle fingers over bottom half.
  - Place apex of mask over bridge of nose, then lower mask over mouth and upper chin.
  - Use ring and little fingers to bring jaw up to mask.
  - Connect flow-restricted, oxygen-powered ventilation device to mask.
  - Trigger the flow-restricted, oxygen-powered ventilation device until chest rises.
  - Repeat every 5 to 6 seconds in the adult patient only.
  - If necessary, consider use of adjuncts.
  - If chest does not rise, reevaluate.
  - If abdomen rises, reposition head.
  - If air is escaping from under the mask, reposition fingers and mask.
  - If chest still does not rise, use alternative method of artificial ventilation such as pocket mask.
  - Check for obstruction.
- *Use when there is suspected neck injury.*
  - After opening airway, attach adult mask.
  - Immobilize head and neck; for example, have an assistant hold head manually or use your knees to prevent movement.
  - Position thumbs over top half of mask, and index and middle fingers over bottom half.
  - Place apex of mask over bridge of nose, then lower mask over mouth and upper chin.
  - Use ring and little fingers to bring jaw up to mask without tilting head or neck.
  - Connect flow-restricted, oxygen-powered ventilation device to mask, if not already done.
  - Trigger the flow-restricted, oxygen-powered ventilation device until chest rises.

- ◦ Repeat every 5 to 6 seconds.
- ◦ If necessary, consider use of adjuncts.
- ◦ If chest does not rise and fall, reevaluate.
- ◦ If chest does not rise and fall, reposition jaw.
- ◦ If air is escaping from under the mask, reposition fingers and mask.
- ◦ If chest still does not rise, use alternative method of artificial ventilation.
- ◦ Check for obstruction.

Bag to Stoma or Tracheotomy Tube

- Tracheotomy—An artificial permanent opening in the trachea.
- If unable to artificially ventilate, try suction, then artificial ventilation through mouth and nose; sealing stoma may improve ability to artificially ventilate from above or may clear obstruction.

Bag-Valve-Mask to Stoma

- Use infant and child mask to make seal. Technique otherwise very similar to artificially ventilating through mouth. Head and neck do not need to be positioned.

AIRWAY ADJUNCTS

Oropharyngeal (Oral) Airways

- Oropharyngeal airways may be used to assist in maintaining an open airway on unresponsive patients without a gag reflex (Fig. 7-8).
  - ◦ Select the proper size—Measure from the corner of the patient's lips to the bottom of the earlobe or angle of jaw.
  - ◦ Open the patient's mouth.
  - ◦ In adults, to avoid obstructing the airway with the tongue, insert the airway upside down, with the tip facing toward the roof of the patient's mouth.
  - ◦ Advance the airway gently until resistance is encountered. Turn the airway 180 degrees so that it comes to rest with the flange on the patient's teeth.
  - ◦ Another method of inserting an oral airway is to insert it right side up, using a tongue depressor to press the tongue down and forward to avoid obstructing the airway. This is the preferred method for airway insertion in an infant or child.

Nasopharyngeal (Nasal) Airways

- Nasopharyngeal airways (Fig. 7-9) are less likely to stimulate vomiting and may be used on patients who are responsive but need assistance keeping the tongue from obstructing the airway. Even though the tube is lubricated, it may be painful.
- Select the proper size—Measure from the tip of the nose to the tip of the patient's ear. Also consider diameter of airway in the nostril.
- Lubricate the airway with a water-soluble lubricant.
- Insert it posteriorly. Bevel should be toward the base of the nostril or toward the septum.
- If the airway cannot be inserted into one nostril, try the other nostril.
- Never force the airway adjunct into the nostril.

▶**Note:**

Patients with an intact gag reflex will gag and vomit.

Figure 7-8A Oropharyngeal airways. *(Used with permission from Peter DiPrima.)*

Figure 7-8B Oropharyngeal airway placed. *(Used with permission from Peter DiPrima.)*

Use of Oxygen Cylinders

- Oxygen cylinders come in different sizes:
    - D cylinder has 350 L (portable cylinder)
    - E cylinder has 625 L (portable cylinder)
    - M cylinder has 3000 L (onboard tank)
    - G cylinder has 5300 L (onboard tank)
    - H cylinder has 6900 L (onboard tank)
- Careful handling of the tanks is required because their contents are under pressure.
- Oxygen is an oxidizer and supports combustion. It is one of the four sides of the fire tetrahedron (oxygen, chemical reaction, fuel, and heat).
- Tanks should be positioned to prevent falling and blows to the valve-gauge assembly, and should always be secured during transport.
- Full tank has approximately 2000 psi. Varies with ambient temperature.

Nasal airways   Oral airways

Figure 7-9   Oral and nasal airways. *(Reprinted with permission from Brunicardi FC, Andersen DK, Billiar TR, et al (eds). Schwartz's Principles of Surgery, 8th ed. New York: McGraw-Hill.)*

- Dry oxygen is typically not harmful short-term; keep in mind certain respiratory emergencies require treatment with humidified oxygen such as smoke inhalation, toxic inhalation, croup (pediatric patients), and asthma patients.

Operating Procedures
- Remove protective seal.
- Burp the tank by quickly opening, and then shutting, the valve.
- Attach regulator-flow meter to tank.
- Attach oxygen device to flow meter.
- Open flow meter to desired setting.
- Apply oxygen device to patient.
- When complete, remove device from patient, then turn off valve and remove all pressure from the regulator.

EQUIPMENT FOR OXYGEN DELIVERY

Nonrebreather Mask
- Preferred method of giving oxygen to pre-hospital patients.
- Up to 90% oxygen can be delivered.
- Nonrebreather bag must be full before mask is placed on patient.
- Flow rate should be adjusted so that when the patient inhales, bag does not collapse.

Indications for Oxygen Administration Using a Nonrebreather
- Patients who are cyanotic, cool, clammy, or short of breath need oxygen. Concerns about the dangers of giving too much oxygen to patients with a history of chronic obstructive pulmonary disease and infants and children

have not been shown to be valid in the pre-hospital setting. Patients with chronic obstructive pulmonary disease and infants and children who require oxygen should receive high-concentration oxygen.

- Masks come in different sizes for adults, children, and infants. Be sure to select the correct mask size.

Contraindications

- None

Special Considerations

- Patients with laryngectomies (stomas).
- A breathing tube may be present. If it is obstructed, suction it.
- Some patients have partial laryngectomies. If, upon artificially ventilating stoma, air escapes from the mouth or nose, close the mouth and pinch the nostrils.
- Pediatric patients:
  - Place head in correct neutral position for the infant and extend a little past neutral for a child.
  - Avoid excessive hyperextension of the head and avoid excessive bag pressure—use only enough to make chest rise.
  - Ventilate with bag-valve-mask until adequate chest rise occurs. Do not use pop-off valve; must be disabled (placed in closed position) in order to adequately ventilate child or infant.
  - Gastric distention is more common in children.
  - An oral or nasal airway may be considered when other procedures fail to provide a clear airway.

Facial Injuries

- Because the blood supply to the face is so rich, blunt injuries to the face frequently result in severe swelling.
- For the same reason, bleeding into the airway from facial injuries can be a challenge to manage.
- Obstructions
  - Ask "are you choking?"
  - Give abdominal thrusts/Heimlich maneuver or chest thrusts for pregnant or obese victims. Repeat abdominal thrusts until patient becomes unresponsive.
  - When the patient becomes unresponsive, begin CPR.
  - Look into mouth when opening the airway during CPR. Use finger sweep only to remove visible foreign body.
- Dental appliances
  - Dentures—Ordinarily dentures should be left in place. Dentures maintain a natural curvature of the face and will assist in proper ventilation. When dentures are removed, ventilation can become difficult due to the anatomical changes in the face.
  - Partial dentures (plates) may become dislodged during an emergency. Leave in place, but be prepared to remove it if it becomes dislodged.

? CHAPTER QUESTIONS

1. The primary function of the respiratory system is:

   a. the transportation of oxygen to the body cells
   b. the transportation of waste products from the cells to the lungs
   c. filtering the air that enters the lungs
   d. taking oxygen from the air and supplying it to the blood

2. A common cause of airway obstruction in the patient with an altered mental status is:

   a. the tongue
   b. food
   c. dentures
   d. secretions

3. Air entering the body through the mouth and nostrils travels into the:

   a. nasopharynx
   b. oropharynx
   c. laryngopharynx
   d. pharynx

4. The trachea is protected by a small flap of tissue called the:

   a. larynx
   b. epiglottis
   c. esophagus
   d. vallecula

5. The patient's vocal chords are contained in the:

   a. epiglottis
   b. larynx
   c. pharynx
   d. Adam's apple

6. The only completely circular cartilaginous ring of the upper airway is the:

   a. laryngeal cartilage
   b. hyoid membrane
   c. thyroid cartilage
   d. cricoid cartilage

7. The trachea descends into the chest cavity and branches into two main tubes, called:

   a. alveoli
   b. bronchioles
   c. bronchi
   d. alveolar ducts

8. The muscle that separates the chest cavity from the abdominal cavity is the:

    a. intercostal muscle

    b. pleura

    c. pectoralis muscle

    d. diaphragm

9. When a patient inhales:

    a. the diaphragm and the intercostal muscles relax

    b. the diaphragm relaxes and the intercostal muscles contract

    c. the diaphragm and the intercostal muscles contract

    d. the diaphragm contracts and the intercostal muscles relax

10. Inadequate oxygen being delivered to the cells is called:

    a. cyanosis

    b. deoxygenation

    c. hypoperfusion

    d. hypoxia

CROSSWORD

Across

1. The device of choice for assisting ventilations during rescue breathing.

4. The trachea bifurcates into the right and left mainstem _____.

5. The maneuver used to open a patient's airway with a suspected spinal injury.

10. Adequate _____ volume for the adult patient is approximately 500 cc.

12. The major muscle that separates the chest cavity from the abdominal cavity.

13. A medication given to all patients.

Down

2. An _____ adjunct is placed in the oropharynx.

3. When testing a suction unit, the minimum required _____ is 300 mm Hg.

6. Another name for the Yankauer suction catheter.

7. The medical term used to describe fluid in the lungs.

8. When lungs' sounds are difficult to hear on one or both sides they are said to be?

9. Portion of the pharynx that extends from the mouth to the oral cavity at the base of the tongue.

11. An artificially created opening that is found in the neck.

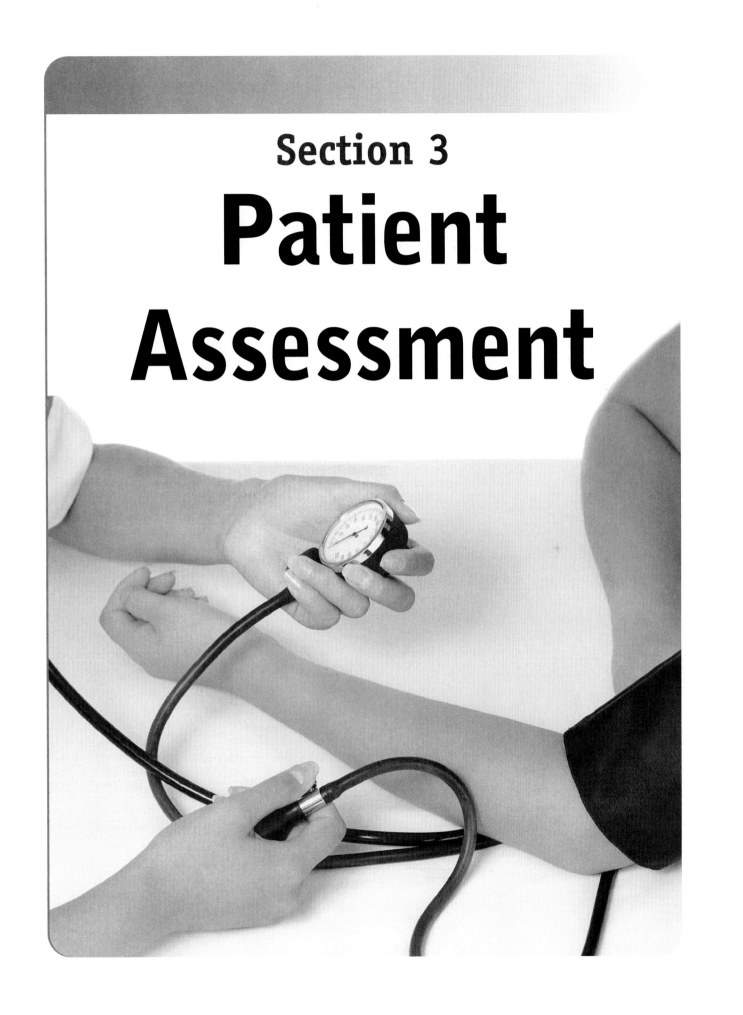

Section 3
Patient
Assessment

Chapter 8
Scene Size-Up/Safety

You arrive on-scene of an overturned vehicle collision (Fig. 8-1), you establish scene safety and begin evaluating a 21-year-old man still in the vehicle, who was the unrestrained driver of a truck that ran into a cement barrier at approximately 50 mph, causing it to overturn. You notice the steering wheel is bent and observe "starring" on the windshield with no skid marks present. The patient has a small amount of blood in his oropharynx. His breathing is labored and tachypneic at 32 breaths per min. His pulse is thready at 154. What do you do next?

SCENE SIZE-UP/ASSESSMENT

The first step in the entire process actually begins before your involvement, with a properly trained dispatcher. The dispatcher, who takes the initial call for help, should collect as much pertinent information as is available, so that the dispatch call is a complete one. Knowing where you are going, a familiarity with the location, and an understanding of the problem, are all "pieces" of information that will help you make a proper "pre-assessment." While responding to the scene, "armed" with the information supplied by the dispatcher and associating that information with your available equipment, your knowledge of the area, and your ability to deal with the upcoming anticipated problems, will better prepare you (mentally and emotionally) to deal with this patient. That preparation will also serve to present an "organized" group of rescuers to on-lookers, family members, and the patient, when your ambulance arrives at the scene, adding to the degree of professionalism perceived by the public.

Body Substance Isolation (BSI)

Body Substance Isolation (BSI)—Assumes all body fluids present a possible risk for infection. Protective equipment includes:

- Latex or vinyl gloves should always be worn
- Eye protection
- Mask
- Gown
- Turnout gear

> **Clinical Significance**
>
> The most important way to prevent infection is to wash your hands after every assignment.

Figure 8-1   Overturned vehicle collision. New York-Presbyterian EMS First Responders. *(Used with permission from Peter DiPrima.)*

Scene safety is an assessment to assure the well-being of the EMT.

- Personal protection—The EMT should ask, "Is it safe to approach the patient?"
  - Crash/rescue scenes.
  - Toxic substances—Low-oxygen areas.
  - Crime scenes—Potential for violence.
  - Unstable surfaces—Slope, ice, water, and the like.
  - Protection of the patient—Environmental considerations.
  - Protection of bystanders—If appropriate, prevent bystanders from becoming patients.
  - If the scene is unsafe, make it safe. Otherwise, do not enter.

Scene size-up is an assessment of the scene and surroundings that will provide valuable information to the EMT.

Mechanism of Injury (MOI)/Nature of Illness (NOI)

- Medical (nature of illness)
  - Nature of illness—Determine from the patient, family, or bystanders why EMS was activated.
  - Determine the total number of patients. If there are more patients than the responding unit can effectively handle, initiate a mass casualty plan.
  - Obtain additional help prior to contact with patients—Law enforcement, fire, rescue, ALS, and utilities. EMT is less likely to call for help if involved in patient care.
  - Begin triage.
- Trauma (mechanism of injury)
  - Mechanism of injury—Determine from the patient, family, or bystanders, and from inspection of the scene what the mechanism of injury is.

○ Determine the total number of patients.
— If there are more patients than the responding unit can effectively handle, initiate a mass casualty plan.
— Obtain additional help prior to contact with patients.
— Begin triage utilizing simple triage and rapid treatment (START).
— If the responding crew can manage the situation, consider spinal precautions and continue care.

? CHAPTER QUESTIONS

1. As an EMT, your initial evaluation of the scene is called the:

a. primary assessment
b. initial assessment
c. hazard assessment
d. scene size-up

2. You have three basic goals during scene size-up. These include all of the following except:

a. determining if additional assistance is needed
b. determining the patient's chief complaint
c. identifying hazards and ensure safety
d. determining what led to your being called to the scene

3. Scene safety should be assessed:

a. during your assessment of the patient
b. when you first make contact with the patient
c. throughout the call
d. when you first arrive at the scene

4. The process of ensuring scene safety should begin with:

a. arrival on-scene
b. dispatch information
c. the arrival of law enforcement
d. first contact with patient

5. EMTs should consider scene safety when responding to:

a. domestic violence calls
b. motor vehicle crashes
c. all EMS responses
d. chest pain calls

Reference

US Department of Transportation, National Highway Traffic Safety Administration. *EMT-Basic National Standard Curriculum*. Washington, DC: US Department of Transportation, National Highway Traffic Safety Administration; 1994.

Chapter 9
Patient Assessment

The emergency medical dispatcher sends you to the scene of a motor-vehicle collision at Avenue Z and Ocean Parkway. The emergency involves a single car that has struck a large boulder. When you arrive at the scene, you do a quick scene size-up. The vehicle has major damage, and no electrical lines are down. First responders from the fire department have secured the scene, and have initiated CPR on a male patient. You notice no obvious signs of trauma on the patient, except a 1-in laceration on the forehead. A police officer on-scene states, "The patient's driver's license indicates he is 24 years old. When we arrived, he was breathing agonally. He then went into cardiac arrest. We extricated him from the vehicle while providing c-spine stabilization and began CPR."

PATIENT ASSESSMENT (MEDICAL) AND PATIENT ASSESSMENT (TRAUMA)

- General impression of the patient (Table 9-1).
  - The general impression is formed to determine priority of care and is based on the EMT's immediate assessment of the environment and the patient's chief complaint.
  - Determine if ill or injured (trauma).
  - If injured, identify mechanism of injury.
  - Age
  - Gender
  - Race
- Assess patient and determine if the patient has a life-threatening condition.
  - If a life-threatening condition is found, treat immediately.
- Assess patient's mental status. Maintain spinal immobilization if needed.
  - Begin by speaking to the patient. Introduce yourself, tell the patient that you are an emergency medical technician, and explain that you are there to help.
  - Assess mental status using AVPU.
    — Alert—Alert to person, place, and time
    — Responds to verbal stimuli
    — Responds to painful stimuli
    — Unresponsive—No gag or cough
- Assess the patient's airway status.
  - Responsive patient—Is the patient able to speak?
    — If yes, assess for adequacy of breathing.
    — If no, open airway. (Remember, jaw-thrust manuever for trauma patients.)

TABLE 9-1: Medical Assessment

Scene Size-up

Take the appropriate body substance isolation (BSI) precautions, is the scene safe? Determine mechanism of injury (MOI) or nature of illness (NOI) and the number of patients. Consider stabilization of cervical spine.

Initial Assessment

General Impression of the Patient: What is the patient's chief complaint? Are they a medical or trauma patient? What is the patient's age, gender and are there any obvious life-threatening problems?

Level of Consciousness: AVPU (Alert, Verbal, Painful stimulus, Unresponsive)

Airway Status Assessment: Responsive patient: Is the patient breathing adequately? Unresponsive patient: Is the Airway open? Suction as needed, insert an oropharyngeal or nasopharyngeal airway as needed.

Breathing Assessment: Responsive patient: If breathing adequately, administer high-concentration oxygen via nonrebreather mask. Unresponsive patient: If breathing adequately, administer high-concentration oxygen via nonrebreather mask. If inadequate, assist ventilations with a bag valve mask with reservoir and high-concentration oxygen. Inspect and palpate the chest, seal and stabilize any flail segments, and auscultate two lung fields.

Circulatory Assessment: Perform a rapid pulse check, is there any bleeding? Assess the skin; color, temperature, and moisture. In children less than 6 y of age assess capillary refill (<2 s is normal).

Identify priority patients; perform transport decision and the need for advanced life support (ALS)

Poor general impression	Difficulty breathing	Chest pain
Unresponsive patient	Hypoperfusion	Uncontrolled bleeding
Altered mental status	Complicated birth	Severe pain

- ○ Unresponsive patient—Is the airway open?
  - — Open the airway.
  - — For medical patients, perform the head-tilt chin-lift.
  - — Suction as necessary.
- ○ For trauma patients or those with an unknown nature of illness, the cervical spine should be stabilized/immobilized and the jaw thrust maneuver performed.
  - — Suction as necessary.
- • Assess the patient's breathing.
  - ○ If breathing is adequate and the patient is responsive, administer high-concentration oxygen via nonrebreather mask.
  - ○ All responsive patients breathing less than 24 breaths per min or greater than 8 breaths per min should receive high-flow oxygen (15 L/min nonrebreather mask).
  - ○ If the patient is unresponsive and the breathing is adequate, open and maintain the airway, and provide high-concentration oxygen via nonrebreather.
  - ○ If the breathing is inadequate, open and maintain the airway, assist the patient's breathing, and utilize ventilatory adjuncts. In all cases, high-concentration oxygen should be used.

- If the patient is not breathing, open and maintain the airway and ventilate using ventilatory adjuncts. In all cases oxygen should be used and rescue breathing should be performed by giving one breath every 5 to 6 seconds.
- Assess the patient's circulation.
  - Assess the patient's pulse.
  - Circulation is assessed by feeling for a radial pulse on a conscious patient.
    — In a patient 1 year old or less, palpate a brachial pulse.
    — If no radial pulse is felt, palpate carotid pulse.
    — According to AHA guidelines, if the patient is pulseless, and it was not a witnessed cardiac arrest, begin CPR by initiating 5 cycles of 30 compressions to 2 ventilations. After the fifth cycle is completed, analyze rhythm utilizing the AED. If a shock is indicated, initiate one shock using the energy setting as outlined by the manufacturer's recommendation (specific to model being used). After the initial shock, initiate another 5 cycles of CPR using the 30:2 ratio of compressions to ventilations. If the cardiac arrest is witnessed, proceed to defibrillation. Initiate one shock using the energy setting as outlined by the manufacturer's recommendations (specific to model being used). After the initial shock, initiate another 5 cycles of CPR using the 30:2 ratio of compressions to ventilations.
  - Assess if major bleeding is present. If bleeding is present, control bleeding.
- Assess the patient's perfusion by evaluating skin color, temperature, and moisture.
  - The patient's skin color is assessed by looking at the nail beds, lips, and eyes.
    — Normal—Pink
    — Abnormal conditions
      Pale
      Cyanotic or blue-gray
      Flushed or red
      Jaundice or yellow
- Assess the patient's skin temperature by feeling the skin.
  - Normal—Warm
  - Abnormal skin temperatures
    — Hot
    — Cool
    — Cold
    — Clammy—Cool and moist (Diaphoresis is profuse sweating.)
- Assess the patient's skin condition. This is an assessment of the amount of moisture on the skin.
  - Normal—Dry
  - Abnormal—Moist or wet
- Assess capillary refill in pediatric patients.
  - Normal capillary refill is less than 2 seconds.
  - Abnormal capillary refill is greater than 2 seconds.

IDENTIFY PRIORITY PATIENTS

- Consider the following:
  - Poor general impression
  - Unresponsive patients—No gag reflex or inability to cough
  - Responsive, but not following commands
  - Difficulty breathing
  - Shock (hypoperfusion)
  - Complicated childbirth
  - Chest pain with BP less than 100 systolic
  - Uncontrolled bleeding
  - Severe pain anywhere
- Expedite transport of the patient. Consider ALS backup as outlined in local/state protocol.
- Proceed to the appropriate focused history and physical examination.

FOCUSED HISTORY, PHYSICAL EXAMINATION, "TRAUMA"

(Tables 9-2 and 9-3)

- Reconsider mechanism of injury.
- Look for injuries that have possibly been overlooked and injuries consistent with asignificant mechanism of injury, such as:
  - Ejectionor or partial ejection from vehicle
  - Death of a patient in the same passenger compartment
  - Extrication time greater than 20 minutes
  - Collision resulting in 12 in of intrusion into the passenger compartment
  - Vehicle rollover with 90 degree rotation or more and unrestrained

Table 9-2: Focused History and Physical Examination (Rapid Assessment)

Mechanism of Injury - TRAUMA	Nature of Illness – MEDICAL
ALL PATIENTS: • Ejection from a vehicle • Death of a passenger from the same vehicle • Fall > 20 ft • Rollover of vehicle • High-speed crash • Vehicle versus pedestrian • Motorcycle crash • Unresponsive or AMS • Penetrations of the head, neck, chest, abdomen • Hidden injuries (seat belt/airbag) INFANTS AND CHILDREN • Falls > 10 ft • Medium-speed vehicle crash • Bicycle crash	Assess complaint, signs and symptoms: (OPQRST): O = Onset-When or How did the symptoms start? P = Provocation-What caused or makes the symptoms change or worsen? Q = Quality-Describe symptoms/sensations/pain. R = Radiation-Does sensation move to other body areas? S = Severity-How severe is the discomfort? Scale of 1-10. T = Time-How long have the symptoms lasted? I = Interventions-Any interventions performed prior to EMS arrival? • If the patient is unresponsive or they are a priority NOI • Reassess airway and protect the airway • Perform Rapid Assessment

TABLE 9-3: Important Considerations for Priority Patients

Respiratory	Cardiac	AMS	Allergic Reaction	Poisoning/ OD	Environmental	Obstetrics	Behavioral
Onset?	Onset?	Description of episode.	History?	Substance?	Source?	Are you pregnant?	How do you feel?
Provocation?	Provocation?	Onset?	What were they exposed to?	When did they get exposed or ingest substance?	Environment?	How long have you been pregnant?	Determine suicidal tendencies?
Quality?	Quality?	Duration?	How?	How much?	Duration?	Pain or contractions?	Is the patient a threat to themselves or others?
Radiation?	Radiation?	Associated symptoms?	Effects?	Over what period?	Loss of consciousness?	Bleeding or discharge?	
Severity?	Severity?	Evidence of trauma?	Progression?	Interventions?	Effects local or general?	Has your water broken?	Is there an underlying medical problem?
Time?	Time?	Interventions?	Interventions?	Patients estimated weight?		Do you feel the urge to push?	
Interventions?	Interventions?	Seizures?				Last menstrual cycle?	Interventions?
		Fever?					

- Falls greater than 20 ft
- Rollover of vehicle
- High-speed vehicle collision
- Vehicle-pedestrian collision
- Motorcycle crash greater than 20 mph
- Unresponsive or altered mental status
- Penetrations of the head, chest, or abdomen
- Look for hidden injuries from
  — Seat belts
    - If buckled, may have produced injuries.
    - If patient had seat belt on, it does not mean they do not have injuries.
  — Air bags
    - May not be effective without seat belt.
    - Patient can hit wheel after deflation.
    - Lift the deployed air bag and look at the steering wheel for deformation.
    - "Lift and look" under the bag after the patient has been removed.
    - Any visible deformation of the steering wheel should be regarded as an indicator of potentially serious internal injury, and appropriate action should be taken.

High-Risk Trauma Patients

- Any patient with a bleeding disorder
- Any patient on anticoagulant therapy
- Any patient that is immunocompromised or has a respiratory or cardiovascular history
- Patients older than 55 years
- Specific MOI involving pediatric patients:
  - Falls greater than 10 ft

- ○ Bicycle collision
- ○ Vehicle in medium-speed collision, restrained, or unrestrained.
  - — Perform rapid trauma assessment on patients with significant mechanism of injury to determine life-threatening injuries. In the responsive patient, symptoms should be sought before and during the trauma assessment.
  - — Consider spinal stabilization.
  - — Consider ALS request, but do not delay transport awaiting arrival of ALS.
  - — Reconsider transport decision (transport to the appropriate 911 receiving hospital such as a trauma center).
  - — Assess mental status.
  - — As you inspect and palpate, look and feel for the following examples of injuries or signs of injury (**DCAP-BTLS**) (Table 9-4):
- ○ **Deformities**
- ○ **Contusions**
- ○ **Abrasions**
- ○ **Punctures/Penetrations**
- ○ **Burns**
- ○ **Tenderness**

TABLE 9-4: Guidelines for Assessment of Trauma Patients

Utilize Rapid Assessment - If unresponsive or priority MOI or NOI. Reassess mental status, perform spinal immobilization as required, and complete a head to toe examination (DCAP-BTLS).

Remember to roll the patient and assess the posterior body.

D=Deformity	B=Burns
C=Contusions	T=Tenderness
A=Abrasions	L=Lacerations
P=Punctures/Penetrations	S=Swelling

Assess Baseline Vital Signs
Breathing: rate, rhythm, depth
Pulse: rate/quality (strong/weak/regular/irregular)
Pupils: size, reactivity to light and are they equal?
Blood Pressure (systolic/diastolic)
Capillary Refill: children <6 y of age

Assess SAMPLE History
S=Signs and Symptoms
A=Allergies (medications, food, bee stings, etc.)
M=Medications (prescribed or over the counter), are they compliant with taking their medications as prescribed?
P=Past pertinent medical history
L=Last oral intake
E=Events leading to history of present illness (HPI)

- ○ Lacerations
- ○ Swelling
- ○ Crepitation
- Assess the *head*, inspect and palpate for injuries, or signs of injury (DCAP-BTLS).
- Assess the *neck*, inspect and palpate for injuries, or signs of injury (DCAP-BTLS).
- Apply cervical spinal immobilization collar (CSIC) (DCAP-BTLS).
- Assess the *chest*, inspect and palpate for injuries, or signs of injury:
  - ○ DCAP-BTLS
  - ○ Paradoxical motion
  - ○ Crepitation
- Breath sounds in the apices, midclavicular line, bilaterally, bases, midaxillary line, and are they:
  - ○ Present?
  - ○ Absent?
  - ○ Equal?
- Assess the *abdomen*, inspect and palpate for injuries, or signs of injury.
  - ○ DCAP-BTLS
  - ○ Firm
  - ○ Soft
  - ○ Distended
- Assess the *pelvis*, inspect and palpate for injuries, or signs of injury.
  - ○ DCAP-BTLS
  - ○ If no pain is noted, gently compress the pelvis to determine tenderness or motion.
- Assess *all four extremities*, inspect and palpate for injuries, or signs of injury.
  - ○ DCAP-BTLS
  - ○ Distal pulse
  - ○ Sensation
  - ○ Motor function
- Roll patient with spinal precautions and assess posterior body, inspect, and palpate, examining for injuries or signs of injury.
- Assess *baseline* vital signs.
- Assess *SAMPLE* history.
- For patients with no significant mechanism of injury:
  - ○ Perform focused history and physical examination of injuries based on the components of the rapid assessment. The focused assessment is performed on the specific injury site.
  - ○ Assess baseline vital signs.
  - ○ Assess *SAMPLE* history.

FOCUSED HISTORY, PHYSICAL EXAMINATION, "MEDICAL"

- Assess history of present illness.
- Assess patient complaint. Signs are what the EMT can physically see. Symptoms are what the patient describes to the EMT such as complaining of nausea, headache, and so on.

- OPQRST
  - *Onset*—What were you doing when the problem began?
  - *Provocation*—What makes the problem better or worse?
  - *Quality*—How would you describe the problem or pain?
  - *Radiation*—Does the pain radiate, or are there associated problems?
  - *Severity*—How intense is the pain on a scale from 1 to 10?
  - *Time*—How long ago did the problem begin?
- Assess *SAMPLE* history.
  - *Signs/symptoms?*
  - *Allergies*—Are you allergic to any medications?
  - *Medications*—Are you taking any prescribed or over-the-counter medications? When did you take them last? Are you compliant with taking your medications?
  - *Past medical problems*—Have you had any past or recent surgeries? Are you under the care of a physician?
  - *Last oral intake*—What have you had to eat or drink in the past 24 hours?
  - *Events* leading to the emergency—What happened, and what were you doing before the incident?
- Perform rapid assessment.
  - Assess the head as needed.
  - Assess the neck as needed.
  - Assess the chest as needed.
  - Assess the abdomen as needed.
  - Assess the pelvis as needed.
  - Assess the extremities as needed.
  - Assess the posterior body as needed.
- Assess *baseline* vital signs.
- Provide emergency medical care based on signs and symptoms in consultation with medical direction.

UNRESPONSIVE MEDICAL PATIENTS

- Position patient to protect airway.
- Perform rapid assessment.
  - Assess the head.
  - Assess the neck.
  - Assess the chest.
  - Assess the abdomen.
  - Assess the pelvis.
  - Assess the extremities.
  - Assess the posterior aspect of the body.
- Assess baseline vital signs.
- Obtain *SAMPLE* history from bystanders, family, and friends prior to leaving.

DETAILED PHYSICAL EXAMINATION

(Table 9-5)

- Patient and injury specific; that is, minor cut finger would not require the detailed physical examination.

TABLE 9-5: Detailed Assessment

Complete head-to-toe assessment: Perform a full body assessment of areas not previously examined. The purpose is to identify previously unknown wounds and injuries and manage secondary problems.

Assess the head: DCAP-BTLS
Assess the neck: DCAP-BTLS, jugular vein distention, and crepitation
Assess the chest: DCAP-BTLS, paradoxical movement, crepitation, and lung sounds
Assess the abdomen: DCAP-BTLS, swelling (firm/soft)
Assess the pelvis: DCAP-BTLS, if there is no pain present-compress
Assess the extremities: DCAP-BTLS (pulse, motor, sensory)
Assess the posterior body: DCAP-BTLS

Performance is patient and injury specific. The detailed assessment is utilized to gather detailed patient information in addition to initial and focused assessments. Patient illness/injury will guide the EMT as to whether to perform this assessment or not.

- Perform a detailed physical examination on the patient to gather additional information.
  - As you inspect and palpate, look and/or feel for the following examples of injuries or signs of injury (DCAP-BTLS).
  - Assess the head, inspect and palpate for injuries or signs of injury (DCAP-BTLS).
  - Assess the face, inspect and palpate for injuries or signs of injury (DCAP-BTLS).
  - Assess the ears, inspect and palpate for injuries or signs of injury (DCAP-BTLS) plus drainage.
  - Assess the eyes, inspect for injuries or signs of injury (DCAP-BTLS) plus discoloration, unequal pupils, foreign bodies, and blood in the anterior chamber.
  - Assess the nose, inspect and palpate for injuries or signs of injury (DCAP-BTLS) plus drainage and bleeding.
  - Assess the mouth, inspect for injuries or signs of injury (DCAP-BTLS) plus teeth, obstructions, swollen or lacerated tongue, odors, and discoloration.
  - Assess the neck, inspect and palpate for injuries or signs of injury (DCAP-BTLS) plus jugular vein distension and crepitus.
  - Assess the chest, inspect and palpate for injuries or signs of injury (DCAP-BTLS) plus crepitus and paradoxical motion.
  - Breath sounds in the apices, midclavicular line, bilaterally, and at the bases, midaxillary line, bilaterally.
    — Check for presence, absence, and whether they are equal.
  - Assess the abdomen, inspect and palpate for injuries or signs of injury (DCAP-BTLS) plus check for a firm, soft, or distended abdomen.
  - Assess the pelvis, inspect and palpate for injuries or signs of injury (DCAP-BTLS). If the patient does not complain of pain or is unresponsive, gently flex and compress the pelvis to determine stability.
  - Assess all four extremities, inspect and palpate for injuries or signs of injury (DCAP-BTLS) plus distal pulses, sensation, and motor function.
  - Roll with spinal precautions and assess posterior aspect of body, inspect and palpate for injuries or signs of injury.

TABLE 9-6: Ongoing Assessment

Repeat the initial assessment: reassess mental status, monitor airway, breathing, and circulatory status, and adjust priorities as needed. Reassess vital signs, repeat focused examination regarding complaint or injuries (HPI). Reassess interventions. *Stable patients repeat every 15 min; unstable patients repeat every 5 min.*

ASSESS BASELINE VITAL SIGNS

(Table 9-6)

- Repeat initial assessment. For a stable patient, repeat and record every 15 minutes. For an unstable patient, repeat and record at a minimum every 5 minutes.
  - Reassess mental status.
  - Maintain open airway.
  - Monitor breathing for rate and quality.
  - Reassess pulse for rate and quality.
  - Monitor skin color and temperature.
  - Reestablish patient priorities.
- Reassess and record vital signs.
- Repeat focused assessment regarding patient complaint or injuries.
- Check interventions such as adequacy of oxygen delivery/artificial ventilation, management of bleeding, and adequacy of other interventions.

? CHAPTER QUESTIONS

1. Mechanism of injury refers to:

   a. the specific injury that the patient has received

   b. how the patient was injured

   c. the degree of your anticipation that the patient has received an injury

   d. injuries specifically caused by machinery or industrial equipment

2. When responding to a motor vehicle crash, significant mechanism of injury would include:

   a. vehicle rollover

   b. deformity to the vehicle greater than 12 in into the passenger compartment

   c. leaking fuel tank

   d. severe side door damage

   e. all of the above

3. Patient assessment has several main purposes. These include:

   a. to obtain the patient's medical insurance information

   b. to diagnose the reason for the patient's symptoms

   c. to monitor the patient's condition

   d. both b and c are correct

4. The main purpose of the initial and rapid assessments is to:

   a. Identify and manage immediately life-threatening injuries or conditions.
   b. Communicate patient information to the medical facility staff.
   c. Determine whether the patient is injured or has a medical illness.
   d. Examine the patient and gather a patient history.

5. The six components of patient assessment include:

   a. the rapid trauma assessment
   b. baseline vitals
   c. the initial assessment
   d. transport
   e. all of the above

6. It is important to form a general impression of every patient you care for, as it provides valuable information about the patient's condition. Forming a general impression includes:

   a. obtaining the patient's chief complaint
   b. assessment of the patient's mental status
   c. estimation of the patient's weight
   d. the application of high-concentration oxygen

7. During the initial assessment you should be looking for conditions that require immediate management as they are found. These may include:

   a. possible internal injuries to the abdomen
   b. possible fractures to the extremities
   c. open wounds to the chest that may disrupt thoracic pressure
   d. capillary bleeding

8. The mnemonic used to assess a patient's mental status is:

   a. DCAP-BTLS
   b. AEIOU-TIPS
   c. AVPU
   d. OPQRST

9. You may need to make adjustments when gauging the mental status of a child or an infant. These include:

   a. knowing that crying may replace speech as a response
   b. watching and listening to the child's reaction to a shout
   c. noting whether the child follows movement with his eyes
   d. all of the above

10. As you approach your patient, he calls out "please help me—my leg hurts really bad." You would classify his level of responsiveness as:

    a. unresponsive
    b. alert
    c. responds to verbal stimulus
    d. responds to painful stimulus

11. During your assessment, the patient no longer responds to you when you speak to him. However, when you pinch the shoulder skin he tries to move away. Which of the following is true regarding his level of responsiveness?

    a. The patient has become unresponsive.

    b. He has responded with purposeful movement to painful stimulus.

    c. His response to the painful stimulus means he is still alert.

    d. He has responded with nonpurposeful movement to painful stimulus.

12. An unresponsive medical patient requires airway management. Which of the following is true regarding airway control of the unresponsive patient?

    a. An airway adjunct should still be used to keep the airway of a conscious, alert patient open.

    b. The head-tilt-chin-lift maneuver can be used on both medical and trauma patients.

    c. Manual airway maneuvers prevent the tongue and epiglottis from blocking the airway of an unresponsive patient.

    d. Manual airway maneuvers are not necessary if you are using an airway adjunct.

13. A gurgling sound may indicate a liquid substance in the airway. You should immediately:

    a. insert an airway adjunct

    b. turn the patient on his side to let the contents drain out of the mouth

    c. open the mouth and suction out the contents

    d. tilt the head back farther to more completely open the airway

14. Which of the following is true regarding crowing and stridor?

    a. Both are rattling sounds produced on exhalation.

    b. Airway adjuncts should be used in a child with suspected infection of the epiglottis.

    c. Both are commonly associated with swelling or muscle spasms of the airway.

    d. They are usually relieved by proper positioning of the airway, and airway adjuncts.

15. As soon as the patient's airway is opened, assess the breathing status to:

    a. determine the need for early oxygen therapy

    b. determine if the breathing is adequate or inadequate

    c. provide positive pressure ventilation with supplemental oxygen if needed

    d. all of the above

Reference

US Department of Transportation, National Highway Traffic Safety Administration. *EMT-Basic National Standard Curriculum.* Washington, DC: US Department of Transportation, National Highway Traffic Safety Administration; 1994.

Chapter 10

Assessment of the Geriatric Patient

You and your partner are called to the scene of a home in a nearby neighborhood. Upon arrival you find an 85-year-old man unconscious, not breathing. His home health-care nurse states the patient "just stopped breathing." He is on home oxygen and has a garbage bag full of medications for COPD. You begin your initial assessment, and attempt to ventilate. You find the patient difficult to ventilate. What would be your next action?

- The elderly population is at a greater risk for nearly all types of injuries and illnesses.
- They present with different signs and symptoms because of the changing physiology of the geriatric body system.
- In the United States, people over 65 make the fastest growing segment of the population.
- Because of the aging process, there can be many subtle differences in how illness and injury present in geriatrics when compared to their younger counterparts.
- Coexisting medical problems further hamper the emergency medical technician (EMT) assessment.
- The aging process is inevitable.
- Physiology starts to change as early as 30 years of age.
- Because of significant advances in medicine, there is an increase in longevity of people with chronic illnesses.
- It is important for the EMT to be able to differentiate chronic changes from aging, and acute changes due to illness or injury.

CARDIOVASCULAR SYSTEM

- Diminished pumping action of the heart due to loss of muscle strength.
- Progressive increases in heart rate, and slow degeneration of the conduction system.
- Loss of elasticity of the vascular system which causes diminished ability to constrict and dilate resulting in a weaker heart that must pump against higher resistance, with slowed electrical conduction within the heart.

RESPIRATORY SYSTEM

- Diminished size and strength of pulmonary musculature.
- Alveolar surfaces degenerate, impairing gas exchange.
- Lung elasticity is lost as ribs also become less pliable.
- The pulmonary system's ability to resist disease and infection decreases.
- Net effect is less gas exchange, increased infection, and a loss of muscle coordination.

MUSCULOSKELETAL SYSTEM

- Loss of minerals to the skeleton due to osteoporosis.
- Increased susceptibility to fractures from bones being brittle.
- Progressive loss of joint flexibility and muscle strength.
- Kyphosis will complicate spinal immobilization.
- In all, elderly patients fall more, fracture bones easier, take longer to heal, and may also be victim to additional medical problems.

NEUROLOGICAL SYSTEM

- Decrease in mass of brain (loss of neurons).
- Slowing of reflexes from nerve cell degeneration.
- Difficulty in being able to perceive body position.
- Decreased night vision and some loss of hearing.
- Deterioration of nervous system contributes to the high incidence of falls, and a general slowing in the body's adaptation to stressors.

GASTROINTESTINAL SYSTEM

- Loss in sense of appetite, smell, and thirst.
- Diminished function of the intestinal tract with less effective peristaltic waves and absorption of nutrients.
- Liver function diminishes, which also hampers digestion.
- Malnutrition and constipation are common results from the change in physiology due to aging.

RENAL SYSTEM

- Loss of nephrons decreases kidney size and function.
- Reduced renal blood flow from progressive stenosis of the renal vasculature.
- Electrolytes normally controlled by the kidneys may become disturbed.
- Overall changes may result in diminished filtration of waste products from the blood, which causes electrolyte disturbances and possible drug toxicity.

INTEGUMENTARY SYSTEM

- Thinning of skin from loss of subcutaneous layer.
- Replacement skin cells develop slower.

- Sense of touch dulled as are other sensory structures.
- Resultant changes include increased fragility of the skin and a loss in the protective barrier as the skin tears more easily.

LEADING CAUSES OF DEATH IN THE ELDERLY

- Cardiovascular diseases
- Cancer
- Fractures and falls
- Pulmonary diseases
- Diabetes
- Misuse of drugs

The manifestation of these emergencies may be altered due to more than one pathological process occurring at once in the body. Those especially at risk are geriatrics who:

- Live alone
- Are incontinent
- Are immobile
- Have recently been hospitalized
- Have recently been bereaved
- Have an altered mental status

ASSESSMENT: SCENE SIZE-UP

- Be attentive to BSI precautions—Especially with concerns of TB in the geriatric population.
- Note the environmental conditions they live in.
- Watch for environmental influences when numerous geriatrics share living quarters.
- The ease in determining the MOI versus NOI is not as clear, as the precipitating event (ie, the fall or the heart attack) may have actually occurred days earlier.

THE INITIAL ASSESSMENT

- Mental status
  - Important to differentiate acute from chronic alteration
- Airway
  - Diminished gag reflex increases risk of airway compromise.
- Breathing
  - Respiratory muscle failure occurs rapidly in light of pulmonary emergencies.
  - Carefully assess respiratory rate *and* tidal volume.
- Circulation
  - Assess central and peripheral pulses (noting rate and rhythm).
  - Indirect measures of circulatory adequacy may include mental status and skin characteristics.

- Skin condition and temperature
  - Dehydration is best assessed by evaluating mucous membranes of the eyes and mouth, rather than the skin.
  - Fever may not be present during infectious processes as this response is blunted in the geriatric patient.

Focused History and Physical Examination

- Based on the assessment findings made during your initial assessment, first determine patient criticality (priority or nonpriority).
- Secondly, decide whether to conduct a focused history and physical examination, or a rapid physical examination.
- In any instance, however, certain characteristics may be present which make assessment difficult. These include failing eyesight and diminished hearing.
- Problems with diminished sight or blindness.
  - Increased anxiety occurs from an inability to see surroundings along with an inability to control the situation.
  - As an EMT, you should talk calmly and be positioned in front of the patient should they have any remaining eyesight.
  - Explain what you are doing fully.
- Problems with diminished hearing or deafness
  - Hearing loss is not a direct result of aging.
  - Ask prior to assuming the geriatric patient is deaf.
  - Ensure hearing aid is turned on if used by the patient.
  - When speaking louder, increase volume rather than pitch of your voice.
  - Consider lip reading or note writing if the patient prefers.

Regarding Geriatric Trauma Patients

- Note mechanism of injury; remember that geriatrics are more prone to falls.
- Maintain a high index of suspicion at all times as the pain experienced by the geriatric patient may be masked.
- Consider a rapid trauma assessment on all trauma patients.
  - Inspect and palpate for DCAP-BTLS (*D*eformities, *C*ontusions, *A*brasions, *P*unctures/*p*enetrations, *B*urns, *T*enderness, *L*acerations, *S*welling, *C*repitation)
- Obtain a baseline set of vitals.
- Complete a SAMPLE (*S*igns/*S*ymptoms, *A*llergies, *M*edications, *P*ast medical problems, *L*ast oral intake, *E*vents) history from the geriatric patient.

Regarding Geriatric Medical Patients

- Remember to determine if presenting conditions are acute changes or chronic findings.
- Obtaining a history may be problematic with geriatrics, so be diligent with your task and patient with their responses.
- Always talk *to* the patient whenever possible instead of *about* the patient with other family members that may be present.

- During the SAMPLE history of a geriatric patient, remember the following points:
  ○ The patient may easily fatigue.
  ○ Clearly explain what you are doing.
  ○ Watch for the patient trying to minimize what is wrong.
  ○ Peripheral pulses may be difficult to assess.
  ○ Watch for symptoms from numerous chronic illnesses.
  ○ Differentiate findings from aging from findings due to an acute illness or injury.
- Questions that may help during your assessment of the geriatric patient:
  ○ Have you had any trouble breathing?
  ○ Have you had a cough lately?
  ○ Have you had any chest pain?
  ○ Have you been dizzy (vertigo)?
  ○ Have you fainted at all (syncopal episodes)?
  ○ Any history of headaches?
  ○ Any change with nutrition habits (eating and drinking)?
  ○ Any alterations in bowel or bladder habits?
  ○ Any recent history of falls?
- Completion of the physical examination considerations:
  ○ Geriatric patients typically dress in layers (you must expose to assess!).
  ○ Perform a rapid medical assessment in cases of altered mental status.
  ○ Time and patient condition allowing, the detailed physical examination may provide additional clues as to what is underlying the patient's complaints.

EMERGENCY MANAGEMENT

- Maintain a patent airway.
- Watch for dentures.
- Suction any excess secretions or fluids.
- Consider a jaw thrust if neck is relatively inflexible.
- Insert a simple mechanical airway.
- Deterioration may occur rapidly.
- Insert an OPA when no gag reflex is present, or an NPA should airway maintenance be warranted in the patient with an intact gag reflex.
- Assess and be prepared to assist ventilations.
  ○ Respiratory muscles fatigue easily.
  ○ When providing positive pressure ventilation (PPV), be cautious not to create excessive airway pressures which may promote gastric insufflation or cause pulmonary injury (barotrauma).
- Ensure adequate oxygenation
  ○ Via nonrebreather (NRB) at 15 L/min with adequate ventilations.
  ○ Via PPV with reservoir attached and liter flow at 15 L/min with inadequate breathing.
- Monitor pulse oximetry constantly.
- Use a nasal cannula at 6 L/min only if the patient has adequate ventilations and cannot tolerate the NRB.

Optimal Patient Position

- Opt for position of comfort (Fowler's probably) if patient's condition allows it.
- Use left lateral recumbent, should an altered mental status or airway aspiration concern exist.
- Full spinal precautions should be taken if there is a need based upon MOI, or if the patient's circumstances are unknown.
- Use extra padding when immobilizing a geriatric with kyphosis of the spine.

Transport

- Perform ongoing assessment en route.
- Be attentive to changes in status as geriatrics can rapidly decompensate.
- Repeat and record assessment findings every 15 minutes if the patient is stable, or every 5 minutes with an unstable patient.

ASSESSMENT OF THE GERIATRIC CARDIOVASCULAR EMERGENCY

Heart Attack (Myocardial Infarction)

- Typical chest pain from an MI may not be present.
- Weakness, fatigue, and dyspnea are common initial findings seen with these "silent heart attacks."
- Common medication that may be prescribed is "nitro," and the EMT-B can assist in the administration if appropriate per medical direction.
- Refer to Chapter 15, Cardiovascular Emergencies, for a thorough discussion.

Congestive Heart Failure (CHF)

- Chronic weakening of the heart which causes blood to back up into the lungs.
- Commonly presents with abnormal breath sounds, JVD, peripheral edema, fatigue, and dyspnea.
- For these patients, ensure high concentrations of oxygen, place them in a Fowler's position, and deliver PPV should their breathing become inadequate.

ASSESSMENT OF THE GERIATRIC RESPIRATORY EMERGENCY

- Dyspnea is an extremely common finding with the geriatric population.
- Since geriatric patients already have diminished pulmonary capacity, any additional disturbance could prove fatal.
- May be the primary symptom, or an associated complaint.

Pulmonary Edema

- Usually due to the heart's inability to pump blood, causing a backup of fluid.
- This results in excess fluid "leaking" into the lungs and severely hampering oxygen and carbon dioxide diffusion.

- May cause crackles, orthopnea, or blood-tinged sputum.
- Requires the administration of high-flow oxygen, Fowler's positioning, and rapid transport.
- Severe cases may necessitate positive pressure ventilation.

Pulmonary Embolism

- Caused by a sudden blockage of a blood vessel carrying blood from the right side of the heart to the lungs (for oxygenation).
- The drop in perfusion to the lungs results in sudden onset of respiratory distress, sharp local chest pain, and possible fainting.
- Like other pulmonary disturbances, the major treatment includes high-flow oxygen, assistance with breathing if necessary, and rapid transport.

Chronic Obstructive Pulmonary Disease (COPD)

- General name given to numerous disease etiologies that result in the deterioration of normal lung tissue.
- As the lung tissue is destroyed, the patient has a harder time maintaining normal oxygenation.
- They characteristically use oxygen at home as the disease advances.
- Pre-hospital management includes assuring adequate oxygenation and ventilation.

ASSESSMENT OF THE GERIATRIC ALTERED MENTAL STATUS PATIENT

- Not a result of aging, but the consequence of pathologic condition(s) within the body.
- Be sure to determine if altered mental status is an acute change in the patient, or a chronic finding.
- Anything that can alter oxygenation, ventilation, perfusion, neuron activity, blood chemistry, and the like could cause an alteration in mental status.
- Although management is essentially the same despite cause, understanding common reasons for altered mental status may show the EMT what else to assess for.

Stroke

- Common medical emergency in the geriatric population.
- Results when a blood vessel in the brain is blocked or ruptures.
- Brain cells die from lack of oxygen and from rising pressure in the skull.
- The region of the brain affected determines the symptoms seen (please refer to Chapter 18, Acute Stroke).
- Key emergency care is identifying the emergency, providing oxygen therapy and airway maintenance, and rapidly transporting the patient.

Transient Ischemic Attack (TIA)

- Also known as a "mini stroke."
- Is caused by a temporary diminishment of blood flow to a region of the brain.

- Region of the brain tissue affected malfunctions, causing the altered mentation and other signs.
- Resolves itself completely within 24 hours (but usually within the first few hours).
- Treatment is the same as recommended for a stroke.

Seizure

- Sudden alteration in the normal mental status of the patient caused by a massive electrical discharge in the brain.
- Results in abnormal muscular contraction which may cause inadequate breathing and airway compromise.
- Treatment goals include close attention to the airway status, suctioning as needed, provision of PPV if breathing is inadequate, and protection from injury if the seizure is still progressing.

Syncope

- "Fainting" episode which is relatively common to geriatrics.
- Usually reverses once patient is again horizontal.
- Any condition that causes a temporary decrease to blood flow in the brain can cause a syncopal episode.
- Treatment is mainly supportive to any lost function of the airway, breathing, or circulatory status.
- Ensure oxygenation, ventilation, and immobilization if warranted.

Drug Toxicity

- Defined as an adverse or toxic reaction to a drug.
- Common emergency also for geriatrics as they tend to be on multiple drugs simultaneously.
- Occasionally they overdose accidentally by forgetting that they previously took the medication.
- Abnormal reactions usually cause inadequate airway, breathing, circulation, or a combination thereof.
- Treatment is geared toward supporting any lost function of the airway, breathing, and circulation.

Dementia

- Irreversible malfunctioning of normal brain activity.
- Occurs in about 15% of the population over the age of 65.
- Results in impaired cognition, memory loss, and abstract thought.
- Could be caused by certain medications, brain tumors, heart disease, urinary retention, and many other underlying disease states.

Alzheimer Disease

- Thought to be the most common cause of dementia in the elderly population.
- Nerve cell disease where the brain tissue progressively deteriorates and dies.

- Results in changes in mental status, which may not be life threatening, but presents as a special challenge to pre-hospital care providers.
- Treatment supportive of airway, breathing, and circulation.

ASSESSMENT FINDING: TRAUMA OR SHOCK

- One of the leading causes of death to the elderly.
- Commonly from blunt trauma as a result of falls, motor vehicle collisions (MVCs), and pedestrians hit by a car.
- If fall related, ascertain if fall was preceded by a moment of dizziness.
- Other than specific treatment for isolated traumatic injuries, any indication of hypoperfusion should be considered as a serious sign of trauma.

ASSESSMENT OF THE GERIATRIC ENVIRONMENTAL EMERGENCY

- Geriatric patients have a harder time regulating normal core body temperature.
- Stay cognizant of environmental temperature when entering the scene of a geriatric patient.
- Remember that hypothermia or hyperthermia may occur in the presence of a normal ambient temperature.
- Refer to Chapter 24, Environmental Emergencies, for more details.

ASSESSMENT OF THE GERIATRIC ABUSE PATIENT

- Incidence of geriatric abuse has risen over the past several years.
- May be found in extended-care facilities or at the home of the individual.
- Abuse could be physical, mental, sexual, or financial.
- If you suspect geriatric abuse, carefully document your objective findings and be sure to notify the ED.

? CHAPTER QUESTIONS

1. Changes in the geriatric body systems include:

   a. increased tendency for respiratory infection
   b. cough power intensifies
   c. frequent fevers with illness
   d. skin becomes tougher

2. Cardiovascular system changes in the geriatric patient include:

   a. widespread arteriosclerosis
   b. a decrease in resting heart rate
   c. an increase of electrical conducting cells
   d. increased elasticity of the arteries

3. You are caring for a 72-year-old female patient. Changes in her respiratory system may include:

   a. the body becoming more sensitive to hypoxia

   b. more air entering and exiting the lungs, and an increase in lung tissue elasticity

   c. calcium deposits where the ribs join the sternum, causing the rib cage to be less pliable

   d. a progressive increase in diffusion of oxygen and carbon dioxide across the alveolar membrane

4. The most significant musculoskeletal change resulting from aging is a loss of minerals in the bones, known as:

   a. osteoarthritis

   b. skeletal hypertrophy

   c. osteoporosis

   d. kyphosis

5. The neurological system becomes impaired by the normal effects of aging. Changes that occur include:

   a. The ability to discern lower frequency sounds is slowly lost.

   b. A decrease in the amount of cerebral spinal fluid in the skull.

   c. Nerve cells begin to degenerate and die as early as the mid-forties.

   d. The elderly have a harder time perceiving their body position.

6. The renal system is affected by the normal aging process. Which of the following are common changes in the elderly patient's renal system?

   a. The kidneys begin retaining more fluid, and increase in size and weight.

   b. There is a buildup of nephrons in the kidneys over time, decreasing their function.

   c. There is a greater amount of blood per minute passing through the kidneys for filtration.

   d. It is common for the elderly to suffer from drug toxicity due to kidney malfunction.

7. As a result of the normal aging process, the response to an illness is altered. Medical problems present with different signs and symptoms. For example:

   a. A slowing respiratory rate, instead of increasing, may indicate respiratory failure rather than improved oxygenation.

   b. A lack of chest pain in a geriatric patient experiencing a heart attack is common.

   c. Because the geriatric patient is predisposed to peripheral vascular diseases, a diminished radial pulse may not be an abnormal sign.

   d. All of the above.

Reference

US Department of Transportation, National Highway Traffic Safety Administration. *EMT-Basic National Standard Curriculum.* Washington, DC: US Department of Transportation, National Highway Traffic Safety Administration; 1994.

Chapter 11
Communications

Upon arriving at the scene of a patient in severe respiratory distress, you begin assessing the patient and determine the respiratory difficulty is secondary to being stung by an hornet. The patient is complaining of respiratory difficulty, urticaria, and angioedema, and the patient is describing a closing sensation of the throat. You and your partner decide the patient requires an intramuscular injection of epinephrine, and begin transport per local protocol. You contact medical control via cellular phone and give your presentation to the physician. The physician orders you to administer 0.3 mg of epinephrine IM using the Epipen. Your communication via cell phone for medication orders from the medical control physician are complete and the patient states the tightness feeling in the throat has subsided. This mode of communication is an example of what type of communication?

COMMUNICATION SYSTEM

System Components

- Base station—A radio which is located at a stationary site such as a hospital, mountaintop, or public safety agency's, tall building.
- Mobile two-way radios (transmitter/receivers).
  - Implies a vehicle-mounted device.
  - Mobile transmitters usually transmit at lower power than base stations (typically 20-50 W).
  - Typical transmission range is 10 to 15 miles over average terrain.
- Portable radios (transmitter/receivers).
  - Handheld device.
  - Typically has a power output of 1 to 5 W, limiting their range.
- Repeater/base station—Receives a transmission from a low-power portable or mobile radio on one frequency and retransmits at a higher power on another frequency.
- Digital radio equipment.
- Cellular telephones.

Radio Communications

- Radio frequencies are assigned and licensed by the Federal Communication Commission (FCC).
- Response to the scene.

- The dispatcher needs to be notified that the call was received (acknowledgment of the assignment).
- Dispatch needs to know that the unit is enroute (response).
- Other agencies, such as a local hospital, should be notified as appropriate.
- Arrival at the scene—The dispatcher must be notified.

Communication with Medical Direction

- In some systems, medical direction is at the receiving facility, and in other systems, medical direction is at a separate site.
- In either case, the emergency medical technician (EMT) may need to contact medical direction for consultation, and to get orders for administration of medications. Radio transmissions need to be organized, concise, and pertinent.
- Since the physician will determine whether to order medications and procedures based on the information given by the EMT, information *must* be accurate.
- After receiving an order for a medication or procedure (or denial of such a request), repeat the order word for word.
- Orders that are unclear or appear to be inappropriate should be questioned.

Communication with Receiving Facilities

- EMTs provide information that allows hospitals to prepare for a patient's arrival by having the right room, equipment, and personnel prepared.

PATIENT REPORTING CONCEPTS

- When speaking on the radio, keep these principles in mind:
  - Radio is on and volume is properly adjusted.
  - Listen to the frequency and ensure it is clear before beginning a transmission.
  - Press the "press-to-talk" (PTT) button on the radio and wait for 1 second before speaking.
  - Speak with lips about 2 to 3 in from the microphone.
  - Address the unit being called, then give the name of the unit (and number if appropriate) where the transmission is originating from.
  - The unit being called will signal that the transmission should start by saying "go ahead" or some other term standard for that area. A response of "stand by" means wait until further notice.
  - Speak clearly and slowly, in a monotone voice.
  - Keep transmissions brief. If, on occasion, a transmission takes longer than 30 seconds, stop at that point and pause for a few seconds so that emergency traffic can use the frequency if necessary.
  - Use clear text.
  - Avoid codes.
  - Avoid meaningless phrases like "be advised."

- Courtesy is assumed, so there is no need to say "please," "thank you," and "you're welcome."
- When transmitting a number that might be confused (eg, a number in the teens), give the number, then give the individual digits.
- The airwaves are public and scanners are popular. Emergency medical services (EMS) transmissions may be overheard by more than just the EMS community. Do not give a patient's name over the air.
- For the same reason, be careful to remain objective and impartial in describing patients. An EMT may be sued for slander if he injures someone's reputation in this way.
- An EMT rarely acts alone—Use *we* instead of *I*.
- Do not use profanity on the air. The FCC takes a dim view of such language and may impose substantial fines.
- Avoid words that are difficult to hear like *yes* and *no*. Use *affirmative* and *negative*.
- Use the standard format for transmission of information.
- When the transmission is finished, indicate this by saying *over*. Get confirmation that the message was received.
- Avoid codes, especially those that are not standardized.
- Avoid offering a diagnosis of the patient's problem.
- Use EMS frequencies only for EMS communication.
- Reduce background noise as much as possible by closing the window.
- Notify the dispatcher when the unit leaves the scene.
- When communicating with medical direction or the receiving facility, a verbal report should be given. The essential elements of such a report, in the order they should be given, are:
  — Identify unit and level of provider (who and what)
  — Estimated time of arrival
  — Patient's age and sex
  — Chief complaint
  — Brief, pertinent history of the present illness
  — Major past illnesses
  — Mental status
  — Baseline vital signs
  — Pertinent findings of the physical examination
  — Emergency medical care given
  — Response to emergency medical care
- After giving this information, the EMT will continue to assess the patient. Additional vital signs may be taken and new information may become available, particularly on long transports. In some systems, this information should be relayed to the hospital (refer to local protocol). Information that must be transmitted includes deterioration in the patient's condition.
- Arrival at the hospital.
  - The dispatcher must be notified.
  - In some systems, the hospital should also be notified.
- Leaving the hospital for the station—The dispatcher should be notified.
- Arrival at the station—The dispatcher should be notified.

Verbal Communication (Transition of Care)

- After arrival at the hospital, give a verbal report to the staff.
- Introduce the patient by name (if known).
- Summarize the information given over the radio:
  - Chief complaint
  - History that was not given previously
  - Additional treatment given en route
  - Additional vital signs taken en route
  - Give additional information that was collected but not transmitted.

Interpersonal Communication

- Make and keep eye contact with the patient.
- When practical, position yourself at a level lower than the patient.
- Be honest with the patient.
- Use language the patient can understand.
- Be aware of your own body language.
- Speak clearly, slowly, and distinctly.
- Use the patient's proper name, either first or last, depending on the circumstances. Ask the patient what he wishes to be called.
- If a patient has difficulty hearing, speak clearly with lips visible.
- Allow the patient enough time to answer a question before asking the next one.
- Act and speak in a calm, confident manner.

Common Communication Issues with Elderly Patients

- Potential for visual deficit
- Potential for auditory deficit

? CHAPTER QUESTIONS

1. In the emergency pre-hospital care communications system, a mobile transmitter/receiver:
   a. is a portable, hand-carried radio useful when working at a distance from your vehicle
   b. is a device that receives transmissions and rebroadcasts them at a higher power
   c. serves as a dispatch and coordination area
   d. is a vehicle-based radio which comes in a variety of power ranges

2. Components of an emergency communications system may include:
   a. cellular phones
   b. a base station
   c. digital equipment
   d. all of the above

3. As an EMT you will be expected to communicate with partners, dispatch, medical direction, and hospitals. The progression of radio transmissions includes:

   a. notifying dispatch of your arrival at the hospital

   b. contacting law enforcement with medical information about the patient

   c. contacting the patient's personal physician while en route to the hospital

   d. notifying dispatch when you are 5 minutes from the scene

4. The ground rules for radio communication include:

   a. using EMS frequencies for all radio traffic, including personal messages

   b. pressing your lips against the microphone for clarity while speaking

   c. pushing the press-to-talk button and waiting for 1 second before speaking

   d. giving the receiving hospital what you feel the patient's diagnosis is

5. When receiving orders from medical direction, the EMT should do all of the following except:

   a. repeat the order(s) word for word

   b. give the patient's name over the radio

   c. ask for clarification of an order you did not understand or feel is inappropriate

   d. avoid phrases such as *please, thank you,* and *you're welcome*

6. When communicating with medical direction, you should provide the following information:

   a. the patient's chief complaint

   b. the patient's marital status

   c. the patient's ethnic origin

   d. the patient's name

7. Once you arrive at the hospital with your patient, it is important to give the ER staff an oral report. This report should include:

   a. personal information about the patient not pertinent to medical care

   b. only new information; it is not necessary to repeat your broadcasted (radio) report

   c. treatment given to the patient en route and his response to it

   d. the patient's billing and insurance information

8. Documentation you assemble as an EMT has a variety of functions. These include:

   a. helping to ensure the continuity of care for the patient

   b. providing data for researchers and scientists

   c. submitting records to insurance companies

   d. all of the above

Reference

US Department of Transportation, National Highway Traffic Safety Administration. *EMT-Basic National Standard Curriculum.* Washington, DC: US Department of Transportation, National Highway Traffic Safety Administration; 1994.

Chapter 12
Documentation

You and your partner have just completed an assignment involving a pedestrian auto accident. Your partner has begun the clean-up process in the ambulance, and you are going to begin documenting the assignment. You sit down in the crew room at the hospital and begin the difficult task of documenting all subjective and objective information. You include the patient's name, address, social security number, and date of birth. What are some of the necessary documentation requirements needed to complete a thorough Pre-Hospital Care Report (PCR)?

DOCUMENTATION

- Minimum documentation requirements that should be on every ambulance call report (Fig. 12-1):
  - Information gathered at time of the emergency medical technician's (EMT's) arrival at scene, at initial contact with patient, following all interventions, and on arrival at facility.
    — Chief complaint
    — Level of consciousness (AVPU [alert, verbal, painful, unresponsive])
    — Mental status
    — Systolic blood pressure for patients greater than 3 years old
    — Skin perfusion (capillary refill) for patients less than 6 years old
    — Skin color and temperature
    — Pulse rate and quality
    — Respiratory rate and effort
  - Administrative information
    — Time incident was reported
    — Time unit was notified
    — Time of arrival at patient side
    — Time unit left scene
    — Time of arrival at destination
    — Time transfer of care occurred

THE PRE-HOSPITAL CARE REPORT (LEGAL MEDICAL DOCUMENT)

- Functions as:
  - Continuity of care (a form that is not read immediately in the emergency department may very well be referred to later for important treatment rendered by EMTs).

MMDDYY RUN NO 5- 2 COPY AGENCY VEH ID

AGENCY NAME

DISPATCH INFORMATION

CALL LOCATION

LOCATION CODE

MILEAGE
END
BEGIN
CODE TOTAL

CALL REC'D
ENROUTE
AT SCENE
FROM SCENE
AT DESTINATION
IN SERVICE
IN QUARTERS

PATIENT INFORMATION

FIRST NAME   LAST NAME

ADDRESS

APPT/UNIT NUMBER   (PHO)NE -

CITY   ST ZIP +4

AGE   D.O.B. MM / DD / YYYY F M SS# - -

○ Residence
○ Health
○ Farm
○ Industrial
○ Other Work
○ Residence
○ Road
○ Other

Call Received as
○ EMERGENCY
○ NON EMERGENCY
○ STANDBY

Physician

CARE IN PROGRESS ON ARRIVAL:
○ None ○ Citizen ○ PD/FD/Other First Responder ○ Other EMS ○ PAD used

MECHANISM OF INJURY
○ MVA (✓ seat belt used →) ○ Fall of ___ feet ○ GSW ○ Machinery
○ Struck by vehicle ○ Unarmed assault ○ Knife ○ ___

○ Extrication required ___ minutes

Seat belt used?
○ Yes ○ No ○ Unknown

Seat Belt Use Reported By
○ Crew ○ Patient
○ Police ○ Other

CHIEF COMPLAINT   **SUBJECTIVE ASSESSMENT**

PRESENTING PROBLEM

Fill in circle
○ Airway Obstruction
○ Respiratory Arrest
○ Respiratory Distress
○ Cardiac Related (Potential)
○ Cardiac Arrest

○ Allergic Reaction
○ Syncope
○ Stroke/CVA
○ General Illness/Malaise
○ Gastro-Intestinal Distress
○ Diabetic Related (Potential)
○ Pain ___

○ Unconscious/Unresp.
○ Seizure
○ Behavioral Disorder
○ Substance Abuse (Potential)
○ Poisoning (Accidental)

○ Shock
○ Head Injury
○ Spinal Injury
○ Fracture/Dislocation
○ Amputation
○ Other ___

○ Major Trauma
○ Trauma-Blunt
○ Trauma-Penetrating
○ Soft Tissue Injury
○ Bleeding/Hemorrhage

○ OB/GYN
○ Burns
Environmental
○ Heat
○ Cold
○ Hazardous Materials
○ Obvious Death

PAST MEDICAL HISTORY
○ None
○ Allergy to ___
○ Hypertension ○ Stroke
○ Seizures ○ Diabetes
○ COPD ○ Cardiac
○ Other (List) ○ Asthma

Current Medications (List)

VITAL SIGNS	TIME	RESP	PULSE	B.P.	LEVEL OF CONSCIOUSNESS	GCS	R	PUPILS	L	SKIN	STATUS
		Rate: ○ Regular ○ Shallow ○ Labored	Rate: ○ Regular ○ Irregular		○ Alert ○ Voice ○ Pain ○ Unresp.		○ ○ ○ ○	Normal Dilated Constricted Sluggish No-Reaction	○ ○ ○ ○	○ Unremarkable ○ Cool ○ Pale ○ Warm ○ Cyanotic ○ Moist ○ Flushed ○ Dry ○ Jaundiced	○ C ○ U ○ P ○ S
		Rate: ○ Regular ○ Shallow ○ Labored	Rate: ○ Regular ○ Irregular		○ Alert ○ Voice ○ Pain ○ Unresp.		○ ○ ○ ○	Normal Dilated Constricted Sluggish No-Reaction	○ ○ ○ ○	○ Unremarkable ○ Cool ○ Pale ○ Warm ○ Cyanotic ○ Moist ○ Flushed ○ Dry ○ Jaundiced	○ C ○ U ○ P ○ S
		Rate: ○ Regular ○ Shallow ○ Labored	Rate: ○ Regular ○ Irregular		○ Alert ○ Voice ○ Pain ○ Unresp.		○ ○ ○ ○	Normal Dilated Constricted Sluggish No-Reaction	○ ○ ○ ○	○ Unremarkable ○ Cool ○ Pale ○ Warm ○ Cyanotic ○ Moist ○ Flushed ○ Dry ○ Jaundiced	○ C ○ U ○ P ○ S

OBJECTIVE PHYSICAL ASSESSMENT

COMMENTS

TREATMENT GIVEN *FILL IN CIRCLE*
○ Moved to ambulance on stretcher/backboard
○ Moved to ambulance on stair chair
○ Walked to ambulance
○ Airway Cleared
○ Oral/Nasal Airway
○ Esophageal Obturator Airway/Esophageal Gastric Tube Airway (EOA/EGTA)
○ EndoTracheal Tube (E/T)
○ Oxygen Administered @ ___ L.P.M., Method ___
○ Suction Used
○ Artificial Ventilation Method ___
○ C.P.R. in progress on arrival by: ○ Citizen ○ PD/FD/Other First Responder ○ Other
○ C.P.R. Started @ Time ___   Time from Arrest Until C.P.R. ___ Minutes
○ EKG Monitored (Attach Tracing) [Rhythm(s) ___]
○ Defibrillation/Cardioversion No. Times ___ ○ Manual ○ Semi-automatic

○ Medication Administered (Use Continuation Form)
○ IV Established Fluid ___ Cath. Gauge ___
○ Mast Inflated @ Time ___)
○ Bleeding/ Hemorrhage Controlled (Method Used: ___)
○ Spinal Immobilization Neck and Back
○ Limb Immobilized by ○ Fixation ○ Traction
○ (Heat) or (Cold) Applied
○ Vomiting Induced @ Time ___ Method ___
○ Restraints Applied, Type ___
○ Baby Delivered @ Time ___ In County ___
  ○ Alive ○ Stillborn ○ Male ○ Female
○ Transported in Trendelenburg position
○ Transported in left lateral recumbent position
○ Transported with head elevated
○ Other ___

DISPOSITION (See list)   **DISP. CODE**   **CONTINUATION FORM USED** YES

CREW	IN CHARGE	DRIVER'S NAME	NAME	NAME
	○ EMT ○ AEMT #	○ CFR ○ EMT ○ AEMT #	○ CFR ○ EMT ○ AEMT #	○ CFR ○ EMT ○ AEMT #

AGENCY COPY

EMS 100 (11/86) provided by NYS-EMS PROGRAM
DOH 3283 (7/02)

Figure 12-1 New York state PCR document.

- Legal document—A good report has documentation of what emergency medical care was provided, the status of the patient on arrival at the scene, and any changes upon arrival at the receiving facility. Information should include objective and subjective information.
  — All documentation should be clear, concise, and legible.
- Educational—Used to demonstrate proper documentation and how to handle unusual or uncommon cases.
- Administrative—Used for billing and service statistical analysis for research.
- Evaluation and continuous quality improvement.

Types of Ambulance Call Reports

- Traditional reports are written forms with check boxes and a section for a narrative.
- Computerized versions are filled in by means of an electronic clipboard or a similar device.
- Sections include date, times, service, unit, names of crew, patient data (patient name, address, date of birth, insurance information, sex, age, nature of call, mechanism of injury, location of patient, treatment administered prior to arrival of EMT, signs and symptoms, care administered, baseline vital signs, SAMPLE [*s*igns/*s*ymptoms, *a*llergies, *m*edications, *p*ast medical problems, *l*ast oral intake, *e*vents] history, and changes in condition).
- Check boxes should be filled in completely.
  - Avoid stray marks.
- Narrative section (if applicable):
  - Describe, don't conclude.
  - Include pertinent negative/positive findings (**Pertinent negative:** absence of a sign or symptom that helps substantiate or identify a patient's condition).
  - Record important observations about the scene, that is, suicide note, weapon, and the like.
  - Avoid radio codes.
  - Use abbreviations only if they are standard medical abbreviations.
  - When information of a sensitive nature is documented, note the source of that information, that is, communicable diseases.
  - State reporting requirements such as child abuse, animal bites, and the like.
  - Be sure to spell words correctly, especially medical words. If you do not know how to spell it, find out or use another word.
  - For every reassessment, record time and findings.
- Confidentiality—The ambulance call report and the information on the form are considered confidential. Be familiar with state laws.
- Distribution—Local/state protocols will determine where the different copies of the form should be distributed.
- Falsification issues:
  - When an error of omission or commission occurs, the EMT should not try to cover it up. Instead, document what did or did not happen and what steps were taken (if any) to correct the situation.
  - Falsification of information on the Pre-Hospital Care Report may lead not only to suspension or revocation of the EMT's certification/license, but also to poor patient care because other health-care providers have a false impression of which assessment findings were discovered or what treatment was given.

- Difficult documentation issues:
  - Vital signs—Document only the vital signs that were actually taken.
  - Treatment—If a treatment like oxygen was overlooked, do not chart that the patient was given oxygen.

DOCUMENTATION OF PATIENT REFUSAL

- Competent adult patients have the *right to refuse* treatment.
- Before the EMT leaves the scene, he/she should:
  - Try again to persuade the patient to go to a hospital.
  - Ensure the patient is able to make a rational, informed decision.
  - Inform the patient why he/she should go and what may happen to him if he does not.
  - Consult medical direction as directed by local protocol.
  - If the patient still refuses, document any assessment findings and emergency medical care given, and then have the patient sign a refusal form.
  - Have a family member, police officer, or bystander sign the form as a witness. If the patient refuses to sign the refusal form, have a family member, police officer, or bystander sign the form verifying that the patient refused to sign.
  - Complete the PCR for a patient refusal.
    — Complete patient assessment.
    — Care EMT wished to provide for the patient.
    — Statement that the EMT explained to the patient the possible consequences of failure to accept care, including potential death.
    — Offer alternative methods of gaining care.
    — State willingness to return even if patient refuses treatment and transport.

SPECIAL SITUATIONS/REPORTS/INCIDENT REPORTING

Correction of Errors

- Draw a single horizontal line through the error, initial it, and write the correct information beside it.
- Do not try to obliterate the error—This may be interpreted as an attempt to cover up a mistake.

Errors Discovered After the Report Form Is Submitted

- Preferably in a different color ink, draw a single line through the error, initial, and date it and add a note with the correct information.
- If information was omitted, add a note with the correct information, the date, and the EMT's initials.

Documentation at Multiple Casualty Incidents

- When there is not enough time to complete the form before the next call, the EMT will need to fill out the report later.
- The local Multiple Casualty Incidents (MCI) plan should have some means of recording important medical information temporarily, that is, triage tag that can be used later to complete the form.
- The standard for completing the form in an MCI is not the same as for a typical call. Your local plan should have guidelines.

Special Situation Reports

- Used to document events that should be reported to local authorities, or to amplify and supplement primary report (Fig. 12-2).
- Should be submitted in timely manner.
- Should be accurate and objective.
- The EMT should keep a copy for his/her own records.
- The report, and copies, if appropriate, should be submitted to the authority described by local protocol.
- Exposure.
- Injury.

Emergency Medical Services Agency
Unusual Occurrence Report
EMS-903

(Refer to The Back of This Form For Directions)

1. Incident Date/Time	2. Provider Agency Name	3. Event #	4. Reporting Date

5. Address or Location of Incident

6. Person Reporting Incident

7. Preferred Method of Contact

Email: Address:

Phone: Fax:

8. Affiliation	9. Unit

10. Type of Incident

11. Incident Description: Be as specific as possible. Include names, addresses, times, dates, etc. Use separate sheets of paper if necessary.

12. Attachments YES / NO # of pages or documents_____

FOR EMS AGENCY USE	EMSA Incident #
Final Disposition:	Date received:
Reviewed By:	Date closed:

Figure 12-2 Emergency Medical Services Agency Unusual Occurrence Report (EMS-903). (*From http://www.sccgov.org/portal/site/ems/.*)

CONTINUOUS QUALITY IMPROVEMENT

- Information gathered from the Pre-Hospital Care Report can be used to analyze various aspects of the EMS system.
- This information can then be used to improve different components of the system and prevent problems from occurring in the future.

? CHAPTER QUESTIONS

1. The medical documentation you prepare has legal and administrative functions. Which of the following is true regarding these uses of your documentation?

   a. Since the documentation is not considered a legal document, you will not be able to refer to it when testifying in court.

   b. Since the EMT is the only person who will read the documentation, legibility and use of abbreviations is not of importance.

   c. The EMTs documentation is generally not used when preparing bills.

   d. The medical documentation you provide typically becomes a part of the patient's permanent hospital record.

2. The Department of Transportation's (DOT) minimum data set for patient information gathered by the EMT includes:

   a. capillary refill for patients less than 1 year old

   b. systolic blood pressure for patients greater than 8 years old

   c. the patient's respiratory rate and effort

   d. the patient's medical insurance information

3. Administrative information in the DOT's minimum date set includes:

   a. the location of the unit prior to responding to the call

   b. the time the unit left the hospital after transferring care

   c. the time the incident was reported ("called in")

   d. the time the EMT radioed the patient report to the hospital

4. An important division of a PCR is the patient's vital signs. Which of the following is true regarding this division of the PCR?

   a. Once the baseline vital signs are assessed, the second set of vital signs can be estimated.

   b. At least two complete sets of vital signs should be taken and recorded.

   c. The exact time the patient's vital signs were taken is not critical.

   d. All of the above.

5. Information that is measurable or verifiable in some way is called:

   a. pertinent negatives

   b. objective information

   c. subjective information

   d. pertinent information

CROSSWORD

Across

1. _____ of injury is the manner in which an injury occurred.
5. Physical _____ is when an EMT performs systematic hands-on approach to evaluating a patient.
8. The mnemonic for performing cervical spinal immobilization.
10. Patient _____.
13. During the general impression it is important to determine the patient's _____.
14. A baseline vital sign _____.
15. The medical term used for the hip.
16. _____ assessment is used for patients with an MOI.
20. A _____ forwards a radio transmission and increases its strength.
21. _____ is the medical term for the absence of breathing.
22. In the mnemonic DCAPBTLS the "B" stands for?

Down

1. Acronym for 1 across.
2. _____ complaint is why the patient called the ambulance.
3. Acronym for nature of illness.

4. The process of evaluating a scene for safety.

6. Medical term that describes two or more rib fractures on each affected rib resulting in paradoxal chest wall movement.

7. A form of presenile dementia that is due to atrophy of the frontal and occipital lobes.

9. A scale used to determine and quantify a level of a patient's coma.

11. Mnemonic used to determine patient history.

12. Head _____ chin lift is a maneuver used to open a patients airway manually.

17. Mnemonic used to evaluate patient's level of consciousness.

18. Mnemonic used for the ambulance call report.

19. When evaluating baseline vitals, the EMT must evaluate _____, pulse rate and quality, respiratory rate and quality, and blood pressure.

Section 4
Medical Emergencies

Chapter 13
General Pharmacology

Your emergency medical services (EMS) unit is dispatched to the staging area of a mass casualty incident (MCI). Upon arrival at the staging area, the staging officer orders you and your partner to wear the appropriate personal protective equipment and report to the treatment sector "cold zone." The report of a possible terrorist attack was confirmed when the first arriving units surveyed the scene and determined there were multiple casualties in a shopping mall which described an explosion and a device that disseminated a gas that has patients experiencing signs and symptoms of SLUDGEM (*s*alivation, *l*acrimation, *u*rination, *d*efecation, *G*I upset—nausea/vomiting/cramps/diarrhea, *e*mesis, *m*uscle twitching).

Report given by the incident commander reveals "a device was disseminated, and a chemical released of what was determined by the haz-mat team to be a nerve agent." You and your partner don the appropriate gear and grab your haz-mat response bag that contains the Mark-I auto-injectors needed to begin treatment. How would you begin treatment using the Mark-I auto-injectors?

As an emergency medical technician (EMT), it is important to understand what medications are used and the dangers associated with their administration.
- Medications typically carried on an EMS unit:
  - Activated charcoal (Fig. 13-1)
  - Oral glucose
  - Oxygen
  - Nebulized medication (ie, albuterol sulfate)
  - Epipen and Epipen Jr (Figs. 13-2, 13-3)
  - Mark-I auto-injector (Fig. 13-4)
  - Aspirin (Fig. 13-5)
  - Nitroglycerin (Fig. 13-6)
- Medication names:
  - Generic—The name listed in the *U.S. Pharmacopeia,* a governmental publication listing all drugs in the United States, and is assigned to the drug before it becomes officially listed. Usually a simple form of the chemical name.
  - Trade (brand)—The name a manufacturer uses in marketing the drug.
- *Indications*—The indication for a drug's use includes the most common uses of the drug in treating a specific illness.

Figure 13-1   Activated charcoal. *(Used with permission from Peter DiPrima.)*

Figure 13-2   Epipen auto-injector. *(Used with permission from Peter DiPrima.)*

Figure 13-3   Epipen Jr auto-injector. *(Used with permission from Peter DiPrima.)*

Figure 13-4   Mark-I auto-injector. *(Used with permission from Peter DiPrima.)*

Figure 13-5 Children's chewable aspirin. *(Used with permission from Peter DiPrima.)*

Figure 13-6 Nitrolingual spray and nitroglycerin tablets. *(Used with permission from Peter DiPrima.)*

- *Contraindications*—Situations in which a drug should not be used because it may cause harm to the patient or offer no effect in improving the patient's condition or illness.
- *Expiration Date*—Date that indicates that the medication is expired and should not be used.

FORMS OF MEDICATIONS

- Compressed powders or tablets—Nitroglycerin
- Liquids for injection—Epinephrine
- Gels—Instaglucose (Fig. 13-7)
- Suspensions—Activated charcoal
- Fine powder for inhalation—Prescribed inhaler
- Gases—Oxygen
- Sublingual spray—Nitroglycerin
- Liquid/vaporized fixed-dose nebulizer
- Dose—State how much of the drug should be given

Figure 13-7 Instaglucose gel. *(Used with permission from Peter DiPrima.)*

►**Note:**

Each drug is in a specific medication form to allow properly controlled concentrations of the drug to enter into the bloodstream where it has an effect on the target body system.

- Administration—State route by which the medication is administered, such as oral, sublingual (under the tongue), injectable, or intramuscular.
- Actions—State desired effects a drug has on the patient and/or his body systems.
- Side effects—State any actions of a drug other than those desired. Some side effects may be predictable.
- Reassessment strategies after the administration of a medication include:
  - Repeat baseline vital signs
  - Part of the on-going patient assessment
  - Documentation of response to intervention

PRE-HOSPITAL MEDICATIONS USED BY EMTS

Activated Charcoal

Class: Adsorbent.

Actions: Adsorbs toxins by chemical binding and prevents gastrointestinal adsorption.

Indications: Poisoning following emesis or when emesis is contraindicated.

Contraindications: None in severe poisoning.

Precautions: Should only be administered following emesis, in cases in which it is so indicated. Use with caution in patients with altered mental status. May adsorb ipecac before emesis. If ipecac is administered, wait at least for 10 minutes to administer activated charcoal.

Side Effects: Nausea, vomiting, and constipation.

Dosage: 1 g/kg (typically 50-75 g) mixed with a glass of water to form slurry.

Routes: Oral.

Pediatric Dosage: 1 g/kg mixed with a glass of water to form slurry.

Oral Glucose

Class: Caloric

Actions: Needed for adequate utilization of amino acids

Indications: Hypoglycemia

Contraindications: Hyperglycemia

Precautions: Renal and hepatic disease

Side Effects: Confusion and dizziness

Dosage: one tube (15-g)

Routes: By mouth (PO)

Oxygen

Class: Gas.

Actions: Necessary for cellular metabolism.

Indications: Hypoxia.

Contraindications: None.

Precautions: Use cautiously in patients with COPD, humidify when providing high-flow rates.

Side Effects: Drying of mucous membranes.

Dosage: Cardiac arrest: 100%. Other critical patients: 100%.

Routes: Inhalation.

Pediatric Dosage: 24% to 100% as required.

Albuterol Sulfate (Proventil, Ventolin)

Class: Relatively selective beta-2 adrenergic bronchodilator.

Description: Albuterol is a sympathomimetic that is selective for beta-2 adrenergic receptors. It relaxes smooth muscles of the bronchial tree and peripheral vasculature by stimulating adrenergic receptors of the sympathetic nervous system.

Onset and Duration: Onset: 5 to 15 minutes after inhalation; 30 minutes PO.

Duration: 3 to 4 hours after inhalation; 4 to 6 hours PO.

Indications: Relief of bronchospasm in patients with reversible obstructive airway disease. Prevention of exercise-induced bronchospasm.

Contraindications: Prior hypersensitivity reaction to albuterol cardiac dysrhythmias associated with tachycardia. Tachycardia caused by digitalis intoxication.

Adverse Reactions: Tachycardia, restlessness, apprehension, headache, dizziness, nausea, palpitations, increase in blood pressure, dysrhythmias, hypokalemia.

Drug Interactions: Sympathomimetics may exacerbate adverse cardiovascular effects. Antidepressants may potentiate the effects on the vasculature. Beta blockers may antagonize albuterol.

How Supplied:

MDI: 90 mcg/metered spray (17-g canister with 200 inhalations)

Solution for aerosolization: 0.5% (5 mg/mL)

Pre-diluted nebulized solution: 2.5 mg in 3 mL NS (0.083%)

Dosage and Administration for Bronchial Asthma

Adult: Albuterol sulfate solution 0.083% (one unit dose bottle of 3.0 mL), by nebulizer, at a flow rate that will deliver the solution over 5 to 15 minutes. May be repeated twice (total of three doses).

Pediatric: Albuterol sulfate 0.083% (one unit dose bottle of 3.0 mL), by nebulizer, at a flow rate that will deliver the solution over 5 to 15 minutes. May be repeated twice during transport (total of three doses).

Special Considerations

Pregnancy Safety: Category C.

May precipitate angina pectoris and dysrhythmias. Should be used with caution in patients with diabetes mellitus, hyperthyroidism, prostatic hypertrophy, or seizure disorder.

Epinephrine

Class: Sympathomimetic.

Description: Epinephrine stimulates alpha, beta-1, and beta-2 adrenergic receptors in dose-related fashion. It is the initial drug of choice for treating bronchoconstriction and hypotension resulting from anaphylaxis.

Indications: Acute allergic reaction.

Contraindications: Hypersensitivity.

Adverse Reactions: Headache, nausea, restlessness, weakness, dysrhythmias, hypertension, precipitation of angina pectoris.

Drug Interactions: Monoamine oxidase (MAO) inhibitors and bretylium may potentiate the effect of epinephrine. Beta-adrenergic antagonists may blunt inotropic response.

How Supplied: Auto-injector (Epipen) 0.5 mg/mL (1:2000).

Dosage and Administration—Anaphylactic Reaction

Adult: 0.3 mg

Pediatric: 0.15 mg

Special Considerations

Pregnancy Safety: Category C

May increase myocardial oxygen demand

Mark-I Auto-Injector

The MARK-I kit contains two separate auto-injectors with the following medications:

AtroPen—*atropine sulfate*, 2 mg in 0.7 mL

ComboPen—*pralidoxime chloride* (2-PAM), 600 mg in 2 mL

Each auto-injector is a disposable, spring-loaded, pressure-activated system prefilled with medication. The Mark-I kit consists of one atropine and one pralidoxime auto-injector linked together with a plastic clip. The atropine is administered first followed by the pralidoxime.

Pralidoxime (2-PAM)

Class: Antidote to cholinesterase inhibitors, organophosphate chemicals, organophosphate pesticides.

Mechanism of Action: Pralidoxime (pra-li-DOX-eem) is used together with another medicine called atropine to treat poisoning caused by organic phosphorus pesticides (ie, diazinon, malathion, mevinphos, parathion, and sarin) and by organophosphate chemicals ("nerve gases") used in chemical warfare. Poisoning with these chemicals causes your muscles, including the muscles that help you breathe, to become weak. Pralidoxime is used to help you get back strength in your muscles. Pralidoxime is to be given only by or under the direct supervision of a doctor or trained military personnel.

Effects: Along with its needed effects, this medicine may cause some unwanted effects. Although not all of these side effects may occur, if they do occur they may need medical attention. Check with your doctor as soon as possible if any of the following side effects occur:

Blurred or double vision, difficulty in focusing your eyes, difficulty in speaking, difficult or rapid breathing, dizziness, fast heartbeat, muscle stiffness or weakness, pain at the place of injection (after injection into a muscle).

Pregnancy

Studies on effects in pregnancy have not been done in either humans or animals.

Children

Although there is no specific information comparing use of pralidoxime in children with use in other age groups, this medicine is not expected to cause different side effects or problems in children than it does in adults.

Common Emergency Indications

When an emergency arises, you will need to know how to inject the pralidoxime auto-injector. It is important that you do not remove the safety cap on the auto-injector until you are ready to use it. This prevents spillage of the medicine from the device during storage and handling.

To Use the Pralidoxime Auto-Injector

1. Remove the gray safety cap.
2. Place the black tip of the device on the thigh, with the injector pointed straight at the thigh.
3. Press hard into the thigh until the auto-injector functions. Hold in place for several seconds.
4. Remove the auto-injector and dispose of it as directed.
5. Massage the injected area for 10 seconds.

Treatment of Organic Phosphorus Chemical Poisoning

Adults

The usual dose is 600 mg injected into a muscle. The dose may be repeated 15 minutes after the first dose and again 15 minutes after the second dose, if needed.

Children

Dose must be determined by your doctor.

Treatment of Overdose of Medicines Used to Treat Myasthenia Gravis in Adults and Teenagers

At first, the dose is 1 to 2 g injected into a vein. Then, the dose is 250 mg injected into a vein every 5 minutes.

Children

Dose must be determined by your medical director.

Precautions While Using This Medicine

This medicine will add to the effects of CNS depressants (medicines that may make you drowsy or less alert). Some examples of CNS depressants are antihistamines or medicine for hay fever, other allergies, or colds; sedatives, tranquilizers, or sleeping medicine; prescription pain medicine or narcotics; barbiturates; medicine for seizures; muscle relaxants or anesthetics, including some dental anesthetics. Check with your doctor before taking any of the above while you are using this medicine.

Atropine

Class: Antimuscarinic, parasympathetic blocker, anticholinergic. It is better to refer to atropine as an antimuscarinic rather than an anticholinergic. The word cholinergic refers to the neurotransmitter acetylcholine (ACh) and therefore, anticholinergic implies antagonism of ACh everywhere. Atropine does not block ACh everywhere. For example, voluntary muscle contraction occurs when ACh (liberated from motor nerves) stimulates nicotinic receptors located in the membranes of skeletal muscle. If atropine was truly anticholinergic, then it would paralyze people, which, of course, it does not. Atropine is antimuscarinic, meaning that it blocks ACh primarily at muscarinic receptor sites. Muscarinic receptors are found predominantly in the heart, lungs, gastrointestinal tract, genitourinary tract, and glands.

Mechanism of Action: Competitively blocks ACh at muscarinic receptor sites by competing for the muscarinic receptors.

Effects: An easy way to learn the effects of atropine is to remember that its effects are opposite to that of parasympathetic nervous system stimulation.

As mentioned, this is because it blocks the action of the ACh liberated from the parasympathetic nerve endings.

Heart: Accelerates HR, conduction velocity, and force of contraction (slightly). The major parasympathetic nerve to the head is the vagus nerve (tenth cranial). When the vagus nerve is stimulated, ACh is liberated and upon combining with the muscarinic receptors of the brain, decreases the HR, conduction velocity, and force of contraction (slightly). Thus, atropine causes the opposite to occur.

Lungs: Inhibits glandular secretion in the respiratory tract. Relaxes smooth muscle in the bronchial tree resulting in bronchodilation. Liberation of ACh from parasympathetic nerves adjacent to respiratory tract structures (nose, mouth, pharynx, and bronchi) results in increased respiratory tract secretions and bronchial smooth muscle contraction. Atropine causes the opposite. The drying of respiratory secretions and the prevention of anesthesia-induced bradycardia are the basis of using atropine preoperatively.

Gastrointestinal Tract: Inhibits gastrointestinal secretions. Decreases gastrointestinal motility. Parasympathetic stimulation of the gastrointestinal tract via ACh combining with muscarinic receptors results in increased gastrointestinal secretions and an increase in gastrointestinal motility. By blocking muscarinic receptors, atropine decreases gastrointestinal secretions and decreases motility. Atropine all but stops the secretion of saliva, which is why it causes a dry mouth with difficulty in swallowing.

Pupils: Pupillary dilation. ACh liberated upon stimulation of parasympathetic nerves adjacent to the sphincter muscle of the iris combines with muscarinic receptors and constricts the pupil. Atropine does the opposite. Atropine is a far more effective mydriatic when instilled directly into the eye rather than when given intravenously. Actually, 0.5 mg of atropine given intravenously has little ocular effects, and atropine administration during cardiac arrest does not cause fixed and dilated pupils.

Genitourinary Tract: Decreases normal bladder tone and intensity of bladder contractions. The effect of ACh on muscarinic receptors of the bladder is to increase bladder tone and the intensity of bladder contractions. In other words, it facilitates urination. Atropine blocks the effects of ACh on muscarinic receptors and thus inhibits bladder motility. This is why atropine-containing drugs can cause urinary retention— especially in elderly males with prostate problems.

Cholinergic Poisonings

Organophosphate poisoning and certain types of mushroom poisonings. The symptoms of cholinergic poisoning result from excessive muscarinic stimulation by acetylcholine or by acetylcholine-like drugs. Atropine is the drug of choice for cholinergic poisoning because it blocks the muscarinic receptor sites and therefore protects the individual from the effects of muscarinic overstimulation. The symptoms of cholinergic poisonings are salivation, lacrimation, urination, abdominal cramps, diarrhea, vomiting, bradycardia, dyspnea (secondary to bronchoconstriction and excessive bronchial secretions), seizures, and death. Atropine may be life-saving in this situation.

Treatment of Organic Phosphorus Chemical Poisoning

For significant organophosphate poisonings, start with 1 to 2 mg IV, may repeat as necessary. Severe organophosphate poisonings may require very little amounts of atropine. Best guide for atropinization is cessation of secretions.

Children

Dose: 0.02 mg/kg IV—may repeat every 3 to 5 minutes to a total dose of mg/kg. Maximum single IV dose in child is 0.5 mg, minimum single IV dose in child is 0.1 mg. May be administered intratracheally at dose of 0.05 mg.

Class: Antimuscarinic, parasympathetic blocker, anticholinergic.

Mechanism of Action: Competitively blocks ACh at muscarinic sites.

Effects: Heart—Accelerates HR, conduction velocity, and force of contraction (slightly). Lungs—Inhibits glandular secretion in the respiratory tract, relaxes smooth muscle in the bronchial tree resulting in bronchodilation.

Gastrointestinal tract (GIT): Inhibits gastrointestinal secretions, decreases gastrointestinal motility.

Pupils: Pupillary dilation.

Genitourinary tract: Decreases normal bladder tone and intensity of bladder contractions.

Common Emergency Indications: Symptomatic bradyarrhythmias, cholinergic poisonings, asystole, refractory bronchospasms. Symptomatic bradyarrhythmias—0.5 to 1 mg IV, may repeat every 3 to 5 minutes, 0.4 mg/kg total dose. Asystole—1 mg IV; may repeat in 3 to 5 minutes to a total dose of 3 mg.

Organophosphate Poisonings: 1 to 2 mg IV prn (best guide is cessation of secretions). Refractory bronchospasm—1 mg combined with a beta-2 agonist via nebulizer.

PEDS: 0.02 mg/kg IV may repeat every 5 minutes to a total dose of 0.04 mg/kg. Max single dose in child 0.5 mg, minimum 0.1 mg.

Side effects: Tachyarrhythmias, exacerbation of glaucoma, precipitation of myocardial ischemia.

Aspirin

Class: Platelet inhibitor/anti-inflammatory

Actions: Blocks platelet aggregation

Contraindications: Patients with history of hypersensitivity to the drug

Precautions: GI bleeding, and upset

Side Effects: Heartburn, nausea, vomiting, wheezing

Dosage: 162 to 325 mg PO or chewed

Routes: PO

Pediatric Dosage: Not recommended

Nitroglycerin

Nitroglycerin Spray (Nitrolingual Spray)

Class: Antianginal/vasodilator.

Actions: Smooth muscle relaxant, decreases cardiac work, dilates coronary arteries, dilates systemic arteries.

Indications: Angina pectoris, chest pain associated with myocardial infarction.

Contraindications: Hypotension.

Precautions: Constantly monitor vital signs. Syncope can occur.

Side Effects: Dizziness, hypotension, headache.

Dosage: One spray administered under the tongue; may be repeated in 10 to 15 minutes; no more than three sprays in a 15 minute period; spray should not be inhaled.

Routes: Sprayed under tongue on mucous membrane.

Pediatric Dosage: Not indicated.

Nitroglycerin (Nitrostat and Others)

Class: Antianginal/vasodilator.

Description: It was originally believed that nitrates and nitrites dilated coronary blood vessels, thereby increasing blood flow to the heart. It is now believed that atherosclerosis limits coronary dilation and that the benefits of nitrates and nitrites result from dilation of arterioles and veins in the periphery. The resulting reduction in preload and to a lesser extent in afterload decreases the workload of the heart and lowers myocardial oxygen demand. Nitroglycerin is a very lipid soluble and is thought to enter the body from the Gl tract through the lymphatics rather than the portal blood.

Onset and Duration: Onset: 1 to 3 minutes; duration: 20 to 30 minutes.

Indications: Ischemic chest pain, hypertension, congestive heart failure.

Contraindications: Hypersensitivity.

Adverse Reactions: Transient headache, postural syncope, reflex tachycardia, hypotension, nausea and vomiting, allergic reaction, muscle twitching, diaphoresis.

Drug Interactions: Other vasodilators may have additive hypotensive effects.

How Supplied:

Tablets (sublingual): 0.15 mg (1/400 g), 0.3 mg (1/200 g), 0.4 mg (1/150 g), 0.6 (1/100 g)

Aerosol (translingual): 0.4-mg metered dose

Parenteral: 0.5 mg/mL, 0.8 mg/mL, and 5.0 mg/mL

Tablets (sustained release): 2.6 mg, 6.5 mg, and 9 mg

Capsules (sustained release): 6.5 mg, 9 mg

Topical: 2% ointment

Dosage and Administration: 1/150 g or spray 0.4 mg, sublingually, every 5 minutes, for a total of three doses.

Special Considerations:

Pregnancy Safety: Category C.

Susceptibility to hypotension in older adults increases.

Nitroglycerin decomposes when exposed to light or heat.

Must be kept in airtight containers. Active ingredient of nitroglycerin "stings" when administered SL.

? CHAPTER QUESTIONS

1. An EMT is permitted, with medical direction, to administer, or assist the patient in administering, all of the following except:

   a. nitroglycerin

   b. oxygen

   c. penicillin

   d. oral glucose

2. Medications administered sublingually are:

   a. swallowed
   b. inhaled
   c. dissolved under the tongue
   d. injected under the skin

3. Which of the following is true regarding medication routes-of-administration?

   a. Most medications administered by the EMT are administered by injection.
   b. All medications are administered by the oral route.
   c. The route that is chosen controls how quickly the medication is absorbed by the body.
   d. Drugs administered by the sublingual route have a relatively slow rate of absorption.

4. A drug administered by EMT-basics, and used for a wide range of medical and traumatic emergencies, is:

   a. Tylenol
   b. glucose
   c. nitroglycerin
   d. oxygen

5. The EMT-b may administer which of the following medications to treat a severe allergic reaction?

   a. Glutose
   b. Adrenalin
   c. Liqui-Char
   d. Alupent

6. A 26-year-old female patient has breathing difficulty, and has been prescribed a bronchodilator. Having met all the requirements to administer the medication, the steps include:

   a. placing the patient on a nasal cannula for convenience
   b. leaving the oxygen off the patient until you can assess if the medication worked
   c. having the patient inhale fully, then place her lips around the mouthpiece
   d. having the patient hold her breath as long as is comfortable after inhaling the medication

7. When administering a metered-dose inhaler, tips for the procedure include:

   a. depressing the canister just before the patient begins inhaling
   b. coaching the patient to hold his breath as long as possible
   c. having the patient breathe in and out quickly
   d. being careful not to shake the canister

References

American Heart Association. 2005 American Heart Association Guidelines for Cardiopulmonary Resuscitation and Emergency Cardiovascular Care.

Halperin HR, Tsitlik JE, Gelfand M, et al. A preliminary study of cardiopulmonary resuscitation by circumferential compression of the chest with use of a pneumatic vest. *N Engl J Med.* 1993;329:762–768.

Paradis NA, Martin GB, Rivers EP, et al. Coronary perfusion pressure and the return of spontaneous circulation in human cardiopulmonary resuscitation. *JAMA.* 1990; 263:1106–1113.

2007 Physicians Desk Refernce. 61st ed PDR. The Thompson Corporation.

US Department of Transportation, National Highway Traffic Safety Administration. *EMT-Basic National Standard Curriculum.* Washington, DC: US Department of Transportation, National Highway Traffic Safety Administration; 1994.

Chapter 14
Respiratory Emergencies

Upon arriving on-scene, you are met by an elderly woman who is screaming, "What took you so long to get here? My husband's inside dying! Hurry! Get in there and help him!" You enter the apartment with caution and determine your scene to be safe. As you enter, you see an elderly man sitting by the window, in a tripod sitting position, in obvious respiratory distress. You hear audible wheezing and the patient is cyanotic. He says, "I...cannot.....breathe!" You and your partner begin your assessment and determine the patient has an extensive medical history, which includes chronic obstructive pulmonary disease. What initial treatment do you want to render?

REVIEW OF THE RESPIRATORY SYSTEM ANATOMY AND PHYSIOLOGY

Figure 14-1 is a schematic diagram showing the anatomy of the respiratory system.

- "Eupnea" describes normal, unlabored breathing.
- "Dyspnea" - difficulty breathing
- "Tachypnea" - rapid breathing
- "Bradypnea" - slow breathing
- "Apnea" - absent breathing
- **Hypoxic drive** is a form of respiratory drive in which the body uses oxygen chemoreceptor's instead of carbon dioxide receptors to regulate the respiratory cycle.

Diaphragm Physiology

- Inhalation (active process)
  - Diaphragm and intercostal muscles contract, increasing the size of the thoracic cavity.
  - Diaphragm moves slightly downward, flares lower portion of rib cage.
  - Ribs move upward/outward.
  - Air flows into the lungs.
- Exhalation (passive process)
  - Diaphragm and intercostal muscles relax, decreasing the size of the thoracic cavity.
  - Diaphragm moves upward.
  - Ribs move downward/inward.
  - Air flows out of the lungs.

> **Clinical Significance**
>
> Over 200,000 people die from respiratory emergencies each year in the United States.

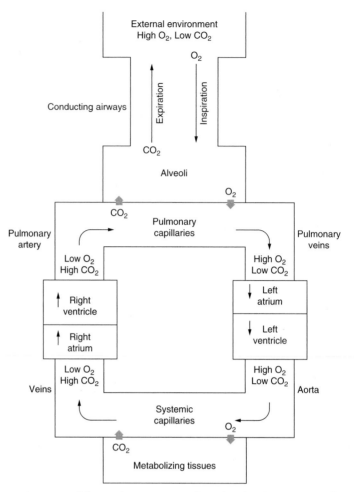

Figure 14-1   Anatomy of the respiratory system. (Reprinted with permission from Levitsky MG. *Pulmonary Physiology.* 7th ed. New York: McGraw-Hill; 2007:3.)

Respiratory Physiology

Alveolar/Capillary Exchange

- Oxygen-rich air enters the alveoli during each inspiration.
- Oxygen-poor blood in the capillaries passes into the alveoli.
- Oxygen enters the capillaries as carbon dioxide enters the alveoli.

Capillary/Cellular Exchange

- Cells give up carbon dioxide to the capillaries.
- Capillaries give up oxygen to the cells.

ASSESSMENT OF THE RESPIRATORY SYSTEM

Initial Assessment

- General impression
  - What is the position the patient was found in?
  - What is the skin color?

- ○ Mental status (alert, verbal, painful, unresponsive [AVPU])
- ○ Ability to speak—Is the patient able to speak in full sentences?
- ○ Respiratory effort—Is breathing labored?

Airway

- Proper ventilation cannot take place without an adequate airway.

Breathing

- Signs of life-threatening problems
- Alterations in mental status
- Severe central cyanosis, pallor, or diaphoresis
- Absent or abnormal breath sounds
- Speaking limited to one or two words
- Tachycardia
- Use of accessory muscles or presence of retractions

Focused History and Physical Examination

- SAMPLE (*s*igns/*s*ymptoms, *a*llergies, *m*edications, *p*ast medical problems, *l*ast oral intake, *e*vents) history
  - ○ Gather a past and present history.
  - ○ OPQRST (onset, provokes, quality, radiates, severity, time) history.
  - ○ Paroxysmal nocturnal dyspnea (sudden onset of dyspnea occurring suddenly at night, usually an hour or two after the individual has fallen asleep) and orthopnea (form of dyspnea in which the person can breathe comfortably only when standing or sitting erect).
  - ○ Coughing and hemoptysis (coughing up blood from the larynx, trachea, brochi, or lungs).
  - ○ Associated chest pain.
  - ○ Smoking history or exposure to secondary smoke.
  - ○ Similar past episodes.

Physical Examination

- Inspection
  - ○ Look for asymmetry, increased diameter, or paradoxical motion of the chest.
- Palpation of the thoracic cavity
  - ○ Feel for subcutaneous emphysema or tracheal deviation in the neck.
  - ○ Percussion.
  - ○ Auscultation.

Normal Breath Sounds

- Bronchial, bronchovesicular, and vesicular

Abnormal Breath Sounds

- Snoring
- Stridor—Sign of an upper airway obstruction and is described as a high-pitched or harsh sound which is heard on inspiration.
- Wheezing—Whistling sound heard during inspiration and/or expiration.

- Rhonchi—Low-pitched squeaking noise heard during auscultation.
- Rales/crackles—Described as fine or coarse and is heard on auscultation. It is produced by air passing over retained secretions.

Extremities

- Look for peripheral cyanosis.
- Look for swelling and redness, indicative of a venous clot.
- Look for finger clubbing, which indicates chronic hypoxia.

Vital Signs

- Heart rate
  - Tachycardia
- Blood pressure
  - Pulsus paradoxus (a pulse that weakens abnormally during inspiration)
- Respiratory rate
  - Observe for trends

Pulse Oximetry

Pulse oximetry is a non invasive monitoring system that provides continuous information about arterial oxygen saturation without subjecting the patient to a painful arterial stick. Using light to measure arterial oxygen saturation (SaO_2), the pulse oximeter tracks the patient's SaO_2 level non invasively and continuously monitors pulse rate and amplitude too. Pulse oximetry works by placing a pulsating arteriolar vascular bed between a dual light (red and infrared) source and a photo detector. The photo detector records the relative amount of each color absorbed by arterial blood and transmits the data to a monitor, which displays the information with each heartbeat. If the SaO_2 level or pulse rate exceeds or drops below user preset limits, visual and audible alarms go off. Normal value for a pulse oximeter is 97% to 100%.

MANAGEMENT OF RESPIRATORY DISORDERS

Basic Principles

- Maintain the airway.
- Protect the cervical spine if trauma is suspected.
- Any patient with respiratory distress should receive high-concentration oxygen.
- Any patient suspected of being hypoxic should receive high-concentration oxygen.
- Oxygen should never be withheld from a patient suspected of suffering from hypoxia.

Common Causes of Airway Compromise

- Tongue, foreign matter, trauma, burns
- Allergic reaction, infection

Assessment

- Differentiate cause, and correct when possible.

EMERGENCY MANAGEMENT OF A PATIENT WITH POSSIBLE AIRWAY COMPROMISE

Conscious Patient

- If the patient is able to speak, encourage coughing.
- If the patient is unable to speak, perform abdominal thrusts.

Unconscious Patient

- Open the airway and attempt to give two ventilations. If they fail, reposition the head and reattempt.
- If they fail, administer cardiopulmonary resuscitation (CPR).
- Attempt finger sweeps only if foreign body is visualized.
- If foreign body is removed, resume ventilation.
- If unsuccessful, continue CPR and finger sweeps if bolus is visualized.

ADULT RESPIRATORY DISTRESS SYNDROME

Common causes of adult respiratory distress syndrome (ARDS) include:

- Sepsis
- Aspiration
- Pneumonia
- Pulmonary injury
- Burns/inhalation injury
- Oxygen toxicity
- Drugs
- High altitude
- Hypothermia
- Near-drowning syndrome
- Head injury
- Pulmonary emboli
- Tumor destruction
- Pancreatitis
- Invasive procedures (bypass, hemodialysis)
- Hypoxia, hypotension, or cardiac arrest

Pathophysiology

- High mortality
- Multiple organ failure
- Affects interstitial fluid
- Causes increase in fluid in the interstitial space, disrupts diffusion and perfusion

Assessment

- Symptoms related to underlying cause
- Abnormal breath sounds heard such as crackles or rales

Management

- Manage the underlying condition.
- Provide supplemental high-concentration oxygen.
- Support respiratory effort.
- Provide positive pressure ventilation if respiratory failure is imminent.
- Monitor vital signs.

TYPES OF OBSTRUCTIVE LUNG DISEASE

- Emphysema
- Chronic bronchitis
- Asthma

Causes

- Genetic disposition
- Smoking and other risk factors

EMPHYSEMA

Pathophysiology

- Exposure to noxious substances. Exposure results in the destruction of the walls of the alveoli. Weakens the walls of the small bronchioles and results in increased residual volume.
- Cor pulmonale—Hypertrophy or failure of the right ventricle.
- Polycythemia—Increase in red blood cells.
- Increased risk of infection and dysrhythmia.

Assessment

- History
  - Recent weight loss, dyspnea with exertion
  - Cigarette and tobacco usage
- Lack of cough
- Physical examination
  - Barrel chest
  - Prolonged expiration and rapid rest phase
  - Thin
  - Pink skin due to extra red cell production
  - Hypertrophy of accessory muscles
  - "Pink puffers"

CHRONIC BRONCHITIS

Pathophysiology

- Results from an increase in mucus-secreting cells in the respiratory tree
- Alveoli relatively unaffected
- Decreased alveolar ventilation

Assessment

History

- Frequent respiratory infections
- Productive cough

Physical Examination

- Often overweight
- Rhonchi present on auscultation
- Jugular vein distention (JVD)
- Ankle edema (pedal edema)
- Hepatic congestion (ascites)
- "Blue bloater"

ASTHMA

- Chronic inflammatory disorder
- Results in widespread but variable air-flow obstruction
- The airway becomes hyperresponsive
- Induced by a trigger, which can vary by individual
- Trigger causes release of histamine, causing bronchoconstriction and bronchial edema
- Approximately 6 to 8 hours later, immune system cells invade the bronchial mucosa and cause additional edema

Assessment

- Identify immediate threats and treat as needed.
- SAMPLE and OPQRST history.
- History of asthma-related hospitalization?
- History of respiratory failure/ventilator use?
- Physical examination
- Presenting signs may include dyspnea, wheezing, and cough.
- Wheezing is not present in all asthmatics.
- Speech may be limited to one to two consecutive words.
- Look for hyperinflation of the chest and accessory muscle use.
- Carefully auscultate breath sounds and measure peak expiratory flow rate.

Management/Treatment Goals

- Correct hypoxia.
- Reverse bronchospasm.
- Maintain the airway.
- Support breathing.
- High-flow oxygen or assisted ventilations as indicated.
- Administer medications such as nebulized albuterol sulfate (per local protocol).

How to administer nebulized medication

1. If using a multi-dose bottle of medicine when you use a nebulizer, use a dropper to administer the correct dosage of medication into the cup with saline solution. If the medicine is in single-use vials, twist the top off the plastic vial and squeeze the contents into the nebulizer cup.

2. Connect the mouthpiece, or mask, to the T-shaped elbow. Fasten the unit to the cup. For children older than 2, using a mouthpiece is recommended because it will deliver more medication than a mask.

3. Connect the nebulizer tubing to the port on the oxygen regulator.

4. Turn the oxygen on to a liter flow of 2 to 4 L/min and check the nebulizer for misting. When using a finger valve, cover the air hole to force air into the nebulizer. If you are not using a finger valve, the nebulizer will mist continually.

5. To administer a nebulizer correctly, hold it in an upright position. This will prevent spillage.

6. When you administer a nebulizer, have the patient sit in a comfortable, upright position. Place the mouthpiece in the patient's mouth between their teeth and have them close their lips around it. When using a mask, be sure it fits well so the mist doesn't get into the patient's eyes.

7. Have the patient gently exhale. As the mist starts, have them inhale slowly through their mouth. Have the patient take over 3 to 5 seconds for each breath while keeping your finger over the valve hole.

8. Have them hold their breath for up to 10 seconds before exhaling. This allows the medication time to deposit in the airway.

9. At the end of a deep breath, uncover the finger valve hole to stop the mist.

10. When you use a nebulizer, occasionally tap the side of the nebulizer to help the medication drop to where it can be misted.

11. Continue until the medicine is gone from the cup. The nebulizer will most likely begin sputtering when it is empty.

Pneumothorax

The presence of air between the outside of the lung and the inside of the chest wall, in an area called the "pleural cavity." Normally the result of trauma! The amount of air present will determine the severity of the pneumothorax and the amount of lung tissue that has "collapsed," which will, in turn, determine the degree of dyspnea experienced by the patient. The source of the air, in the pleural cavity can be external or internal (a hole in the chest wall or a hole in the lungs). If from a hole in the lungs, the hole may be secondary to some disease process (without trauma) and in such cases the pneumothorax is referred to as a "spontaneous pneumothorax." The hole (whether internal or external) may have a flap of tissue attached to its perimeter, creating a valve that will permit the movement of air in only one direction. This may lead to a condition called "tension pneumothorax," an immediate life-threatening condition. Tension pneumothorax at its most threatening stage, is indicated by tracheal shift, as the tension pushes the lungs to one side or the other and the lungs drag the trachea over to the same side. A "life threat" is created when the mediastinum is also dragged to one side, which shifts the heart and may cause a "crimp" in the aorta and/or the vena cava, disrupting blood flow to or from the heart. If you observe tracheal shift, left or right of center, notify an advanced life support provider. Patients with pneumothorax will complain of mild to severe dyspnea (depending on the amount of collapsed lung tissue) with either a gradual or sudden onset (depending on the "size of the hole"). Breath sounds will either be diminished or absent over the site of the pneumothorax. For any patient with suspect pneumothorax, be alert to any change in tracheal position.

Pleural Effusion

A collection of fluid in the pleural cavity. It may be the result of irritation, infection, or some other disease process. The presence of the fluid limits the movement of the lungs, and, if the amount of fluid is significant enough, may cause a "collapsed lung" or partial "collapse," in the area of the fluid. Patients will report dyspnea, lung sounds may be "distant" in the area of the effusion.

Pulmonary Embolism

An embolus is an obstruction in the circulatory system that interrupts blood flow. A pulmonary embolus is an "obstruction" (interruption) of blood flow to the lungs. Pulmonary embolism is a process where a blood clot (thrombus) breaks loose from it origin (usually the site of a "deep vein thrombosis" [DVT] in the leg) and becomes an embolus. This "traveling thrombus" (embolus) makes its way through the vena cava to the right side of the heart, and is immediately pumped out of the heart to the lungs through the pulmonary artery. This artery becomes smaller and smaller until the embolus is eventually lodged "in place" and interrupts the blood flow to the lungs. The patient reports a very sudden onset of dyspnea and acute pleuritic pain. You may observe cyanosis and/or tachypnea.

Hyperventilation Syndrome

Hyperventilation is a condition resulting in blood chemistry where arterial carbon dioxide levels fall below normal. It can be the result of fast shallow breathing (tachypnea,) as might be the case in aspirin (ASA) overdose, or slow deep breathing (bradypnea) as might be presented in some type of head injury. It is usually caused by some disease process, and as such, is to be considered an indicator of some major, life-threatening illness. Hyperventilation syndrome occurs in the absence of any other associated disease process and is usually the result of some psychological influence. The patient usually presents tachypneic, and reports dyspnea, in spite of the tachypnea. The determination of the underlying cause is *not* one that should be made in the field. This patient should be treated with high-concentration oxygen, as with any other patient in respiratory distress, and the diagnosis left to the professional health-care providers at the advanced level. If, however, you are convinced through a thorough history taking, that this event is psychologically triggered, and would like to try to "talk the patient" through the event, please feel free to do so, while the patient is being treated with high-flow oxygen. By encouraging the patient to breathe normally you may be able to break the psychological trigger, and hyper-oxygenated air, inhaled (and exhaled) normally during a hyperventilation syndrome event, will not otherwise exacerbate the syndrome condition. Breathing into paper bags, or using oxygen masks without the oxygen flowing, is inappropriate at this level of care.

There are a several other medical conditions that may present as dyspnea, and they warrant mention here. They include:

1. The **common cold.** A condition that may lead to mild to moderate dyspnea.

2. **Pneumonia.** A bacterial or viral infection, usually with an associated fever, where fluid accumulates in the interstitial space between the alveolus and its capillary, resulting in an ineffective exchange of oxygen and carbon dioxide. This patient will most likely present with moderate dyspnea and tachypnea.

3. **Croup.** An inflammation of the lining of the larynx, typically seen in children less than 3 years of age. It is characterized by a "seal bark" type cough and responds well to the administration of humidified air (oxygen).

4. **Epiglottitis.** A bacterial infection of the epiglottis that can produce moderate to severe swelling. When encountered in children (up to 12 years of age) can significantly threaten a patent airway, because of the degree of swelling compared to the size of the adolescent airway anatomy. Patients in this age range need to be approached cautiously because any action (by the provider) perceived as "threatening" by the patient, may exacerbate the condition beyond the ability of the basic life support provider to maintain a patent airway. A thorough history prior to approaching any child, when practical, will help avoid the problem.

? CHAPTER QUESTIONS

Your patient is a 69-year-old man who presents sitting at the kitchen table in moderate respiratory distress. His elbows are on the table allowing him to be seated in a tripod position, and he appears to be really working at breathing. Although this problem came on gradually today, his family states that he has had lung disease for a long time. He is a lifetime smoker and is on home oxygen at 2 L/min via nasal cannula. He takes the following medications:

- Atrovent MDI
- Proventil MDI

He appears very thin and barrel chested with a pink complexion. You immediately notice pronounced accessory muscles in his neck and chest along with retractions. He labors to breathe, pursing his lips during exhalation. His vital signs are pulse 90 regular, BP 140/80, respiratory rate of 40 labored, skin warm and pink, diffuse wheezes, and his SpO_2 is 90%.

1. Your pre-hospital diagnosis is:

   a. asthma
   b. congestive heart failure
   c. chronic bronchitis
   d. emphysema

2. This disease is characterized by:

   a. alveolar wall destruction
   b. hyper mucous secretion
   c. decreased left ventricular function
   d. decreased tidal volume

3. His pink complexion is caused by:

   a. decreased carbon dioxide
   b. increased oxygen levels
   c. increased production of red blood cells
   d. decreased tidal volume

4. Immediate management of this patient includes:

   a. continued oxygen at 2 L/min via nasal cannula
   b. bronchodilation
   c. IV fluid replacement with NS
   d. all of the above

Chapter 15
Cardiovascular Emergencies

While evaluating a 55-year-old man complaining of crushing substernal chest pressure, the patient states he feels like he is going to "black out." The patient is pale, cool, and diaphoretic. He describes a feeling of impending doom. You summon an advanced life support unit through emergency medical services (EMS) dispatch and they have a 10 minute arrival time. The patient is placed in the supine position and you begin your initial assessment. What is your treatment regimen for this cardiac patient?

REVIEW OF CIRCULATORY SYSTEM—ANATOMY AND PHYSIOLOGY

Circulatory (Cardiovascular)

- Heart structure/function (Fig. 15-1)
  - Atrium
    — Right—Receives blood from the veins of the body and the heart and pumps oxygen-poor blood to the right ventricle.
    — Left—Receives blood from the pulmonary veins (lungs) and pumps oxygen-rich blood to the left ventricle.
  - Ventricle
    — Right—Pumps blood to the lungs.
    — Left—Pumps blood to the body.
  - Valves prevent backflow of blood.

Cardiac Conduction System

- Electrical impulses travel through the electrical conduction system (Fig. 15-2).
- Our heart is more than just a muscle.
- The heart has specialized contractile and conductive tissue:
  - *Automaticity*—Ability to generate an electrical impulse without stimulation from another source
  - *Excitability*—Ability to respond to an electrical stimulus (this is a property of all myocardial cells)
  - *Conductivity*—Ability to propagate an impulse from cell to cell

Sinoatrial (SA) Node (Dominant Pacemaker of the Heart)

- Located in the right atrium near the entrance of the superior vena cava.
- Intrinsic rate *60 to 100* beats per minute.

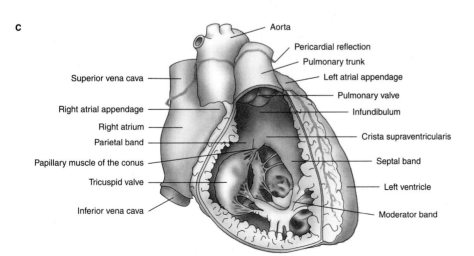

Figure 15-1 A-E Anatomy of the heart. (*Reprinted with permission from Cheitlin MD, Sokolow M, McIllroy MB. Clinical Cardiology. 6th ed. Originally published by Appleton & Lange. Copyright 1993 by The McGraw-Hill Companies, Inc.*)

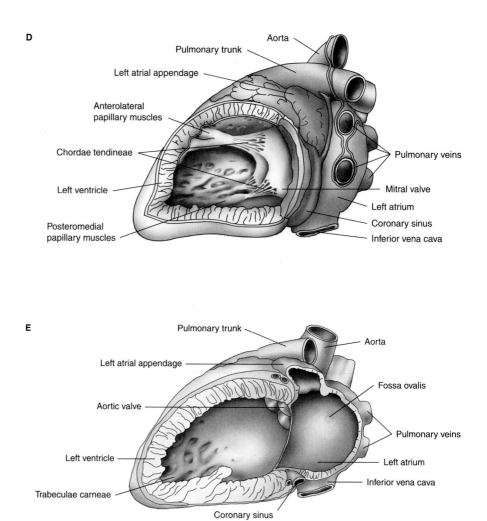

Figure 15-1 A-E *(Continued)*

Atrioventricular Node

- Responsible for creating a slight delay in conduction before sending the impulse to the ventricles.
- Impulse travel time 0.08 to 0.16 seconds.
- No pacemaking properties in the node itself.
- Atrioventricular (AV) junction tissue has an intrinsic rate of *40 to 60* beats per minute.

Bundle of His

- Bundle of fibers coming off the AV node, located at the top of the interventricular septum.
- Considered part of the AV junction.
- Makes the electrical connection between the atria and ventricles.

Bundle Branches

- Created by the bifurcation of the bundle of His into left and right bundle branches.

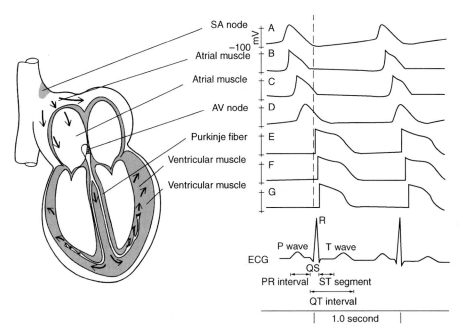

Figure 15-2 Cardiac conduction system. *(Reprinted with permission from Mohrman DE, Heller LJ. Cardiovascular Physiology. 6th ed. New York: McGraw-Hill; 30.)*

- Carry electrical impulse at high velocity to the interventricular septum and each ventricle simultaneously.
- Rate of *20 to 40* per minute.

Purkinje Fibers

- Terminal ends of the bundle branches.
- Network of fibers helping to spread the impulse throughout the ventricular walls.
- Rapid impulse 0.08 to 0.09 seconds.
- Rate of *20 to 40* per minutes.

Blood Vessels

Arteries

- Function—Carry blood away from the heart to the rest of the body.
- Major arteries of the cardiovascular system include:
  - Coronary arteries—Vessels that supply the heart with blood
  - Aorta
    - Major artery originating from the heart and lying in front of the spine in the thoracic and abdominal cavities
    - Divides at the level of the navel into the iliac arteries
  - Pulmonary
    - Artery originating at the right ventricle
    - Carries oxygen-poor blood to the lungs

- Carotid
  — Major artery of the neck.
  — Supplies the head with blood.
  — Pulsations can be palpated on either side of the neck.
- Femoral
  — The major artery of the thigh.
  — Supplies the groin and the lower extremities with blood.
  — Pulsations can be palpated in the groin area.
- Radial
  — Major artery of the lower hand.
  — Pulsations can be palpated at the wrist thumb side.
- Brachial
  — An artery of the upper arm.
  — Pulsations can be palpated on the inside of the arm between the elbow and the shoulder.
  — Used when determining a blood pressure (BP) using a BP cuff (sphygmomanometer) and a stethoscope.
- Posterior tibial—Pulsations can be palpated on the posterior surface of the medial malleolus.
  — Dorsalis pedis
  — An artery in the foot.
  — Pulsations can be palpated on the anterior surface of the foot.
- Arterioles—The smallest branches of an artery leading to the capillaries.

Capillaries

- Tiny blood vessels that connect arterioles to venules
- Found in all parts of the body
- Allows for the exchange of nutrients and waste at the cellular level

Veins

- Function—Vessels that carry blood back to the heart
- Major veins:
  - Pulmonary vein—Carries oxygen-rich blood from the lungs to the left atrium
  - Venae cavae
    — Superior
    — Inferior
    — Carries oxygen-poor blood back to the right atrium
- Venules—The smallest branches of the veins leading to the capillaries

Blood Composition

- Red blood cells
  - Give the blood its color
  - Carry oxygen to organs
  - Carry carbon dioxide away from organs
- White blood cells—Part of the body's defense against infections
- Plasma—Fluid that carries the blood cells and nutrients
- Platelets—Essential for the formation of blood clots

Physiology

Pulse

- Left ventricle contracts sending a wave of blood through the arteries.
- Can be palpated anywhere an artery simultaneously passes near the skin surface and over a bone.
- Peripheral pulses can be located at:
    - Radial
    - Brachial
    - Posterior tibial
    - Dorsalis pedis
- Central pulses can be located at:
    - Carotid
    - Femoral

Blood Pressure

- Systolic—The pressure exerted against the walls of the artery when the left ventricle contracts
- Diastolic—The pressure exerted against the walls of the artery when the left ventricle is at rest

Inadequate Circulation

- Shock (hypoperfusion)—A state of profound depression of the vital processes of the body
- Characterized by signs and symptoms such as pale, cyanotic, cool clammy skin, rapid but weak pulse, rapid and shallow breathing, restlessness, anxiety or mental dullness, nausea and vomiting, reduction in total blood volume, low or decreasing blood pressure, and subnormal temperature

SIGNS/SYMPTOMS OF CARDIAC COMPROMISE

- Squeezing, dull pressure, chest pain commonly radiating down the arms or to the jaw
- Sudden onset of sweating (this in and of itself is a significant finding)
- Difficulty breathing (dyspnea)
- Anxiety, irritability
- Feeling of impending doom
- Abnormal pulse rate (may be irregular)
- Abnormal blood pressure
- Epigastric pain
- Nausea/vomiting

EMERGENCY MANAGEMENT—INITIAL PATIENT ASSESSMENT OF A CARDIAC PATIENT

Circulation—If Pulse Is Absent

- Effective chest compressions produce blood flow during cardiopulmonary resuscitation (CPR). The American Heart Association (AHA) guidelines note the following about chest compressions during CPR:

- To give effective chest compressions, all rescuers should "push hard and push fast."
- Compress the chest at a rate of about 100 compressions per minute for all victims (except newborns).
- Allow the chest to recoil (return to normal position) completely after each compression, and use approximately equal compression and relaxation times.
- Try to limit interruptions in chest compressions. Every time you stop chest compressions, blood flow stops.
- The AHA recommends a compression-to-ventilation ratio of 30:2 for all lone (single) rescuers to use for all victims from infants (excluding newborns) through adults. This recommendation applies to all lay rescuers and to all health-care providers who perform one-rescuer CPR.
- When attempting defibrillation, all rescuers should deliver one shock followed by immediate CPR, beginning with chest compressions. All rescuers should check the victim's rhythm after giving about five cycles (about 2 minutes) of CPR. Once automated external defibrillators (AEDs) are reprogrammed by the manufacturers, they should prompt rescuers to allow a rhythm check every 2 minutes.
- AEDs are recommended for use in children 1 year of age and older. The evidence is insufficient to recommend for or against the use of AEDs in infants under 1 year of age. For sudden witnessed collapse in a child, use the AED as soon as it is available. For unwitnessed cardiac arrest in the out-of-hospital setting, use the AED after about five cycles (about 2 minutes) of CPR. Ideally the AED should be proven (via published studies) to accurately and reliably recognize pediatric shockable rhythms and be capable of delivering a *child* energy dose. Many AEDs are now equipped to deliver smaller doses through the use of smaller child pads or a key or other means. If you are giving CPR to a child (older than 1 year) and the available AED does not have child pads or a way to deliver a smaller dose, use a regular AED with adult pads. *Do not* use child pads or a child dose for adult victims of cardiac arrest.
- Health-care provider *child* CPR guidelines now apply to victims from 1 year to the onset of puberty.
- Lone health-care providers should tailor their sequence of actions for the most likely cause of arrest in victims of all ages.
- *CPR first* (provide about five cycles or 2 minutes of CPR before activating the emergency response number) for unresponsive infants and children (except infants and children with sudden, witnessed collapse) and for all victims of likely *hypoxic* (asphyxial) arrest (ie, drowning, injury, drug overdose).
- Opening the airway remains a priority for an unresponsive trauma victim with suspected cervical spine injury; if a jaw thrust without head extension does not open the airway, health-care providers should use the head-tilt-chin-lift maneuver.
- Basic health-care providers check for "adequate" breathing in adults and presence or absence of breathing in infants and children before giving rescue breaths. Advanced providers will look for "adequate" breathing in victims of all ages and be prepared to support oxygenation and ventilation.

- Chest compressions are recommended if the infant's or child's heart rate is less than 60 per minute with signs of poor perfusion despite adequate oxygenation and ventilation.
- Rescuers must provide compressions of adequate rate and depth and allow adequate chest recoil with minimal interruptions in chest compressions.
- Use one or two hands to give chest compressions for a child, press on the sternum at the nipple line. For the infant, press on the sternum just below the nipple line.
- During two-rescuer infant CPR, the technique using two thumbs encircling hands should include a thoracic squeeze.
- Health-care providers should use a 30:2 compression-to-ventilation ratio for one-rescuer CPR for victims of all ages and for two-rescuer CPR for adults. Health-care providers should use a 15:2 compression-to-ventilation ratio for two-rescuer CPR for infants and children.
- During two-rescuer CPR with an advanced airway in place, rescuers no longer provide cycles of compressions with pauses for ventilation. The compressor provides continuous compressions and the rescuer providing rescue breaths gives 8 to 10 breaths per minute (1 breath about every 6-8 seconds).
- When two or more health-care providers are present during CPR, rescuers should rotate the compressor role every 2 minute.

Responsive Patient with a Known History—Cardiac

- Perform initial assessment.
- Perform focused history and physical examination.
- Place patient in position of comfort.
- Cardiac:
  - Complains of chest pain/discomfort.
  - Administer high-concentration oxygen.
  - Assess baseline vital signs.
  - Important questions to ask:
    — Onset (Did the chest pain or discomfort occur during rest or exertion?)
    — Provocation (Does anything make the pain better or worse?)
    — Quality (Have the patient describe the discomfort—Dull, sharp, tearing, and so on. Remember not to ask leading questions.)
    — Radiation (Does the pain travel anywhere?)
    — Severity (Scale from 1 to 10.)
    — Time (How long has the patient been complaining of chest discomfort?)

Has the patient been prescribed nitroglycerin (NTG), and is the NTG with the patient? If so, is the blood pressure greater than 100 systolic?

- Administer one dose, repeat in 3 to 5 minutes if no relief and if authorized by medical direction (maximum of three doses).
- Reassess vital signs and chest pain after each dose.
- If the blood pressure is less than 100 systolic, continue with elements of focused assessment and transport promptly!

? CHAPTER QUESTIONS

1. When assessing a responsive adult patient with possible cardiac compromise, you should:

   a. insert an airway adjunct

   b. apply oxygen at 15 L/min via nonrebreather mask

   c. ventilate with high-concentration oxygen

   d. begin CPR

2. The mnemonic used to obtain a description of the patient's chest pain is:

   a. SAMPLE

   b. AVPU

   c. DCAP-BTLS

   d. OPQRST

3. When asking about the quality of chest pain, you are asking:

   a. if the pain is sharp, dull, burning, or squeezing

   b. what the patient was doing at the time the pain began

   c. for the patient to rate the pain on a scale of 1 to 10

   d. if the pain travels to any other part of the body

4. When using the mnemonic OPQRST, the "P" stands for:

   a. pressure

   b. pallor

   c. perspiration

   d. provocation

5. You assess your cardiac compromise patient for peripheral edema because:

   a. This condition suggests heart failure.

   b. The patient might be going into shock from fluid shifting.

   c. This may indicate cardiac tamponade.

   d. This condition indicates hypoxia.

6. When caring for a patient with cardiac compromise, you should place him in:

   a. a position of most comfort to him

   b. the Trendelenburg position

   c. the left lateral recumbent position

   d. a supine position

7. NTG eases chest pain by:

   a. constricting blood vessels and sending more blood back to the heart

   b. increasing the amount of oxygen absorbed by the blood in the lungs

   c. increasing the diameter of blood vessels and decreasing the workload of the heart

   d. relaxing the patient and reducing anxiety

8. Which of the following is true regarding the administration of nitroglycerin?

   a. Nitroglycerin is contraindicated if the patient's systolic BP is below 100 mm Hg.

   b. After the first dose, give two tablets for the second dose 3 to 5 minutes later.

   c. You may need to double the dose of nitroglycerin for patients taking Viagra.

   d. Even if the patient has taken several nitroglycerin tablets prior to your arrival, you may give up to three more doses.

9. When assisting a patient in taking nitroglycerin tablets for chest pain, you must make sure:

   a. The patient swallows the tablet with water.

   b. You have contacted the patient's doctor.

   c. The medication has not expired.

   d. The medication is prescribed to another family member.

10. You must reassess your patient within 2 minutes after administering nitroglycerin as one of the side effects is:

    a. a brief feeling of shortness of breath

    b. a sudden decrease in heart rate

    c. a decrease in blood pressure

    d. numbness and tingling in the extremities

11. When comparing angina pectoris and myocardial infarction (MI), remember:

    a. Nitroglycerin may give incomplete or no relief of MI pain.

    b. Pain from an MI radiates, while pain from angina does not.

    c. Angina usually includes other symptoms such as pale, sweaty skin.

    d. Pain from both usually subsides within 10 minutes, or after activity stops.

Reference

1. ECC Committee, Subcommittees and Task Forces of the American Heart Association. 2005 American Heart Association Guidelines for Cardiopulmonary Resuscitation and Emergency Cardiovascular Care. *Circulation*. 2005; 112(24).

Chapter 16
Automated External Defibrillation

You are called to the scene of a commercial dwelling where a 68-year-old patient has gone unconscious. When you arrive at the scene, a man comes frantically running out to the ambulance and says, "Please hurry. Bob was at a board meeting when he suddenly collapsed. The guys are inside doing cardiopulmonary resuscitation (CPR), and our manager is getting the automated external defibrillator (AED)!" You enter the board room and find two people performing CPR. One of the workers says they just defibrillated the patient and returned performing CPR.

What would be your next step in this resuscitation?

IMPORTANCE OF AUTOMATED EXTERNAL DEFIBRILLATION TO THE EMT

- Fundamentals of early defibrillation—Successful resuscitation of out-of-hospital arrest depends on a series of critical interventions known as the chain of survival as outlined by the American Heart Association (AHA):
  ○ Early access
  ○ Early CPR
  ○ Early defibrillation
  ○ Early ACLS
  ○ Integrated post-cardiac arrest care

DEFIBRILLATION

- Immediate defibrillation is appropriate for all rescuers responding to sudden *witnessed* collapse with an AED (Fig. 16-1) on site (for victims ≥ 1 year of age). Compression before defibrillation should occur for 2 minutes or five cycles if cardiac arrest is not witnessed.
- One shock followed by immediate CPR, beginning with chest compressions. The rhythm is analyzed after five cycles of CPR or 2 minutes.
- For attempted defibrillation of children 1 to 8 years of age with an AED, the rescuer should use a pediatric dose-attenuator system if one is available. If the rescuer provides CPR to a child in cardiac arrest and does not have an AED with a pediatric dose-attenuator system, the rescuer should use a standard AED. For infants (<1 year of age), a manual defibrillator is preferred. If a manual defibrillator is not available, an AED with pediatric dose attenuation is desirable. If neither is available, an AED without a dose attenuator may be used.

Figure 16-1   Examples of AEDs.

Overview of Automated External Defibrillators

- Types of automated external defibrillators
  - Fully automated defibrillator operates without action by emergency medical technician (EMT), except to turn on power (used in public access defibrillation).
  - Semi-automated defibrillator uses a computer voice synthesizer to advise EMT as to what steps to take based upon its analysis of the patient's cardiac rhythm.

ANALYSIS OF CARDIAC RHYTHMS

- Defibrillator computer microprocessor evaluates the patient's rhythm and confirms the presence of a rhythm for which a shock is indicated.
- Accuracy of devices in rhythm analysis has been high both in detecting rhythms needing shocks and rhythms not needing shocks.
- Analysis is dependent on properly charged defibrillator batteries.

Causes of Inappropriate Delivery of Shocks

- Human error
- Mechanical error (machine failure)

LETHAL SHOCKABLE RYTHMS

Ventricular Tachycardia

- Attach defibrillator to unresponsive, pulseless, nonbreathing patients to avoid delivering inappropriate shocks (Fig. 16-2).

> **Clinical Significance**
> Studies have shown an increased rate of resuscitation when patients received $1^1/_2$ to 3 minutes of CPR prior to defibrillation.

Figure 16-2   Ventricular tachycardia.

Interruption of CPR

- No person should be touching the patient when rhythm is being analyzed and when shocks are delivered.
- Chest compressions and artificial ventilations are stopped when the rhythm is being analyzed and when shocks are delivered.

ADVANTAGES OF AUTOMATED EXTERNAL DEFIBRILLATION

- Easier to learn than CPR; however, must memorize treatment sequence.
- EMS delivery system should have:
  - Necessary links in chain of survival.
  - Medical direction.
  - EMS system with audit and/or quality improvement program in place.
  - Mandatory continuing education with skill competency review for EMS providers.
  - Continuing competency skill review every 3 months for EMTs.
  - Remote defibrillation through adhesive pads:
    — Defibrillation is "hands-off"
    — Safer method
    — Better electrode placement
    — Has larger pad surface area
    — Provokes less anxiety in EMT
  - Rhythm monitoring—Option on some defibrillator models.

USE OF AUTOMATED EXTERNAL DEFIBRILLATORS DURING RESUSCITATION ATTEMPTS

- Operational steps for a nonwitnessed cardiac arrest:
  - Take infection-control precautions—Should be done en route to scene.
  - Arrive on-scene and perform initial assessment.
  - Stop CPR if in progress.
  - Verify pulselessness and apnea.
  - Have partner resume CPR five cycles of 30:2.
  - Attach device.
  - Turn on defibrillator power.
  - Begin narrative if machine has tape recorder.
  - Stop CPR.
  - Clear patient.
  - Initiate analysis of rhythm.
    — Machine advises shock.
      - Deliver shock.
      - Resume CPR for five cycles.
      - Reanalyze rhythm.
- Check pulse.
- If pulse, check breathing.
- If breathing adequately, give high-concentration oxygen by nonrebreather mask and transport.
- If not breathing adequately, artificially ventilate with high-concentration oxygen and transport.

- If no pulse, resume CPR for 2 minutes (five cycles).
  - Reanalyze
  - Transport
- If, after any rhythm analysis, the machine advises no shock.
  - Continue with five cycles of CPR.

STANDARD OPERATIONAL PROCEDURES

- Assuming no on-scene ALS, the patient should be transported when one of the following occurs:
  - The patient regains a pulse.
  - The patient is packaged and ready for transport.
- One EMT operates defibrillator, one does CPR.
- EMT must be familiar with device used in operational EMS setting.
- All contact with patient must be avoided during analysis of rhythm.
- State "clear the patient" before delivering shocks.
- No defibrillator is capable of working without properly functioning batteries. Check batteries at beginning of shift. Carry extra batteries.

Age and Weight Guideline

- Airway and artificial ventilation is of prime importance.
- Automated external defibrillation is not used in cardiac arrest in children under 1 year of age.

Recurrent Ventricular Fibrillation

- Defibrillation with no available ACLS (Fig. 16-3).
- If pulse is not present:
  - Stop vehicle.
  - Start CPR if defibrillator is not immediately ready.
  - Analyze rhythm.
  - Deliver shock if indicated.
  - Continue resuscitation as per protocol.
- If transporting to hospital with a conscious patient having chest pain, who then becomes unconscious, pulseless, and apneic:
  - Stop vehicle.
  - Attach AED and turn defibrillator on, follow prompts.
  - Start CPR if defibrillator is not immediately ready.
  - Analyze rhythm.
  - Deliver one shock, if prompted by the AED.
  - Continue resuscitation as per AHA guidelines.

Figure 16-3 Ventricular fibrillation.

- If "no shock" message is delivered and no pulse is present:
  - Start or resume CPR.
  - Continue or begin transport.

WITNESSED ARREST

- Defibrillation is initial step; CPR should be performed if defibrillator is unavailable. (Follow 2005 AHA guidelines.)
  - Pulse checks should not occur during rhythm analysis.
  - Coordination of advanced life support (ALS) personnel or EMT-paramedics when EMTs are using automated external defibrillators.
    - — EMS system design establishes protocols.
    - — AED usage does not require ALS on-scene.
    - — ALS should be notified of arrest events as soon as possible.
    - — Considerations for EMT transporting the patient or waiting for ALS to arrive on the scene to transport should be in local protocols established by medical direction.
  - Safety considerations
    - — Water—Rain, pool, and the like
    - — Metal
  - Post resuscitation care
    - — After automated external defibrillation protocol is completed, patient may:
      - Have pulses
      - Have no pulse with machine indicating "no shock indicated"
      - Have no pulse with machine indicating shock

DEFIBRILLATOR MAINTENANCE

- Regular maintenance of defibrillators is necessary as outlined in the manufacturer's directions.
- EMS Shift Checklist for automated defibrillators must be accomplished on a daily basis by EMTs.
- Defibrillator failure is most frequently related to improper device maintenance; most common is battery failure. EMTs must assure proper battery maintenance and battery replacement schedules.

Training and Sources of Information

The AHA publishes a variety of guidelines and additional information on automated external defibrillation.

Maintenance of Skills

Most systems permit a maximum of 90 days between practice drills to reassess competency in usage of AEDs.

Medical Direction

- Successful completion of AED training in an EMT course does not permit usage of the device without approval by state laws/rules and local medical direction authority.

- Every event in which an AED is used must be reviewed by the medical director or a designated representative.
- Reviews of events using AEDs may be accomplished by:
  - Written report.
  - Review of voice-ECG (electrocardiogram) tape recorders attached to AEDs.
  - Solid-state memory sections and magnetic tape recordings stored in device.

Quality Improvement

Involves both individuals using AEDs and the EMS system in which the AEDs are used.

TABLE 16-1: Summary of Key BLS Components for Adults, Children, and Infants

COMPONENT	RECOMMENDATIONS		
	ADULTS	**CHILDREN**	**INFANTS**
Recognition	Unresponsive (for all ages)		
	No breathing or no normal breathing (ie, only gasping)	No breathing or only gasping	
	No pulse palpated within 10 s for all pages (HCP only)		
CPR sequence	C-A-B		
Compression rate	At least 100/min		
Compression depth	At least 2 in (5 cm)	At least ⅓ AP diameter About 2 in (5 cm)	At least ⅓ AP diameter About 1½ in (4 cm)
Chest wall recoil	Allow complete recoil between compressions HCPs rotate compressors every 2 min		
Compression interruptions	Minimize interruptions in chest compressions Attempt to limit interruptions to <10 s		
Airway	Head tilt-chin lift (HCP suspected trauma: jaw thrust)		
Compression-to-ventilation ratio (until advanced) airway placed)	30:2 1 or 2 rescuers	30:2 single rescuer 15:2 2 HCP rescuers	
Ventilations: when rescuer untrained or trained and not proficient	Compressions only		
Ventilations with advanced airway (HCP)	1 breath every 6-8 s (8-10 breaths/min) Asynchronous with chest compressions About 1 s per breath Visible chest rise		
Defibrillation	Attach and use AED as soon as available. Minimize interruptions in chest compressions before and after shock; resume CPR beginning with compressions immediately after each shock.		

Abbreviations: AED, automated external defibrillator; AP, anterior-posterior; CPR, cardiopulmonary rescuscitation; HCP, healthcare provider.
*Excluding the newly born, in whom the etiology of an arrest is nearly always asphyxial.
Reprinted with permission from *2010 American Heart Association Guidelines for Cardiopulmonary Resuscitation and Emergency Cardiovascular Care. Part 4: CPR Overview. Circulation.* 2010;122(suppl 3):S676-S684. © 2010 American Heart Association, Inc.

? CHAPTER QUESTIONS

1. Which of the following is true regarding AEDs?

   a. Manual defibrillators can deliver the first shock more quickly than AEDs.
   b. The AED operator must know how to recognize various heart rhythms.
   c. AEDs allow "hands-free" defibrillation, which is safer for EMS personnel.
   d. AEDs require paramedics to operate them.

2. On which of the following patients would the AED *not* be applied?

   a. A traumatic cardiac arrest patient involved in a motor vehicle crash
   b. A 54-year-old female patient, pulseless, apneic, who collapsed in the kitchen
   c. A 64-year-old man, conscious and breathing, with a heart rate of 188 per min
   d. A 6-year-old girl electrocuted with no pulse and no breathing

3. As soon as you find your adult patient is in cardiac arrest, and you establish the patient has been down for 5 minutes, you should immediately:

   a. apply the AED and begin the defibrillation process
   b. obtain the patient's history from family or bystanders if possible
   c. begin ventilating the patient with high-concentration oxygen and start chest compressions at a ratio of 30 compressions to 2 ventilations
   d. manage the airway by inserting an oropharyngeal airway

4. While transporting a patient with no pulse, remember:

   a. to arrange for an advanced life support rendezvous if possible
   b. if the patient regains a pulse, then goes back into cardiac arrest, you may administer the maximum number of shocks allowed again
   c. no matter what the maximum number of shocks you may give per protocol, medical control can order you to make additional attempts at defibrillation
   d. all of the above

References

Circulation. 2005; 112 (Suppl I): IV-51–IV-57; published online before print November 28, 2005, doi:10.1161/CIRCULATIONAHA.105.166556.

Circulation. 2005; 112 (Suppl I): IV-58–IV-66; published online before print November 28, 2005, doi:10.1161/CIRCULATIONAHA.105.166557.

Circulation. 2005; 112 (Suppl I): IV-67–IV-77; published online before print November 28, 2005, doi:10.1161/CIRCULATIONAHA.105.166558.

Circulation. 2005; 112 (Suppl I): IV-84–IV-88; published online before print November 28, 2005, doi:10.1161/CIRCULATIONAHA.105.166560.

US Department of Transportation, National Highway Traffic Safety Administration. *EMT-Basic National Standard Curriculum.* Washington, DC: US Department of Transportation, National Highway Traffic Safety Administration; 1994.

Chapter 17
Altered Mental Status and Diabetic Emergencies

A call comes into the local emergency medical services (EMS) system for an adult male diabetic emergency at 2144 Motorcycle Parkway. This address is known by both police and EMS for a diabetic patient who has uncontrolled diabetes. When he becomes hypoglycemic, he becomes very belligerent and violent. EMS and police arrive at this location to find the patient's son on the front lawn yelling into the front door of the premises. His son tells the police that his dad is hypoglycemic, violent, and is "tearing the house apart."

Police secures the scene and EMS is allowed to enter the premises. The 55-year-old man is found handcuffed on the floor, flailing around making incomprehensible noises. He is pale, cool, diaphoretic, and has an obviously altered mental status. You ask EMS dispatch to have an advanced life support unit respond, and you begin to evaluate the patient. High-concentration oxygen is administered via a nonrebreather. The patient's vital signs are as follows: blood pressure 158/72; pulse rate 102, strong/bounding; respiratory rate 16; equal/full, skin pale, cool, and diaphoretic. You begin to package the patient and determine the patient has an intact gag reflex. Your partner hands you the Insta-glucose, and you administer the gel buccally (between the cheek and gums).

What is your next treatment modality, and is the treatment rendered *so* far correct?

ANATOMY AND PHYSIOLOGY OF THE ENDOCRINE SYSTEM

What Is a Hormone?
- A substance secreted by an endocrine gland that has effects upon other glands or systems of the body (Fig. 17-1)
- Greatly influenced by stress

Pituitary Gland
- Located at the base of the brain (Fig. 17-2)
- Has two endocrine glands (regulatory)
- Master gland of the body
- Regulates function of most other endocrine glands by hormone secretion

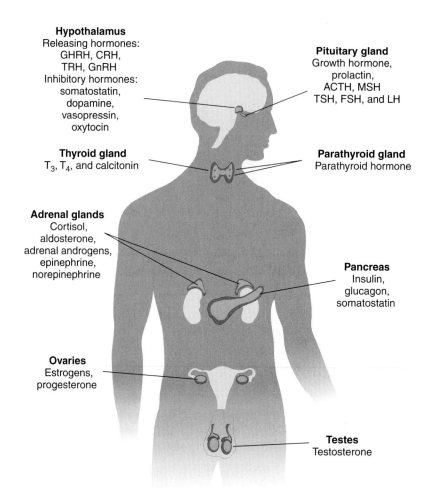

Figure 17-1   Endocrine system. *(Reprinted with permission from Molina PE. Endocrine Physiology. 2nd ed. McGraw-Hill. Fig. 1-1. 2006:2.)*

Thyroid Gland

- Located in the neck
- Anterior and lateral to the trachea
- Below the larynx
- Secretes thyroid hormones which regulate metabolic rate

Parathyroid Gland

- Four small pea-sized glands on the posterior surface of the thyroid glands
- Controls metabolism of calcium and phosphorus

Adrenal Gland

- Located on top of the kidneys
- Two glands that function as separate endocrine glands

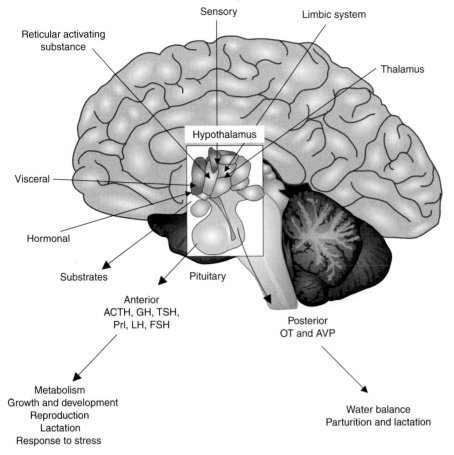

Figure 17-2 Effects of specific endocrine hormones secreted from the anterior and posterior pituitary gland. *(Reprinted from Molina PE. Endocrine Physiology. 2nd ed. McGraw-Hill. Fig. 2-1. 2006:2.)*

Adrenal Cortex

- Secretes glucocorticoids, mineral corticoids, and small amounts of sex hormones

Adrenal Medulla

- Produces epinephrine and norepinephrine

Ovaries

- Paired in the pelvic cavity
- Reproduction

Estrogen

- Promotes monthly formation of inner uterine lining
- Promotes breast development during adolescence

Progesterone

- Aids in promotion of monthly formation of inner uterine lining
- Causes sodium/water retention

Testes

- Located in the scrotum
- Secretes testosterone
- Promotes growth
- Develops and maintains secondary sexual characteristics

Pancreas

- Located retroperitoneal adjacent to the duodenum on the right and extends to the spleen on the left
- Endocrine and exocrine gland
- Islets of Langerhans secrete two regulating hormones:
  - Insulin from beta cells (decreases blood sugar)
  - Glucagon from alpha cells (increases blood sugar)

Glucagon

- While fasting for a few hours, or a moderate decrease in blood glucose level, stimulates alpha cells to secrete glucagon
- Increases liver glycogenolysis
- Increases blood glucose levels
- Allows for stabilization of sugar levels

Insulin

- Secretion of insulin from the beta cells is stimulated by high blood sugar
- Increases glucose transport into the cells
- Increases glucose metabolism by cells; increases liver glycogenesis
- Decreases blood glucose concentration toward normal levels (60-120 mg/dL)

PATHOPHYSIOLOGY OF DIABETES

Diabetes mellitus is defined as the inability of the pancreas to secrete insulin or the inability to produce enough insulin to control blood glucose levels.
- Diabetes mellitus, type I—Insulin dependent (1 in 10 diabetics):
  - Occurs after birth
  - Juvenile may suffer more severe consequences/effects
- Diabetes mellitus, type II—Noninsulin dependent:
  - Obesity predisposes this form of diabetes
  - Normally occurs in adults
  - May be controlled with diet
  - Some insulin may be produced but is ineffective in controlling blood sugar

EFFECTS OF DIABETES

Osmotic Diuresis

- Glucose is filtered in the kidneys causing increased levels of glucose to be spilled into the urine.
- Secretion of glucose molecules in the urine eventually causes dehydration.

Ketone Body Formation (Body Begins to Go into Starvation Mode)

- Fat breakdown increases to provide alternate energy.
- Fat breakdown products are called ketoacids/ketone bodies.

Renal Secretion of Ketoacids

- When more ketoacids are produced than the kidneys can excrete, they accumulate and produce metabolic acidosis (ketoacidosis).

Long-Term Effects

- Kidney disease in 10% of diabetics
- Blindness in about 5000 diabetics each year
- Peripheral neuropathy
- Heart disease—two to four times more likely than nondiabetics
- Stroke—two to six times more likely than nondiabetics

Signs/Symptoms of Diabetes

- Polydipsia—Abnormal thirst
- Polyphagia—Excessive hunger
- Polyuria—Excessive urination

HYPOGLYCEMIA

Pathophysiology

- Insulin lowers serum glucose by enhancing transfer into cells and by stimulating deposits of glycogen.
- Epinephrine tends to cause hypoglycemia by stimulating the breakdown of glycogen, by interfering with the utilization of glucose at the cell level.
- Glucose cannot enter muscle and fat cells.
- Glucose accumulates in blood, which increases blood osmotic pressure.
- Kidneys increase urine output.

Precipitating Factors

- Fasting or decreased food intake
- Chronic alcoholism—Alcohol depletes liver glycogen stores
- Tumor of the pancreas—Cancer
- Unusual physical activity
- Emotional stress
- Too much insulin or oral hypoglycemic medication
- Sepsis
- Administration of beta blockers
- Overdose of salicylates
- Malnutrition
- Liver disease
- Adrenal gland dysfunction

Onset of Hypoglycemia/Signs/Symptoms

- Develops rapidly
- Weak rapid pulse
- Cold, clammy skin
- Weakness and uncoordinated movements
- Headache
- Irritable, bizarre behavior (may appear intoxicated)
- Seizures and coma in severe cases
- Normal or shallow breathing

HYPOGLYCEMIA VERSUS HYPERGLYCEMIA

Pathophysiology of Diabetic Ketoacidosis

- Blood sugar is too high.
- Insulin dose is too small.
- Patient has not taken insulin:
  - When insulin levels are low, glucose cannot enter the cell and accumulates in the blood.
  - May be triggered by significant emotional stress, infection, excess alcohol, pregnancy, or trauma.
- Onset of hyperglycemia progresses slowly, 12 to 24 hours.

Signs/Symptoms

- Polyuria, polydipsia, polyphagia
- Nausea/vomiting
- Tachycardia, deep rapid respiration
- Warm, dry skin, fruity odor breath
- Fever, abdominal pain, and decreased consciousness

Compensatory Mechanism

- Deep rapid respiration in an attempt to blow off excess acids by CO_2 elimination (Kussmaul breathing)

Emergency Management of the Diabetic Patient

- Monitor and maintain the airway
- Oral glucose (if the patient has an intact gag reflex)
- Call for ALS
- Monitor vital signs
- Transport

COMA

Pathophysiology

- An abnormally deep state of unconsciousness from which the patient cannot be aroused by external stimuli.

Possible Causes of Coma (AEIOU-TIPS)

- *A*cidosis, alcohol
- *E*pilepsy
- *I*nfection
- *O*verdose
- *U*remia
- *T*rauma
- *I*nsulin related
- *P*sychosis
- *S*troke

Assessment of the coma patient includes eliciting specific information:

- Length of coma
- Onset—Sudden or gradual
- History of recent head trauma
- Under medical care
- Alcohol or drug abuse
- Complaints or symptoms prior to coma state
- Medic alert tag present

GLASCOW COMA SCALE (GCS)

- The Glasgow Coma Scale (Table 17-1) is used to determine a patient's level of consciousness. The patient is rated using a scale from 3 to 15. Specific evaluations of neurological function include eye opening, verbal response, and motor response. A score of 3 is the lowest score and a score of 15 is a normal score. This scale is used specifically to evaluate a patient's neurological function and is used in evaluating trauma, stroke, and AMS patients.

TABLE 17-1: Glascow Coma Scale

Eye opening	Spontaneously	4
	To speech	3
	To pain	2
	None	1
Verbal response	Oriented	5
	Confused	4
	Inappropriate	3
	Incomprehensible	2
	None	1
Motor response	Obeys command	6
	Localizes pain	5
	Withdraws from pain	4
	Flexion to pain	3
	Extension to pain	2
	None	1
Maximum score		15

? CHAPTER QUESTIONS

1. A change in a patient's mental status is an indication that the central nervous system has been affected in some manner. Causes may include:

   a. brain injury due to trauma
   b. alteration in the patient's blood oxygen level
   c. alteration in the patient's blood sugar level
   d. any of the above

2. During your assessment of a patient with altered mental status, you note lacerations to the tongue. You should become suspicious of:

   a. a physical attack on the patient
   b. seizure activity
   c. loose dentures and possible airway compromise
   d. a suicide attempt

3. A high level of glucose in the blood is caused by:

   a. a lack of insulin to take glucose into the cells
   b. an adequate amount of insulin, but too much glucose in the blood
   c. too much glucose entering the cells of the body
   d. too much insulin leaving too much glucose in the blood

4. Contraindications to the use of glucose in a patient with altered mental status and a history of medication-controlled diabetes include:

   a. if it is unknown if the patient has taken insulin today
   b. the patient taking insulin today, but not eating
   c. a history of type II diabetes
   d. the patient being unable to swallow

Chapter 18
Acute Stroke

You respond to an assignment involving an elderly male with altered mental status. His wife called emergency medical services (EMS) because the patient has had an abrupt change in mental status. You try to evaluate the patient but he is having a difficult time speaking.

Evaluating this patient who is exhibiting signs and symptoms of a stroke, what three signs/symptoms are evaluated using the Cincinnati Stroke Scale?

STROKE FACTS

- Third leading cause of death in the United States.
- 700,000 people in the United States suffer a stroke.
- Number-one cause of disability in the United States.

Your brain has *three* main components (Fig. 18-1):

1. Cerebrum (which consists of the left and right cerebral hemispheres)
2. Cerebellum
3. The brain stem

The cerebral hemispheres of the brain make up the largest part of the brain. The cerebellum is the structure located behind the brain stem, and the brain stem is the lowest section of the brain and is connected to the spinal cord.

STROKE

- Sudden interruption of blood flow to the brain
- Also known as *cerebral vascular accident (CVA)* or "brain attack"
- Prior risk factors are:
  - Hypertension (HTN)
  - Cigarette smoking
  - TIA (transient ischemic attack)
  - Diabetes mellitus
  - Hypercoagulopathy
  - Carotid bruit
  - High red blood cell count
  - Age, gender, race
  - Prior stroke
  - Heredity

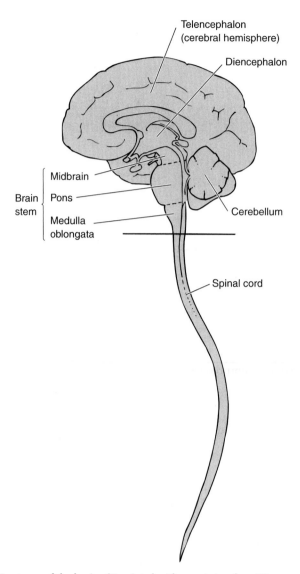

Figure 18-1   Anatomy of the brain. *(Reprinted with permission from Waxman SG. Clinical Neuroanatomy. 25th ed. McGraw-Hill; 2003:2.)*

WARNING SIGNS OF A STROKE

- Numbness, weakness, or paralysis of the face, arm, or leg
- Vision that suddenly blurs or decreases (in one or both eyes)
- Trouble speaking or understanding, or sudden confusion
- Dizziness, loss of balance, or an unexplained fall
- Difficulty swallowing
- Sudden, severe headache that is unexplained

STROKE CLASSIFICATION

Stroke can be divided into two main classifications (Table 18-1).

Ischemic Stroke

- Caused by blood clots. Accounts for 85% of all strokes.
- Only type of stroke that fibrinolytics are administered.

TABLE 18-1: Comparison of Strokes

Ischemic Strokes	Hemorrhagic Strokes
Most common	Least common
Cause: Usually the result of an atherosclerosis or tumor	Cause: Usually the result of a cerebral aneurysm, AV malformation, HTN
Develop slowly	Develop abruptly
Long history of vessel disease	Commonly occur during stress or exercise
May be associated with valvular heart disease, and atrial fibrillation	Associated with cocaine use, and other sympathomimetic amines
History of angina, previous strokes	May be asymptomatic before rupture

- Ischemic strokes are divided into two classes:
  - Cerebral thrombosis
  - Cerebral embolism

Hemorrhagic Stroke

- Caused by a ruptured vessel.
- There are two classes or subcategories:
  - Intracerebral hemorrhage
  - Subarachnoid hemorrhage
- Hemorrhagic stroke accounts for approximately one out of five strokes and is caused by a blood vessel breaking and leaking blood into or around the brain. This type of stroke is generally more serious than an ischemic stroke (one caused by a blocked blood vessel). The nerve cells normally nourished by the hemorrhaging blood vessel, deprived of oxygen and other nutrients, can perish very quickly. The death of these cells leads to varying states of disability.
- *Intracerebral hemorrhage (ICH)*—Refers to the bleeding that occurs into the substance of the brain itself. Intracerebral hemorrhage accounts for 10% of all strokes. Over 30% of patients with ICH will die. About 80% of hemorrhagic strokes are associated with a past medical history of chronic hypertension. Patients that survive an ICH often have a poor morbidity.
- *Subarachnoid hemorrhage (SAH)*—SAH is referred to as bleeding into the fluid that surrounds the brain. The cerebral spinal fluid (CSF) circulates around the subarachnoid space and serves to cushion the brain from injury. SAH accounts for 5% of strokes; 20% die.

Symptoms from Blockage in the Carotid Arteries

The carotid arteries stem off of the *aorta* (the primary artery leading from the heart) and lead up through the neck around the windpipe and on into the brain. When TIAs or stroke occur from blockage in the carotid artery, which they often do, symptoms may occur in either the retina of the eye or the cerebral hemisphere (the large top part of the brain). Symptoms include the following:

- When oxygen to the eye is reduced, people describe the visual effect as a shade being pulled down. People may develop poor night vision. About 35% of TIAs are associated with temporary lost vision in one eye. Although such events are risk factors for future stroke, they pose a lower risk for a stroke and its complications than more widespread TIA symptoms.

- When the cerebral hemisphere is affected, a person can experience problems with speech and partial and temporary paralysis, drooping eyelid, tingling, and numbness, usually on one side of the body. The stroke victim may be unable to express thoughts verbally or to understand spoken words. If the stroke injuries are on the right side of the brain, the symptoms will develop on the left side of the body and vice versa.
- Uncommonly, patients may experience seizures.

Symptoms from Blockage in the Basilar Artery

The other major site of trouble, the basilar artery, is formed at the base of the skull from the vertebral arteries, which run up along the spine and join at the back of the head. When stroke or TIAs occur here, both hemispheres of the brain may be affected so that symptoms occur on both sides of the body. The following symptoms may develop:

- Temporarily dim, gray, blurry, or lost vision
- Tingling or numbness in the mouth, cheeks, or gums
- Headache, usually in the back of the head
- Dizziness
- Nausea and vomiting
- Difficulty swallowing
- Weakness in the arms and legs, sometimes causing a sudden fall

Such strokes usually occur in the brain stem, which can have profound effects on breathing, blood pressure, heart rate, and other vital functions, but does not affect thinking or language.

Signs and Symptoms of Hemorrhagic Stroke

Cerebral Hemorrhage

Symptoms of a cerebral, or parenchymal, hemorrhage typically begins very suddenly and evolve over several hours and include:

- Headache
- Nausea and vomiting
- Altered mental states
- Seizures

Subarachnoid Hemorrhage

When the hemorrhage is subarachnoid in nature, warning signs may occur from the leaky blood vessel a few days to a month before the aneurysm fully develops and ruptures. Warning signs may include:

- Abrupt headaches
- Nausea and vomiting
- Sensitivity to light
- Various neurologic abnormalities (seizures, eg, occur in about 8% of patients)

When the aneurysm ruptures, the stroke victim may experience the following:

- A terrible headache
- Neck stiffness
- Vomiting

- Altered states of consciousness
- Eyes may become fixed in one direction or lose vision
- Stupor, rigidity, and coma

MANAGEMENT GOALS FOR STROKE PATIENTS

- Rapid identification using the Cincinnati Stroke Scale or Los Angeles Prehospital Stroke Scale (Table 18-2)
- Initial assessment
  - Airway
  - Breathing
  - Circulation
- Transport to the closest stroke center
- Alert hospital (stroke notification)
- Check glucose level, if it is appropriate for local protocol

TABLE 18-2: Cincinnati Prehospital Stroke Scale (CPSS)

Sign/Symptom	How Tested	Normal	Abnormal
Facial droop	Have the patient show their teeth or smile	Both sides of the face move equally	One side of the face does not move as well as the other
Arm drift	The patient closes their eyes and extends both arms straight out for 10 s	Both arms move the same, or both do not move at all	One arm either does not move, or one arm drifts downward compared to the other
Speech	The patient repeats "The sky is blue in Cincinnati"	The patient says correct words with no slurring of words	The patient slurs words, says the wrong words, or is unable to speak

Data from American Heart Association and Kothari RU, Pancioli A, Liu T, Brott T, Broderick J. Cincinnati Prehospital Stroke Scale: reproducibility and validity. *Ann Emerg Med.* 1999 Apr;33(4):373-378.

? CHAPTER QUESTIONS

1. Signs and symptoms of neurological deficit include:

   a. chest pain

   b. cool, clammy skin

   c. paralysis or weakness

   d. deep, regular respirations

2. General signs and symptoms of stroke include:

   a. severe headache

   b. sudden weakness or paralysis of face, arm, or leg

   c. difficulty speaking or slurred speech

   d. all of the above

3. Which of the following is correct regarding stroke, or CVA?

    a. The cause is very different from that of a heart attack.

    b. Stroke may cause loss of bladder or bowel control, nausea, and vomiting.

    c. About 25% of all stroke victims die.

    d. The onset of the signs and symptoms is usually gradual, sometimes over days.

4. Which of the following statements is true regarding paralysis caused by stroke?

    a. It is common for both sides of the body to be paralyzed from stroke.

    b. It is difficult to distinguish stroke from spinal injury, as both can cause paralysis to both legs.

    c. Typically, paralysis from strokes affects only one side of the body.

    d. It is a good sign when weakness is only experienced in the extremities, as these patients will not deteriorate further.

References

American Heart Association. *Circulation.* 2005; 112 (Suppl I): IV-111–IV-120; published online before print November, 28 2005, doi:10.1161/CIRCULATIONAHA.105.166562. Accessed May 12, 2007.

US Department of Transportation, National Highway Traffic Safety Administration. *EMT-Basic National Standard Curriculum.* Washington, DC: US Department of Transportation, National Highway Traffic Safety Administration; 1994.

Chapter 19
Seizures and Syncope

At a local café a 32-year-old man begins to have a seizure while waiting to be seated for dinner. A waiter calls 911 and summons help from other staff to clear the chairs and tables away from the patient who has now fallen on the floor. Two minutes go by and you and your partner arrive on-scene. The patient is found in the lobby supine, and presently having a generalized tonic-clonic seizure. What actions should you take initially in caring for this patient?

SEIZURE STATISTICS

According to the American Society of Epilepsy, more than 2 million people in the United States, and over 50 million people worldwide, suffer from epilepsy. In the United States, more than 300,000 people with epilepsy are under the age of 15, and more than 500,000 are over the age of 65. Epilepsy is the third most common neurological disorder in the United States after Alzheimer and stroke.

- Seizure is the sudden and temporary alteration in brain activity caused by a massive electrical discharge in a specific area of the brain.
  - Produces change in mental activity and behavior
  - Convulsions
  - Trancelike periods
- Most common cause of seizures is epilepsy.
- Most common form of epileptic seizure is the grand mal or generalized tonic-clonic seizure.
- Recovery period is referred to as "postictal".

TYPES OF SEIZURES

The international classification of epileptic seizure identifies seizure types by the site of origin in the brain. The two main categories of seizures include partial seizures and generalized seizures. A partial seizure can evolve to a generalized seizure. There are several subtypes of each. Only the most common are described here.

Partial Seizures

- The site of origin is a localized or discreet area in one hemisphere of the brain.
- The two most common types of partial seizure are simple partial and complex partial.

Simple Partial

These produce symptoms associated with the area of abnormal neural activity in the brain—Motor signs, sensory symptoms, autonomic signs and symptoms (involuntary activity controlled by autonomic nervous system), and psychic symptoms (altered states of consciousness). There is no impairment of consciousness in simple partial seizures.

Complex Partial

Impairment of consciousness, characteristic of complex partial seizures (CPS), results in the inability to respond to or carry out simple commands or to execute willed movement, and a lack of awareness of one's surroundings and events. Automatisms may occur. An automatism is a more or less coordinated, involuntary motor activity. A simple complex seizure may begin as a simple partial seizure.

Generalized Seizures

At the onset, seizure activity occurs simultaneously in large areas of the brain, often in both hemispheres. Seizures can be convulsive or nonconvulsive. The two most common types are tonic-clonic and absence.

Tonic-Clonic (Grand Mal)

There is loss of consciousness during the seizure. The tonic phase, consisting of increased muscle tone (rigidity), is followed by the clonic phase, which involves jerking of the extremities. Autonomic symptoms may also be present.

Absence (Petit Mal)

This type occurs most often in children, usually beginning between the ages of 5 and 12 years and often stopping spontaneously in the teens.
The loss of consciousness is so brief that the child usually does not even change position. Most absence seizures last 10 seconds or less. There is no postictal state, but the person usually lacks awareness of what occurs during the seizure.

Myoclonic

These seizures are so brief that they may go unnoticed. They involve sudden muscle contractions that occur much more rapidly than clonic activity and are often confused with tics. Myoclonic seizures occur at all ages and are associated with epileptic syndromes such as West syndrome and Lennox-Gastaut syndrome.

SYNDROME- AND SITUATION-RELATED EPILEPSY

Pediatric epilepsy is one of several symptoms that occur in West syndrome and Lennox-Gastaut syndrome.

West Syndrome

- Also called infantile spasm, is a rare disorder of infancy and early childhood.
- Epilepsy, hydrocephalus, congenital anomalies, and mental retardation characterize it.

Lennox-Gastaut Syndrome

- Usually develops between the ages of 1 and 8 years and is characterized by atonic, absence, and myoclonic seizures. Many of these children are developmentally delayed and have behavioral problems.
- In adults, several medical conditions may precipitate epilepsy, notably withdrawal from chronic alcohol and drug abuse, eclampsia, and stroke.

COMMON CAUSES OF SEIZURES

- Epilepsy
- Head injury
- Medical conditions other than epilepsy
- High fever (more prevalent in pediatric patients)
- Infection
- Poisoning
- Hypoglycemia
- Hyperglycemia
- Hypoxia
- Stroke
- Drug/alcohol withdrawal
- Dysrhythmia
- Hypertension
- Eclampsia
- Electrolyte imbalances
- Idiopathic (unknown)

STATUS EPILEPTICUS ("TRUE EMERGENCY")

- Classified as a seizure lasting greater than 10 minutes without a lucid interval
- Signs/symptoms include (five stages of a generalized tonic-clonic seizure)
  - *Aura*—Warning a seizure is going to happen
  - Tonic—*Muscle rigidity*
  - *Hypertonic*—Severe or extreme muscle rigidity
  - Clonic—*Convulsion*
  - *Postictal*—Recovery period

COMMON PHYSICIAN-PRESCRIBED MEDICATIONS

- Tegretol or Carbatrol (carbamazepine)—First choice for partial, generalized tonic-clonic and mixed seizures.
  - Common adverse effects include fatigue, vision changes, nausea, dizziness, and rash.
- Zarontin (ethosuximide).
  - Adverse effects include nausea, vomiting, decreased appetite, and weight loss.
- Felbatol—Used to treat partial and some generalized seizures.
  - Side effects include decreased appetite, weight loss, inability to sleep, headache, and depression. The drug can rarely cause bone marrow or liver failure. Therefore, the use of the drug is limited, and patients taking it must have blood cell counts and liver tests done regularly during therapy.

- Gabitril—Used with other epilepsy drugs to treat seizures.
  - Common side effects include dizziness, fatigue, weakness, irritability, anxiety, and confusion.
- Keppra—Used with other epilepsy drugs to treat partial seizures.
  - Side effects include tiredness, weakness, and behavioral changes.
- Lamictal—Used to treat partial and some generalized seizures.
  - Has few side effects, but rarely people report dizziness, insomnia, or rash.
- Lyrica—Used to treat partial seizures.
  - Side effects include dizziness, sleepiness (somnolence), dry mouth, peripheral edema, blurred vision, weight gain, and difficulty with concentration/attention.
- Neurontin—Used with other epilepsy drugs to treat partial and some generalized seizures.
  - Few lasting side effects. During the first weeks of treatment you may experience tiredness and dizziness.
- Phenytoin—Used to control partial seizures and generalized tonic-clonic seizures. Can also be given by vein (intravenously) in the hospital to rapidly control active seizures.
  - Side effects include dizziness, fatigue, slurred speech, acne, rash, and increased hair (hirsutism). Over the long term the drug can cause bone thinning.
- Topamax—Used with other medications to treat partial or generalized tonic-clonic seizures.
  - Side effects include sleepiness, dizziness, speech problems, nervousness, memory problems, vision problems, and weight loss.
- Trileptal—Used to treat partial seizures.
  - Most common side effects are fatigue, dizziness, headache, blurred vision, or double vision.
- Depakene, Depakote (valproate, valproic acid)—Used to treat partial, absence, and generalized tonic-clonic seizures.
  - Common side effects include dizziness, nausea, vomiting, tremor, hair loss, weight gain, depression in adults, irritability in children, reduced attention, and a decrease in thinking speed. Over the long term, the drug can cause bone thinning, swelling of the ankles, and irregular menstrual periods. More rare and dangerous effects include hearing loss, liver damage, decreased platelets (clotting cells), and pancreas problems.
- Zonegran—Used with other medications to treat partial seizures.
  - Adverse effects include drowsiness, dizziness, unsteady gait, kidney stones, abdominal discomfort, headache, and rash.
- Valium and similar tranquilizers such as Klonopin or Tranxene—Also prescribed in an emergency setting. Effective in short-term treatment of all seizures. Used often in the emergency room to stop a seizure.
  - Side effects include tiredness, unsteady walking, nausea, depression, and loss of appetite. In children, they can cause drooling and hyperactivity.

EMERGENCY MANAGEMENT

- Position patient and protect from injury
- Maintain airway

- Suction as needed
- Assist breathing as needed
- Prevent injury
- Administer high-concentration oxygen
- Call for ALS (advanced life-saving)
- Begin transport

EMS is summoned to a local professional golf shop for an adult male who passed out. Upon arrival, EMS assesses the scene and determines the scene to be safe. They enter the store and find a 57-year-old morbidly obese patient sitting Fowler's against the wall. He is pale, cool, and extremely diaphoretic. Past/present medical history is gathered and the following is revealed:

Past Medical History
- Carotid endarterectomy
- Hypertension
- Previous syncopal episode

Present Medical History
- Denies chest pain
- Denies shortness of breath
- Patient is complaining of nausea and dizziness

Vital Signs
- Blood pressure: 86/52
- Heart rate: 32 regular
- Respiratory rate: 16 normal, not labored

How should this EMS crew begin treating this patient?

SYNCOPE

- Sudden temporary loss of consciousness. Commonly confused by bystanders as a seizure because the patient usually experiences a convulsion-like activity for a short period.
- Temporary lack of blood flow to the brain.
- Usually occurs when the patient is upright.
- Patient usually regains consciousness when they become horizontal.
- *Look for an underlying cause; syncope could be a sign of serious underlying illness.*

CAUSES OF SYNCOPE

- Syncope is most commonly caused by conditions that do not directly involve the heart.

Noncardiac Causes

- Orthostatic hypotension
- Dehydration
- Blood pressure medications leading to low blood pressure
- Diabetes
- Parkinson
- High altitude
- Stroke
- Migraine
- Situational syncope, such as fainting from blood drawing, micturition syncope (urinating), defecating, coughing, and swallowing. This triggers a reflex of the involuntary nervous system (vasovagal stimulation) that slows the heart rate and dilates blood vessels in the legs causing one to feel nausea, sweating, or weakness prior to passing out.

Cardiac Causes

- Abnormal heart rhythms
- Abnormalities of the heart valves
- High blood pressure
- Tears in the aorta
- Cardiomyopathy

EMERGENCY MANAGEMENT

- Place patient in the supine position or recovery position.
- Administer high-concentration oxygen via nonrebreather or bag-valve-mask.
- Consider immobilization.

? CHAPTER QUESTIONS

1. Seizure patients should be classified as a priority for transport if:

   a. The patient has a history of epilepsy and has not taken antiseizure medication for more than 24 hours.

   b. The seizure lasts longer than 5 minutes.

   c. A second seizure occurs without a period of responsiveness between the seizure episodes.

   d. The patient is still in the postictal state upon your arrival.

2. Medications commonly used in the treatment of epilepsy include:

   a. Nitrostat

   b. Proventil

   c. Epinephrine

   d. Phenobarbital

3. If a seizure patient has been seizing for over 10 minutes, you should:

a. apply high-concentration oxygen by nonrebreather mask and transport immediately

b. insert a nasopharyngeal airway and begin positive pressure ventilation

c. protect the patient from injuring himself until the seizure stops

d. begin CPR and transport immediately

4. A sudden, temporary loss of consciousness due to a temporary lack of blood flow to the brain is called:

a. syncope

b. a seizure

c. stroke

d. a TIA

Reference

US Department of Transportation, National Highway Traffic Safety Administration. *EMT-Basic National Standard Curriculum.* Washington, DC: US Department of Transportation, National Highway Traffic Safety Administration; 1994.

Chapter 20
Allergic Reactions

You have just administered 0.3 mg from an epinephrine preloaded auto-injector to a patient having a severe allergic reaction to shellfish. What are some of the side effects you should see after the administration of this medication?

Allergic reaction is a defense mechanism the body has that provides an exaggerated immune response to any substance. This is a true emergency. The allergic reaction can present with mild symptoms to severe (cardiac arrest).

- The foreign substance is known as an antigen.
- After the antigen is destroyed, the body produces antibodies and the patient becomes sensitized.
- Antibodies are proteins that circulate throughout the body in the blood.
- The primary function is to recognize any future exposure.
- Initial sensitization may have occurred hours, days, months, or years before the patient develops an antigen/antibody reaction.

Pathways for allergens to enter the body:

- Injection—Introduced by a bite, sting, needle, or infusion
- Ingestion—Introduced through the stomach
- Inhalation—Introduced through the respiratory tract
- Absorption—Introduced through the skin

ANAPHYLAXIS

Anaphylaxis is a severe systemic allergic reaction, generally acute in onset, but depends on individual sensitivity, dose, and rate of administration.

- Most anaphylactic episodes are mediated by immunoglobulin E (IgE) antibodies.
- Prior to the anaphylactic event, a sensitization stage must occur.
- The sensitization stage includes:
  - Antigen exposure.
  - Plasma cells produce IgE antibodies against the allergen.
  - IgE antibodies attach to mast cells and basophils.
  - More of the same allergen invades the body.
  - Allergen combines with IgE and attaches to the mast cells and basophils which trigger degranulation. This degranulation causes a release of histamine and other chemical mediators.

- Together these chemicals induce an inflammatory response producing:
  — Increased vascular permeability
  — Vasodilation
  — Smooth muscle contraction
  — Myocardial depression

All of these are responsible for the manifestation of hives (urticaria), edema, bronchospasm, and shock (hypoperfusion).

Possible Causes of an Allergic Reaction

- Venom from insect bites/stings—Bees, wasps, and the like (40-100 deaths occur each year from insect stings)
- Food—Nuts, crustaceans, peanuts, and so on
- Plants, pollen
- Medications (most common penicillin [PCN])
- Others substances such as latex
- Assessment includes:
  - Headache
  - Decreased mental status
  - Skin
    — Patient may state they have a warm tingling feeling in the face, mouth, chest, feet, and hands
    — Itching (pruritus)
    — Hives (urticaria)
    — Red skin (flushing, erythema)
    — Swelling to face, neck, hands, feet, and/or tongue
  - Respiratory system
    — Patient may state they feel a tightness in their throat (angio edema) or chest
    — Cough
    — Rapid breathing
    — Labored breathing
    — Noisy breathing
    — Hoarseness (losing the voice)—"ominous symptom"
    — Stridor
    — Wheezing (audible without stethoscope) secondary to severe bronchospasm
    — Runny nose (rhinorhea)
  - Cardiac
    — Increased heart rate
    — Decreased blood pressure
    — Sense of impending doom

Assessment findings that reveal shock (hypoperfusion) or respiratory distress indicate the presence of a severe allergic reaction.

Emergency Management

Patient has come in contact with the substance that caused past allergic reaction and complains of respiratory distress or exhibits signs and symptoms of shock (hypoperfusion).

Clinical Significance

Insects most commonly associated with triggering severe allergic reactions are members of the hymenoptera class; these include bees, wasps, yellow jackets, hornets, and fire ants.

Clinical Significance

During a severe reaction any delay in care could result in death.

- Perform initial assessment.
- Perform focused history and physical examination.
- Common questions asked:
    - History of allergies?
    - What was patient exposed to?
    - How were they exposed?
    - What effects (signs/symptoms)?
    - Progression?
    - Interventions prior to EMS arrival?
- Assess baseline vital signs and SAMPLE history.
- Administer high-concentration oxygen if not already done in the initial assessment.
- Determine if patient has prescribed preloaded epinephrine available. Facilitate administration of preloaded epinephrine.
- Contact medical direction.
- Record and reassess in 2 minutes.
- Record reassessment findings.
- If patient does not have epinephrine auto-injector available, transport immediately, contact medical direction, and proceed with the administration of epinephrine (preloaded). Follow local protocol.
- Patient has contact with substance that causes allergic reaction without signs of respiratory distress or shock (hypoperfusion).
    - Continue with focused assessment.
    - Patient not wheezing or without signs of respiratory compromise or hypotension should not receive epinephrine.

Relationship to Airway Management

- These patients may initially present with airway/respiratory compromise, or airway/respiratory compromise may develop as the allergic reaction progresses.
- The airway should be managed according to the principles identified in the airway management lesson presented in Chapter 7.

Medications

Epinephrine Auto-injector

- Medication name:
    - Generic—Epinephrine
    - Trade—Adrenalin
- Indications—Must meet the following three criteria:
    - Emergency management of the patient exhibiting the assessment findings of an allergic reaction.
    - Medication is prescribed for this patient by a physician.
    - Medical direction authorizes use for this patient, or standing orders dependent on local protocol.
- Contraindications—There are no contraindications when used in a life-threatening situation.
- Medication form—Liquid administered via an automatically injectable needle and syringe system.

- Dosage:
  - Adult—One adult auto-injector (0.3 mg)
  - Infant and child—One infant/child auto-injector (0.15 mg)
- Administration:
  - Obtain order from medical direction either on-line or off-line.
  - Obtain patient's prescribed auto-injector. Ensure:
    — Prescription is written for the patient experiencing allergic reactions.
    — Medication is not discolored (if able to see).
  - Remove safety cap from the auto-injector.
  - Place tip of auto-injector against the patient's thigh.
    — Lateral portion of the thigh. Midway between the waist and the knee.
  - Push the injector firmly against the thigh until the injector activates.
  - Hold the injector in place until the medication is injected.
  - Record activity and time.
  - Dispose of injector in biohazard container.
- Actions:
  - Dilates the bronchioles.
  - Constricts peripheral blood vessels.
- Side effects (mimics a sympathetic nervous discharge):
  - Increases heart rate
  - Pallor
  - Dizziness
  - Chest pain
  - Headache
  - Nausea
  - Vomiting
  - Excitability, anxiousness
- Reassessment strategies
  - Transport
  - Continue focused assessment, monitor the airway and breathing, and look for circulatory collapse.

? CHAPTER QUESTIONS

1. Anaphylactic shock is brought about by:

   a. fluid loss due to tissue swelling

   b. massive systemic vasodilatation

   c. decreased contractility of the heart

   d. pulmonary hemorrhage

2. An allergen may enter the body through:

   a. the respiratory tract

   b. skin

   c. the GI tract

   d. any of the above

3. During your initial assessment of a patient with an allergic reaction, you may find:

   a. a slow, bounding pulse

   b. strong distal pulses in the feet

   c. edema of the face, neck, lips, hands, and feet

   d. tiny bruises from ruptured capillaries

4. Once epinephrine has been administered to a patient, you should:

   a. Routinely administer a second dose after 10 minutes, if available.

   b. Administer an over-the-counter antihistamine for long-term relief.

   c. See marked improvement and allow the patient to remain at home if he wants.

   d. Reassess the patient after 2 minutes.

5. Epinephrine is the drug of choice for the emergency treatment of severe allergic reactions and:

   a. comes packaged in a vial with a separate syringe and needle

   b. quickly causes vasoconstriction and relaxes the smooth muscles in the lungs to improve breathing

   c. the same dose is administered to both children and adults

   d. works immediately and lasts for up to 2 hours

6. Steps included in administering epinephrine by auto-injector include:

   a. drawing up the medication into the syringe

   b. pushing the injector firmly into the patient's buttocks until the needle is deployed, and the medication is delivered

   c. holding the injector in place until all the medication has been injected

   d. placing the injector back into its container for reuse

Reference

US Department of Transportation, National Highway Traffic Safety Administration. *EMT-Basic National Standard Curriculum*. Washington, DC: US Department of Transportation, National Highway Traffic Safety Administration; 1994.

Chapter 21

Poisoning and Overdose Emergencies

A man calls 911 after arriving at his father's home and finding him unconscious in his car in an enclosed garage. The elderly man, suffering from terminal liver cancer, had written a suicide note, turned on his vehicle in the closed garage, and then remained in his car.

The patient's son removed the patient from the garage and placed the patient outside. The son began resuscitative efforts with the assistance of the emergency 911 operator. Upon arrival, the scene is determined to be safe by the local fire department and you notice firefighters performing rescue breathing via bag-valve-mask.

What are some of the signs and symptoms you would see during a thorough patient assessment?

Thousands of people die each year from accidental or intentional poisonings each year.

EMERGENCY MANAGEMENT OF A POISONING/OVERDOSE

Important questions to consider asking the patient:

- What was the substance?
- When did you ingest/become exposed?
- If ingestion, how much did you ingest?
- Over what time period?
- Were there any interventions?
- How much do you weigh?

Signs, Symptoms, and History of an Ingested Poisoning

- History of ingestion
- Nausea
- Vomiting
- Diarrhea
- Altered mental status

- Abdominal pain
- Chemical burns around the mouth
- Different breath odors

Emergency Management

- Remove pills, tablets, or fragments with gloves from patient's mouth, as needed, without injuring oneself.
- Consult medical direction for administration of activated charcoal.
- Bring all containers, bottles, labels, and the like of poisonous agents to receiving facility.

Signs and Symptoms of an Inhaled Poisoning

- History of inhalation of toxic substance
- Difficulty breathing
- Chest pain
- Cough
- Hoarseness
- Dizziness
- Headache
- Confusion
- Seizures
- Altered mental status

Emergency Management

- Have trained rescuers remove patient from poisonous toxic environment.
- Maintain airway.
- Give high-concentration oxygen, provide rescue breathing when necessary.
- Bring all containers, bottles, labels, and the like of poisonous agents to receiving facility.

Signs and Symptoms of a *Toxic Injection* Poisoning

- Weakness
- Dizziness
- Chills
- Fever
- Nausea
- Vomiting

Emergency Management

- Maintain airway and administer high-concentration oxygen.
- Be alert for vomiting, have suction available.
- Bring all containers, bottles, labels, and the like of poisonous agents to receiving facility.

Signs and Symptoms of an *Absorbed* Poisoning

- History of exposure
- Does the patient have liquid or powder on their skin?
- Burns
- Itching
- Irritation
- Redness

Emergency Management

- Skin—Remove contaminated clothing while protecting oneself from contamination.
- Powder—Brush powder off patient, and then continue as for other absorbed poisons.
- Liquid—Irrigate with clean water for at least 20 minute (and continue en route to facility if possible).
- Eye—Irrigate with clean water away from affected eye for at least 20 minute and continue en route to facility if possible.

Relationship to Airway Management

A patient's condition may deteriorate, so continue to assess patient for airway difficulties and manage as learned previously.

Medications Used for the Treatment of Poisoning

Medication Name: Activated Charcoal (Fig. 21-1)

- Generic—Activated charcoal
- Trade
  - SuperChar
  - Insta-Char
  - Actidose
  - Liqui-Char
- Indications—Poisoning by mouth
- Contraindications
  - Altered mental status
  - Ingestion of acids or alkalis
  - Unable to swallow

Figure 21-1 Activated charcoal. *(Used with permission from Peter DiPrima.)*

- Medication form
  - Premixed in water, frequently available in plastic bottle containing 12.5 g activated charcoal
  - Powder should be avoided in field
- Dosage
  - Adults and children: 1 g activated charcoal/kg of body weight
  - Usual adult dose: 25 to 50 g
  - Usual infant/child dose: 12.5 to 25 g
- Administration
  - Obtain order from medical direction either on-line or off-line.
  - Container must be shaken thoroughly.
  - Since medication looks like mud, patient may need to be persuaded to drink it.
  - A covered container and a straw may improve patient compliance since the patient cannot see the medication this way.
  - If patient takes a long time to drink the medication, the charcoal will settle and will need to be shaken or stirred again.
  - Record activity and time.
- Actions
  - Binds to certain poisons and prevents them from being absorbed into the body.
  - Not all brands of activated charcoal are the same; some bind much more poison than others, so consult medical direction about the brand to use.
- Side effects
  - Black stools.
  - Some patients, particularly those who have ingested poisons that cause nausea, may vomit.
  - If the patient vomits, the dose should be repeated once.
  - Reassessment strategies—The emergency medical technician (EMT) should be prepared for the patient to vomit or further deteriorate.

CARBON MONOXIDE POISONING

- Carbon monoxide (CO) "the silent killer" is a product of incomplete combustion (Fig. 21-2).
  - Colorless gas
  - Odorless gas
  - Tasteless gas
- Carbon monoxide has a greater affinity to hemoglobin than oxygen. This binding of carbon monoxide to hemoglobin is known as carboxyhemoglobin (COHb).

Stages of CO Poisoning

1. 20% to 30% COHb produces headache, weariness, drunken feeling.
2. 30% to 40% COHb produces an increased pulse, increased respiration, ataxia (poor coordination), vomiting, change in vision.

Figure 21-2 Firefighters operating without a self-contained breathing apparatus is a common cause of carbon monoxide poisoning in firefighters. *(Used with permission from Peter DiPrima.)*

3. 40% to 60% COHb produces weakness, amnesia, short attention span.
4. Greater than 60% COHb produces unconsciousness, convulsions, and often is fatal.

ACUTE CYANIDE POISONING

Signs/Symptoms

- Shuts down cellular respiration
- Rapid breathing
- Restlessness
- Dizziness
- Weakness
- Headache
- Nausea/vomiting
- Rapid heart rate
- Convulsions
- Decreased blood pressure
- Loss of consciousness
- Lung injury
- Respiratory failure leading to death

Treatment and Management

- Personal protective equipment
- Decontamination by trained personnel
- Airway
- Breathing
- Circulation

? CHAPTER QUESTION

1. Emergency management for an inhalation poisoning includes:

   a. starting PPV with supplemental O_2 immediately if breathing is inadequate

   b. applying O_2 via nonrebreather mask for apneic patients

   c. decontaminating completely with water from head to toe

   d. transporting the patient in the Trendelenburg position to facilitate blood flow to the brain

Chapter 22
Drug and Alcohol Emergencies

You are called to scene of a local bar for a patron who is acting irrational, belligerent, and starting a fight with other patrons in the bar. Upon arrival, what scene safety issues should be observed prior to making any patient contact?

Drug abuse is the self-administration of a drug in a manner that is not in accordance with medical or social patterns.

STREET DRUGS OF ABUSE

1. *Gamma hydroxy butyrate (GHB).*
   - Central nervous system (CNS) depressant and hypnotic drug
   - Taken by mouth
   - Signs/symptoms—Headache, confusion, ataxia, hallucinations, delirium, euphoria, dizziness, ⇓ HR, ⇓ RR, extra pyramidal effects, seizure-like activity, and coma
   - Onset—15 to 30 minutes
   - Duration—1 to 2 hours with full recovery in about 8 hours
   - Management—Treat symptoms, airway control, restrain as patient will come up combative
   - Names—Gamma hydroxybutyric acid, Verve, Rejoov, Remforce, furanone, Blue Nitro
2. *Methamphetamines and amphetamines*—Strong CNS stimulants that influence and accelerate certain body functions such as increased heart and respiratory rate.
   - Sympathetic excitation
   - Signs/symptoms—Agitation, hypertension (HTN), mydriasis, trismus, diaphoresis, ⇑ Temp, ⇑ HR, ⇑ RR, arrhythmias, seizures
   - Onset—20 to 60 minutes
   - Duration—9 to 19 hours
   - Management—Treat symptoms
   - Names—Ecstasy, X, Crystal, Ice, Meth, Glass, MDMA, Ritalin, Dexedrine, Adderall

3. *Cocaine*—Strong CNS stimulants that influence and accelerate certain body functions such as increased heart and respiratory rate.
   - Local anesthetic, CNS and cardiac stimulant
   - Taken by mouth (PO), main-line, intranasal, rectal, vaginal
   - Signs/symptoms—Similar to amphetamines, CNS ⇑ → CNS ⇓, ⇑ Temp = ⇑ fatality HTN & ⇑ HR → ⇓ BP/shock, ⇑ RR, mydriasis, seizures, acute myocardial infarction (AMI), cardiovascular disease (CVA)
   - Onset—5 to 60 minutes
   - Duration—1 to 2 hours
   - Management—Treat symptoms
   - Names—Coke, crack, rock

4. *Heroin*—An opiate narcotic that is illegal and highly addictive
   - CNS depressant, analgesic
   - Taken PO, main-line, intranasal, intradermal
   - Signs/symptoms—Miosis, ⇓ RR, ⇓ LOC, ⇓ HR, euphoria, lethargy
   - Onset—Rapid
   - Duration—Several hours
   - Management—Naloxone or a new longer acting narcotic antagonist, consider a drip to maintain airway control
   - Names—Smack, black tar, horse

5. *Hallucinogens*—Chemical substances classified in this group are known as psychotomimetic and refer to drugs that mimic a psychological or psychotic state. *Hallucinogen* refers to the hallucinations that these types of drugs produce. This drug group has the ability to induce visual and/or auditory hallucinations.
   - CNS stimulants
   - Taken PO, inhalation
   - Signs/symptoms—⇑⇑ activity, miosis or mydriasis, omnipotence, nystagmus, ⇑ BP, ⇑ HR, hallucinations, paranoia, increased activity and strength, seizures
   - Onset—Rapid
   - Duration—Several hours to days
   - Management—Treat symptoms
   - Names—PCP (phencyclidine), peyote, LSD (lysergic acid diethylamide), mescaline, Jimson weed, nutmeg

6. *Inhalants*—*Huffing* refers to deliberately breathing certain volatile substances which can intoxicate an individual.
   - Short-term effects of inhalant abuse
     - Headaches
     - Rashes around the nose and mouth
     - Weight loss
     - Irregular heart beat
     - Lack of appetite
     - Runny nose
     - Upper respiratory problems
     - Night sweats
     - Shortness of breath
     - Signs of acute poisoning

- Long-term effects of inhalant abuse
  - Brain damage
  - Liver damage

7. *Imidazolines*
   - Alpha-2 stimulant similar to clonidine that inhibits the release of norepinephrine
   - Taken PO
   - Signs/symptoms—Lethargy, $\Downarrow$ BP, shock, $\Downarrow$ HR, $\Downarrow$ RR, coma, possible seizures
   - Onset—30 to 60 minutes
   - Duration—12 to 36 hours
   - Management—Activated charcoal, treat symptoms
   - Names—Visine, Murine, Afrin, Clonidine

8. *Serotonin Syndrome*
   - Adverse reaction to several types of medications
   - Signs/symptoms—*Must include at least three of the following:* mental status changes, agitation, myoclonus, hyperreflexia diaphoresis, shivering, tremor, diarrhea, incoordination, $\Uparrow$ temperature
   - Additional signs/symptoms—$\Uparrow$ HR/RR, mydriasis, HTN, trismus, opisthotonus, flushing, $\Downarrow$ BP, abdominal pain, salivation, seizures, insomnia
   - Onset—Varies
   - Duration—Varies
   - Management—Treat symptoms
   - Names—Amphetamine, cocaine, ecstasy

9. *Other Current Drugs*
   - *Coricidin HBP (CCC)*—Antihistamine for anticholinergic effects—hallucinations, tachycardia, lethargy, seizures (seizure), dry mouth, mydriasis
   - *Robitussin DM*—CNS depressant, similar to narcotics, attaches to narcotic receptor sites in brain; consider naloxone or a new longer acting narcotic antagonist—Agent Lemon/Lemonade/Robofire = Robitussin DM with ammonia, lighter fluid, and lemon flavor
   - *Vicks VapoRub*—Used to bring down the effects of an Ecstacy high or just for camphor effects—CNS stimulant; leads to seizure and CNS depression—usually occur within 90 minutes; treat symptoms
   - *Ritalin*—Used by non-attention deficit hyperactivity disorder (ADHD persons)—crush and snort it—amphetamine signs/symptoms
   - *Prescription Narcotics*—Readily abused and often crushed and snorted for a different high

DRUG WITHDRAWAL

- Symptoms peak 24 to 72 hours
- Seizures possible
- Inadequate breathing
- Hypoperfusion
- Anxiety/agitation
- Confusion

- Tremors
- Profuse sweating
- Tachycardia
- Hypertension
- Hallucinations
- Nausea/vomiting
- Abdominal cramping

ALCOHOL

- *Alcohol* is a depressant, which means it slows the function of the central nervous system.
- Alcohol actually blocks some of the messages trying to get to the brain. This alters a person's perceptions, emotions, movement, vision, and hearing.
- In very small amounts, alcohol can help a person feel more relaxed or less anxious. More alcohol causes greater changes in the brain, resulting in intoxication. People who have overused alcohol may stagger, lose their coordination, and slur their speech. They will probably be confused and disoriented. Depending on the person, intoxication can make someone very friendly and talkative or very aggressive and angry. Reaction times are slowed dramatically, which is why people are told not to drink and drive. People who are intoxicated may think they are moving properly when they are not. They may act totally out of character.
- When large amounts of alcohol are consumed in a short period of time, alcohol poisoning can result. Alcohol poisoning is exactly what it sounds like—The body has become poisoned by large amounts of alcohol. Violent vomiting is usually the first symptom of alcohol poisoning, as the body tries to rid itself of the alcohol. Extreme sleepiness, unconsciousness, difficulty breathing, dangerously low blood sugar, seizures, and even death may result.

DELIRIUM TREMENS

- Life threatening, 5% to 15% mortality
- Suspect in any patient with delirium of unknown cause

Symptoms most commonly occur within 72 hours after the last drink, but may occur up to 7 to 10 days after the last drink. Symptoms may get worse rapidly, and can include:

- Body tremors
- Mental status changes
  - Agitation, irritability
  - Confusion, disorientation
  - Decreased attention span
  - Decreased mental status
    - Deep sleep that persists for a day or longer
    - Stupor, sleepiness, lethargy
    - Usually occurs after acute symptoms
  - Delirium (severe, acute loss of mental functions)
  - Excitement
  - Fear
  - Hallucinations (such as seeing or feeling things that are not present are most common)

- ○ Highly sensitive to light, sound, touch
- ○ Increased activity
- ○ Mood changes rapidly
- ○ Restlessness, excitement
- Seizures
  - ○ Most common in first 24 to 48 hours after last drink
  - ○ Most common in people with previous complications from alcohol withdrawal
  - ○ Usually generalized tonic-clonic seizures
- Symptoms of alcohol withdrawal
  - ○ Anxiety
  - ○ Depression
  - ○ Difficulty thinking clearly
  - ○ Fatigue
  - ○ Feeling jumpy or nervous
  - ○ Feeling shaky
  - ○ Headache, general, pulsating
  - ○ Insomnia (difficulty falling and staying asleep)
  - ○ Irritability or easily excited
  - ○ Loss of appetite
  - ○ Nausea
  - ○ Pale skin
  - ○ Palpitations (sensation of feeling the heart beat)
  - ○ Rapid emotional changes
  - ○ Sweating, especially the palms of the hands or the face
  - ○ Vomiting

EMERGENCY MANAGEMENT

- Administer high-concentration oxygen via nonrebreather if breathing is adequate, or positive pressure ventilation if breathing is inadequate.
- Position patient, maintain high index of suspicion for C-spine injuries.
- Maintain body temperature.
- Access blood glucose.
- Request ALS.
- Access the need for restraints for combative patients per local protocol.
- Transport.

? CHAPTER QUESTIONS

1. Friends of your patient tell you that at a college fraternity party, he drank 15 shots of tequila without stopping. Friends called 911 when he wouldn't respond when they tried to wake him up. You expect your findings to include:

   a. hypoventilation, cyanosis, and coma

   b. diaphoresis, vomiting, and hyperthermia

   c. a 0.350 mg/dL blood alcohol level, seizure activity, and hypertension

   d. pulmonary edema, dysrhythmias, and dilated pupils

2. All of the following are patterns of alcohol abuse except:

a. drinking early in the day

b. drinking alone or in secret

c. admitting a problem with alcohol when confronted

d. denial of any inference of a drinking problem

Reference

US Department of Transportation, National Highway Traffic Safety Administration. *EMT-Basic National Standard Curriculum.* Washington, DC: US Department of Transportation, National Highway Traffic Safety Administration; 1994.

Chapter 23
Acute Abdominal Pain

Upon arriving at the scene, you find an elderly woman who states, "My granddaughter is sick. I don't know what's wrong with her." She then asks you to follow her upstairs to her bedroom. As you enter the room you find a 7-year-old girl lying in bed guarding her abdomen complaining of severe abdominal pain.

What type of questions should you ask the patient and her guardian?

ANATOMY OF THE ABDOMEN GASTROINTESTINAL SYSTEM EMERGENCIES

Figure 23-1 is a schematic diagram showing the anatomy of the abdomen.

- Esophageal varices—Swollen veins in the lower third of esophagus
  - Caused by increased pressure in portal circulation
  - Most common presentation—Painless gastrointestinal (GI) bleeding
- Gastritis—Stomach lining inflammation
  - Caused by increased gastric secretion associated with alcohol, drugs, stress
  - Presents with epigastric pain, belching, indigestion
  - Can lead to gastric ulcer
  - Treatment involves administration of antacids and histamine$_2$-blocking drugs, such as cimetidine
- Peptic ulcer disease—Ulcerations in the stomach, esophagus, or duodenum
  - Caused by excess secretion of hydrochloric acid
  - Also caused by breakdown of mucous lining by drugs or alcohol
  - Presents with epigastric or upper left quadrant pain
  - Pain often improves following meals or antacids
  - If left untreated, can erode entire lining of the organ
- Diverticulitis—Inflammation of the diverticuli
  - Diverticula—Pouches on the large intestine
  - Can become inflamed as with appendicitis
  - Presents like a left-sided appendicitis with abdominal pain, fever, vomiting, anorexia, tenderness
  - Treatment includes antibiotics, diet modification, and surgery
- Bleeding diverticulosis
  - Bleeding from diverticuli on the large intestine
  - Presents with painless rectal bleeding or with some left-side abdominal pain

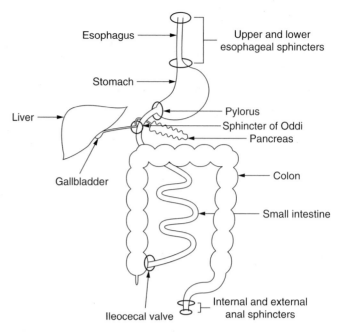

Figure 23-1   Abdominal anatomy simplified. *(Reprinted with permission from Barrett KE. Gastrointestinal Physiology. New York: McGraw-Hill; 2006:7.)*

- Carcinoma of the colon—Malignant growth in the colon
  - Diverse presentation including painless rectal bleeding, weight loss, or abdominal pain
- Appendicitis—Inflammation of the appendix from obstruction or from undetermined cause
  - Patient often complains of acute onset of right lower quadrant pain beginning around the umbilicus with associated nausea, vomiting, fever, and anorexia
  - Rupture can cause peritonitis characterized by guarding, rebound tenderness, and rigid abdomen
  - Treatment includes prevention of shock and transport for surgical removal of appendix
- Perforated abdominal viscus—Perforation of a hollow abdominal organ causing loss of stomach or intestine contents into the abdominal cavity.
  - Produces inflammation and infection of peritoneum and other organs
  - Most common causes are perforated ulcers or diverticulum
  - Presents with sudden-onset abdominal pain and generalized tenderness; rebound often present; abdomen can be rigid
- Bowel obstruction—Intestinal blockage
  - Common causes include tumors, foreign bodies, prior surgery
  - Presents with history of progressive anorexia, abdominal bloating, diffuse abdominal pain, nausea, vomiting, fever, chills
- Upper GI hemorrhage
  - Bleeding from esophagus, stomach, duodenum
  - Common causes include peptic ulcer disease, gastritis, esophagitis, tumors, esophageal varices

- Signs/symptoms include hematemesis, dark stools, frequent diarrhea, orthostatic vital signs
- Treatment—Supplemental O$_2$ and rapid transport
- Lower GI hemorrhage
  - Bleeding from distal small intestine, colon, rectum
  - Common causes include tumors, diverticulosis, hemorrhoids, rectal fissures
  - Signs/symptoms include rectal bleeding (wine colored or bright red), increased stool frequency, crampy diffuse pain, orthostatic vital signs
- Pancreatitis
  - Inflammation of the pancreas
  - Caused by alcoholism or elevated blood fats
  - Presents with sudden onset of midabdominal pain that radiates to the back and shoulders, nausea, and vomiting
  - Treatment includes supportive care and transport
- Cholecystitis
  - Inflammation of the gallbladder
  - Caused by gallstones lodging in duct that drains the bladder or in bile duct, causing liver or pancreatic congestion
  - Presents with colicky pain in the upper right quadrant that worsens following meals and is unrelieved by antacids
  - Treatment—Surgical removal of gallbladder
- Hepatitis
  - Inflammation or infection of the liver
  - Results from viral infections and alcohol or substance abuse
  - Presents with dull right upper quadrant tenderness unrelated to food digestion and often with malaise, decreased appetite, clay-colored stools, jaundice
  - Treatment in nonviral cases involves removing offending agent, while in viral cases patient is observed and treated symptomatically
- Aortic aneurysm
  - Weakness in the wall of the descending aorta creates ballooning in wall which can increase in size and rupture
  - Patient complains of diffuse abdominal pain and severe back pain or tearing sensation if the artery is dissecting
- Kidney stones
  - Result from crystal aggregation in the collecting system of the kidney; crystallized urinary salts held together by organic matter
  - Most common in men 20 to 50 years old
  - Most often seen in spring and fall
  - Presenting symptoms can include excruciating flank pain, difficulty in urinating, hematuria, nausea, and vomiting
  - Predisposing factors
    — Urinary tract infections
    — Immobilization
    — Metabolic disorders (hypercalcemia)
    — Gout (increased uric acid)
    — Tumors

- Complications
  - — Inflammation, infection
  - — Partial or total urinary obstruction
- Urinary tract infections (UTIs)
  - Bladder infection (cystitis) is most common.
  - Most common in sexually active females.
  - Can cause kidney infection.
  - Symptoms include fever, flank pain, chills; dysuria (painful or burning urination); discolored urine; and lower abdominal pain (especially during urination).
- Pyelonephritis
  - Kidney infection/inflammation
  - Often from infection ascending from bladder
  - Most common in women
  - Patients typically febrile, with lower back or flank pain, chills, possible urinary burning
- Acute renal failure—Rapid deterioration of kidney function, potentially reversible
  - Causes
    - — Reduced renal blood flow due to shock, dehydration, vasopressor agents.
    - — Kidney injury from trauma, nephrotoxic drugs, infection.
    - — Urine flow obstruction due to enlarged prostate or tumor.
    - — Metabolic waste products accumulate.
    - — Uremia is present.
- Chronic renal failure—Long-standing failure associated with loss of nephron mass, usually irreversible
  - Complications of renal failure
    - — Elevated potassium levels
    - — Uremic pericarditis and encephalopathy
    - — Pericardial tamponade
    - — Subject to drug toxicity—Failure to eliminate medications
    - — Fluid overload and noncardiac pulmonary edema
- Presentation with severe renal failure includes severe dyspnea, jugular vein distention (JVD), ascites, rales at lung bases
- Presentation with chronic renal failure includes wasted appearance, pasty yellow skin, thin extremities; frostlike appearance of skin in later stages, edema, jaundice, oliguria

REPRODUCTIVE SYSTEM EMERGENCIES—FEMALE

- Pelvic inflammatory disease (PID)
  - Infection of the female reproductive organs
  - Presentation includes lower abdominal pain, pain during movement, vaginal discharge, fever, chills
- Ovarian cyst
  - Fluid-filled sac which forms on the ovaries; can rupture causing pain and tenderness
  - Often presents with lower abdominal pain—Sudden or gradual onset

- Mittelschmerz
  - Abdominal pain accompanying ovulation
  - Associated with release of ovum from ovary
  - Can cause severe pain
- Ectopic pregnancy
  - Implantation of a developing fetus outside of the uterus, most commonly in the fallopian tube
  - If tube ruptures, significant bleeding can follow
  - History of missed menses or irregular periods
  - Presents with low abdominal pain on either side, associated with vaginal bleeding and often pallor and weak pulse
  - Pre-hospital treatment includes supplemental oxygen, prevention of shock, and rapid transport

REPRODUCTIVE SYSTEM EMERGENCIES—MALE

- Testicular torsion
  - Part of a blood vessel becomes twisted or rotated stopping blood flow to testicle
  - More common in younger males and children
  - Presents with severe testicular pain, possibly associated lower abdominal pain and swollen, tender testicle
- Epididymitis
  - Inflammation of the epididymis
  - Secondary to gonorrhea, syphilis, TB, mumps, prostatitis, urethritis, or following prolonged use of indwelling catheter
  - Presents with chills, fever, inguinal pain, swollen epididymus
- Prostatitis
  - Infection of the prostate
  - Presents with urinary frequency, burning pain with ejaculation, occasional pain with defecation, fever and chills, nausea, and vomiting

ASSESSMENT OF THE ACUTE ABDOMEN DIALYSIS PATIENT

- Hemodialysis
  - Waste products removed by machine.
  - Renal failure patients (2-3 times per week).
  - Many patients have home dialysis units.
  - Osmotic mechanism.
  - Patient's blood comes in contact with dialysate which normalizes electrolytes and eliminates wastes.
- Peritoneal dialysis
  - Uses lining of the peritoneal cavity for dialysis.
  - Dialysate is introduced into the peritoneum.
  - Remains there for 1 to 2 hours before removal.
  - Major complication is peritonitis.

- Complications of dialysis
  - Hypotension from dehydration, blood loss, sepsis
  - Chest pain/dysrhythmias from hyperkalemia or ischemia
  - Disequilibrium syndrome from rapid electrolyte and osmotic changes
  - Air embolism from tube opening
  - Clotting of shunt or fistula
  - Hemorrhage from rupture of fistula or shunt
- Management of dialysis patient
  - Use arm opposite shunt for blood pressure
  - Treat medical emergencies
  - Remove patient from dialysis machine by:
    — Turning off dialysis machine
    — Clamping shunt tubing ends
    — Controlling shunt hemorrhage

? CHAPTER QUESTIONS

1. Abdominal pain is considered serious and a high priority when:

   a. There is a sudden, severe onset.
   b. It is accompanied by syncope and hypotension.
   c. It has lasted for more than an hour.
   d. It is accompanied by fever and vomiting.

2. A 59-year-old woman describes a sudden onset of severe, constant abdominal pain that radiates to her lower back. The pain is described as "tearing." On physical examination, you note a pulsating abdominal mass upon palpation of the area. You suspect:

   a. esophageal varices
   b. intestinal obstruction
   c. abdominal aortic aneurysm
   d. ulcer

Chapter 24
Environmental Emergencies

It is the beginning of a very hot summer day. The temperature outside is 99°F, with a heat index of 110°F. An elderly woman is complaining of dizziness, nausea, vomiting, and an episode of syncope. Her husband determines she cannot withstand the extreme heat and summons emergency medical services (EMS). You arrive on-scene, determine the scene is safe, and enter the house. You establish the cause of the patient's complaints is from the house having no ventilation. You look on the wall to see a thermometer reading 112°F. The patient is pale, warm, and extremely diaphoretic. She denies chest discomfort and shortness of breath. She states, "I feel like I am going to pass out!" What is your next course of action?

TEMPERATURE REGULATION

Regulation of temperature is based on heat loss versus heat gained.

When heat loss exceeds heat gained, the result is *hypothermia* (low body temperature). Heat loss occurs by:

- Radiation—Transfer of heat from the surface of one object to another without physical contact.
- Convection—Body heat is lost to surrounding air.
- Conduction—Body heat is lost to surrounding objects through direct physical contact.
- Evaporation—Body heat causes perspiration, which is lost from the surface of the body when changed from liquid to vapor.
- Respiration—Heat loss through the process of breathing.

EMTs must be aware of methods of heat loss when treating patients with hypothermia to prevent further heat loss. When heat gained exceeds heat lost, the result is *hyperthermia* (high body core temperature).

Important questions to ask patients exposed to the environment:

- What is the source?
- How is the environment the patient is in?
- Any loss of consciousness?
- Effects
  - General versus local injury or illness

EXPOSURE TO COLD

Figure 24-1 shows NOAA's National Weather Service windchill chart.

New windchill chart
Wind (mph)

Calm	5	10	15	20	25	30	35	40	45	50	55	60
40	36	34	32	30	29	28	28	27	26	26	25	25
35	31	27	25	24	23	22	21	20	19	19	18	17
30	25	21	19	17	16	15	14	13	12	12	11	10
25	19	15	13	11	9	8	7	6	5	4	4	3
20	13	9	6	4	3	1	0	−1	−2	−3	−3	−4
15	7	3	0	−2	−4	−5	−7	−8	−9	−10	−11	−11
10	1	−4	−7	−9	−11	−12	−14	−15	−16	−17	−18	−19
5	−5	−10	−13	−15	−17	−19	−21	−22	−23	−24	−25	−26
0	−11	−16	−19	−22	−24	−26	−27	−29	−30	−31	−32	−33
−5	−16	−22	−26	−29	−31	−33	−34	−36	−37	−38	−39	−40
−10	−22	−28	−32	−35	−37	−39	−41	−43	−44	−45	−46	−48
−15	−28	−35	−39	−42	−44	−46	−48	−50	−51	−52	−54	−55
−20	−34	−41	−45	−48	−51	−53	−55	−57	−58	−60	−61	−62
−25	−40	−47	−51	−55	−58	−60	−62	−64	−65	−67	−68	−69
−30	−46	−53	−58	−61	−64	−67	−69	−71	−72	−74	−75	−76
−35	−52	−59	−64	−68	−74	−73	−76	−78	−79	−81	−82	−84
−40	−57	−66	−71	−74	−78	−80	−82	−84	−86	−88	−89	−91
−45	−63	−72	−77	−81	−84	−87	−89	−91	−93	−95	−97	−98

Temperature (°F)

Frostbite occurs in 15 minutes or less

$$\text{Wind Chill (°F)} = 35.74 + 0.6215T - 35.75(V^{0.16}) + 0.4275T(V^{0.16})$$

Where, T = Air temperature (°F)
V = Wind speed (mph)

Figure 24-1 NOAA's National Weather Service Wind Chill chart (effective 11/1/2001). (*From http://www.weather.gov/os/windchill/index.shtml.*)

Generalized Cold Emergency—Generalized Hypothermia

Hypothermia occurs when the body loses more heat than it can produce!

- Predisposing risk factors include:
  - Cold environment
  - Immersion
  - Age (extreme ages)
    — Pediatric patients have a large surface area compared to their overall size.
    — Small muscle mass, and the ability to shiver are not well developed in pediatric patients.
    — Children and infants have less body fat.
    — Younger children need help to protect themselves; they cannot put on or take off their clothes.
- Medical conditions that affect body temperature:
  - Shock (hypoperfusion)
  - Head injury

- Burns
- Generalized infection
- Injuries to the spinal cord
- Diabetes and hypoglycemia
- Certain drugs/poisons
- Environmental conditions of cold exposure
  - Obvious exposure
  - Subtle exposure
  - Ethanol ingestion
  - Underlying illness
  - Overdose/poisoning
  - Major trauma
  - Outdoor resuscitation
  - Ambient temperature decreased (home of elderly patient)

Signs and Symptoms of Generalized Hypothermia

- Cool/cold skin temperature—The EMT should place the back of his hand between the clothing and the patient's abdomen to assess the general temperature of the patient. The patient experiencing a generalized cold emergency will present with cool abdominal skin temperature.
- Decreasing mental status or motor function—Correlates with the degree of hypothermia
- Poor coordination
- Memory disturbances
- Reduced or loss of sensation to touch
- Mood changes
- Less communicative
- Dizziness
- Speech difficulty
- Stiff or rigid posture
- Muscular rigidity
- Shivering may be present or absent
- Breathing variations:
  - Early—Rapid breathing
  - Late—Shallow, slow, or even absent breathing
- Slowly responding pupils (sluggish)
- Pulse:
  - Early—Rapid
  - Late—Slow and barely palpable and/or irregular, or completely absent
- Low to absent blood pressure
- Poor judgment/poor coordination—Patient may actually remove clothing
- Complaints of joint/muscle stiffness
- Skin:
  - Red—Early
  - Pale
  - Cyanotic—Blue-gray
  - Stiff/hard

Emergency Management for Generalized Hypothermia

- Remove the patient from the environment and protect the patient from further heat loss.
- Remove wet clothing and cover with a dry warm blanket.
- Handle the patient gently. Avoid rough handling.
- Do not allow the patient to walk or exert him/herself.
- Administer oxygen if not already done as part of the initial assessment—Oxygen administered should be warm and humidified, if possible.
- Assess pulses for 45 to 60 seconds before starting cardiopulmonary resuscitation (CPR).
- If the patient is alert and responding appropriately, actively rewarm.
  - Warm blankets.
  - Apply heat packs or hot water bottles to the groin, axillary, and cervical regions.
  - Turn the heat up high in the patient compartment of the ambulance.
- If the patient is unresponsive or not responding appropriately, rewarm passively:
  - Warm blankets.
  - Turn the heat up high in the patient compartment of the ambulance.
  - Do not allow the patient to eat or drink stimulants.
  - Do not massage extremities.

Local Cold Injuries–Localized to Specific Area of Body

- Look for predisposing factors.
- Tend to occur on the distal end of extremities such as exposed ears, nose, and face.

Signs and Symptoms of Local Cold Injuries

- Local injury with clear demarcation of cold injury site.
- Early or superficial injury:
  - Blanching of the skin—Palpation of the skin in which normal color does not return.
  - Loss of feeling and sensation in the injured area.
  - Skin remains soft.
  - If rewarmed, tingling sensation.
- Late or deep injury:
  - White, waxy skin.
  - Firm to frozen feeling upon palpation.
  - Swelling may be present.
  - Blisters may be present.
  - If thawed or partially thawed, the skin may appear flushed with areas of purple and blanching or mottled and cyanotic.

Emergency Management for Local Cold Injuries

- Remove the patient from the environment.
- Protect the cold injured extremity from further injury.
- Administer oxygen if not already done as part of the initial assessment.

- Remove wet or restrictive clothing.
- If early or superficial injury, splint and cover the extremity.
- Do not rub or massage.
- Do not reexpose to the cold.
- If late or deep cold injury:
  ○ Remove jewelry.
  ○ Cover with dry clothing or dressings.

Do Not

- Break blisters
- Rub or massage area
- Apply heat directly to the extremity
- Allow the patient to walk on the affected extremity

When an extremely long or delayed transport is inevitable, active rapid rewarming should be done.

- Immerse the affected part in a warm water bath (100°F-110°F).
- Monitor the water to ensure it does not cool from the frozen part.
- Continuously stir water.
- Continue until the body part is soft, and color and sensation return.
- Dress the area with dry sterile dressings. If hand or foot, place dry sterile dressings between fingers or toes.
- Protect against refreezing the warmed part.
- Expect the patient to complain of severe pain.

EXPOSURE TO HEAT

Figure 24-2 shows NOAA's National Weather Service heat index.

Temperature (°F)

Relative humidity (%)	80	82	84	86	88	90	92	94	96	98	100	102	104	106	108	110
40	80	81	83	85	88	91	94	97	101	105	109	114	119	124	130	136
45	80	82	84	87	89	93	96	100	104	109	114	119	124	130	137	
50	81	83	85	88	91	95	99	103	108	113	118	124	131	137		
55	81	84	86	89	93	97	101	106	112	117	124	130	137			
60	82	84	88	91	95	100	105	110	116	123	129	137				
65	82	85	89	93	98	103	108	114	121	128	126					
70	83	86	90	95	100	105	112	119	126	134						
75	84	88	92	97	103	109	116	124	132							
80	84	89	94	100	106	113	121	129								
85	85	90	96	102	110	117	126	135								
90	86	91	98	105	113	122	131									
95	86	93	100	108	117	127										
100	87	95	103	112	121	132										

Likelihood of heat disorders with prolonged exposure or strenuous activity

☐ Caution   ☐ Extreme caution   ☐ Danger   ☐ Extreme danger

Figure 24-2   NOAA's National Weather Service heat index.
(From http://www.weather.gov/om/heat/index.shtml (effective 11/1/2001).

- Predisposing factors
  - Climate.
  - High ambient temperature reduces the body's ability to lose heat by radiation.
  - High relative humidity reduces the body's ability to lose heat through evaporation.
- Exercise and activity
  - Can lose more than 1 L of sweat per hour.
  - Loss of electrolytes (sodium, chloride, and fluid through sweat).
- Factors regarding age
  - Elderly
    — Poor thermoregulation
    — Certain medications (beta blockers) affect ability to respond to heat.
    — Lack of mobility—Cannot escape hot environment.
  - Newborn/infants
    — Poor thermoregulation
    — Cannot remove own clothing
- Preexisting illness and/or conditions that may affect the patient who is experiencing a heat emergency:
  - Heart disease
  - Dehydration
  - Obesity
  - Fever
  - Fatigue
  - Diabetes
  - Drugs/medications

Signs and Symptoms
- Muscular cramps
- Weakness or exhaustion
- Dizziness or faintness
- Skin:
  - Moist, pale; normal to cool temperature
  - Hot, dry, or moist—"True emergency"
- Rapid heart rate
- Altered mental status to unresponsive

Emergency Management of Heat Emergencies
- Patient with moist, pale skin; normal to cool skin temperature *(heat exhaustion)*
  - Remove the patient from the hot environment and place in a cool environment (back of air-conditioned ambulance).
  - Administer oxygen if not already done during the initial assessment.
  - Loosen or remove clothing.
  - Cool patient by fanning.
  - Put in supine position with legs elevated.
  - If patient is responsive and is not nauseated, have the patient drink water.
  - If the patient is unresponsive or is vomiting, transport to the hospital with patient on his left side.

- Patient with hot, dry or moist skin *(heat stroke)*
  - Remove the patient from the hot environment and place in a cool environment (back of air-conditioned ambulance with air conditioner running on high).
  - Remove clothing.
  - Administer oxygen if not already done during the initial assessment.
  - Apply cool packs to neck, groin, and armpits.
  - Keep the skin wet by applying water by sponge or wet towels.
  - Fan aggressively.
  - Transport immediately.

BITES AND STINGS

Humans can be injured by the bites or stings of many kinds of animals, including mammals such as dogs, cats, and fellow humans; arthropods such as spiders, bees, and wasps; snakes; and marine animals such as jellyfish and stingrays.

It is a very warm summer night. The streets are full of people celebrating a national holiday. The time is 8 p.m. when EMS is summoned to respond to a private address for a victim with an animal bite. As EMS arrives on-scene, the local police department has secured the site. The police officer approaches the ambulance and states, "You have one to go. She is in front of the location. Apparently the neighbor's bull mastiff attacked her when she entered the neighbor's backyard."

As you approach the patient, you witness bystanders upset about what has occurred. The patient, a young 25-year-old woman, conscious, is complaining of severe pain to her right forearm and left leg. You notice bright red blood on a towel the neighbor was using to control the bleeding. The patient has an obvious deformity to her right forearm, and bleeding appears to be controlled.

What steps should be performed while evaluating and treating this patient?

Mammals

Dogs

In the United States, where the dog population exceeds 50 million, dogs surpass all other mammals in the number of bites inflicted on humans. However, most dog-bite injuries are minor. Each year, about 10 to 20 Americans, mostly children under 10 years of age, are killed by dogs.

Dog bites result in an estimated 340,000 emergency-room visits annually throughout the United States. More than half of the bites seen by emergency departments occur at home. Children under 10 years old, especially boys between 5 and 9 years of age, are more likely than older people to visit an emergency room for bite treatment. Children under 10 years old were also much more liable to be bitten on the face, neck, and head. Nearly all of the injuries suffered by people seeking treatment in emergency rooms were of "low severity," and most were treated and released without being admitted to a hospital or sent to another facility. Many of the bites resulted from people attempting to break up fights between animals.

Cats

Although cats are found in nearly a third of US households, cat bites are far less common than dog bites. The tissue damage caused by cat bites is usually limited, but they carry a high risk of infection. Whereas the infection rate for dog-bite injuries is 15% to 20%, the infection rate for cat bites is 30% to 40%. A typical person who has been bitten is a young girl playing with a pet.

Humans

Bites from mammals other than dogs and cats are uncommon, with one exception—human bites. There are approximately 70,000 human bites each year in the United States. Because the human mouth contains a multitude of potentially harmful microorganisms, human bites are more infectious than those of most other animals.

Arthropods

Arthropods are invertebrates belonging to the phylum *Arthropoda*, which includes insects, arachnids, crustaceans, and other subgroups. There are more than 700,000 species in all. The list of arthropods that bite or sting humans is extensive and includes lice, bedbugs, fleas, mosquitoes, black flies, ants, chiggers, ticks, centipedes, scorpions, and other species. Spiders, bees, and wasps are the three kinds of arthropod that most often bite people.

Spiders

In the United States, only two kinds of venomous spider are truly dangerous: black widow spiders and brown (violin or fiddle) recluse spiders. The black widow, which is found in every state but Alaska, is probably the most notorious spider. It prefers dark, dry places such as barns, garages, and outhouses, and also lives under rocks and logs. Disturbing a female black widow or its web may provoke a bite. Brown recluse spiders also prefer sheltered places, including clothing, and may bite if disturbed.

Bees and Wasps

Bees and wasps will sting to defend their nests or if they are disturbed. Species common to the United States include honeybees, bumblebees, yellow jackets, bald-faced hornets, brown hornets, and paper wasps. Of note also are Africanized bee species, also called "killer bees," that have been found in the United States since 1990. More than 50 Americans die each year after being stung by a bee, wasp, or ant. Almost all of those deaths are the result of allergic reactions, and not of exposure to the venom itself.

Snakes

There are 20 species of venomous snakes in the United States. These snakes are found in every state except Maine, Alaska, and Hawaii. Each year about 8000 Americans receive a venomous snakebite, but no more than about 15 die, mostly from rattlesnake bites.

The venomous snakes of the United States are divided into two families, the *Crotalidae* (pit vipers) and the *Elapidae.* Pit vipers, named after the small heat-sensing pit that lies between each eye and nostril, are responsible for about 99% of the venomous snakebites suffered by Americans. Rattlesnakes, copperheads, and cottonmouths (also called water moccasins) are pit vipers. This family of snakes delivers its venom through two long, hinged fangs in the upper jaw. Some pit vipers carry potent venom that can threaten the brain and spinal cord. The venom of others, such as the copperheads, is less harmful.

The *Elapidae* family includes two kinds of venomous coral snakes indigenous to the southern and western states. Because coral snakes are bashful creatures that come out only at night, they almost never bite humans, and are responsible for approximately 25 bites a year in the United States. Coral snakes also have short fangs and a small mouth, which lowers the risk of a bite actually forcing venom into a person's body. However, their venom is quite poisonous.

Marine Animals

Several varieties of marine animals may bite or sting. Jellyfish and stingrays are two kinds that pose a threat to people who live or vacation in coastal communities.

Signs and Symptoms

Dogs

A typical dog bite results in a laceration, tear, puncture, or crush injury. Bites from large, powerful dogs may even cause fractures and dangerous internal injuries. Also, dogs trained to attack may bite repeatedly during a single episode. Infected bites usually cause pain, cellulitis (inflammation of the connective tissues), and a pus-filled discharge at the wound site within 8 to 24 hours. Most infections are confined to the wound site, but many of the microorganisms in the mouths of dogs can cause systemic and possibly life-threatening infections. Examples are bacteremia and meningitis, especially severe in people diagnosed with acquired immunodeficiency syndrome (AIDS) or other health condition that increases their susceptibility to infection. Rabies is rare among pet dogs in the United States, most of which have been vaccinated against the disease. Tetanus is also rare but can be transmitted by a dog bite if the victim is not immunized.

Cats

The mouths of cats and dogs contain many of the same microorganisms. Cat scratches and bites are also capable of transmitting the *Bartonella henselae* bacterium, which can lead to cat-scratch disease, an unpleasant but usually not life-threatening illness.

Cat bites are mostly found on the arms and hands. Sharp cat teeth typically leave behind a deep puncture wound that can reach muscles, tendons, and bones, which are vulnerable to infection because of their comparatively poor blood supply. This is why cat bites are much more likely to become infected than dog bites. Also, people are less inclined to view cat bites as dangerous and requiring immediate attention; the risk that infection has set in by the time a medical professional is consulted is thus greater.

Humans

Human bites result from fights, sexual activity, medical and dental treatment, and seizures. Bites also raise the possibility of spousal or child abuse. Children often bite other children, but those bites are hardly ever severe. Human bites are capable of transmitting a wide range of dangerous diseases, including hepatitis B, syphilis, and tuberculosis.

Human bites fall into two categories: occlusion (true) bites and clenched-fist injuries. The former presents a lower risk of infection. The latter, which are very infectious and can permanently damage the hand, usually result from a fist hitting teeth during a fight. People often wait before seeking treatment for a clenched-fist injury, with the result that about half of such injuries are infected by the time they are seen by a medical professional.

Spiders

As a rule, people rarely see a black widow bite, nor do they feel the bite as it occurs. The first (and possibly only) evidence that a person has been bitten may be a mild swelling of the injured area and two red puncture marks. Within a short time, however, some victims begin to experience severe muscle cramps and rigidity of the abdominal muscles. Other possible symptoms include excessive sweating, nausea, vomiting, headaches, and vertigo as well as breathing, vision, and speech problems.

A brown recluse spider's bite can lead to necrotic arachnidism, in which the tissue in an area of up to several inches around the bite becomes necrotic (dies), producing an open sore that can take months or years to disappear. In most cases, however, the bite simply produces a hard, painful, itchy, and discolored area that heals without treatment in 2 to 3 days. The bite may also be accompanied by a fever, chills, edema (an accumulation of excess tissue fluid), nausea and vomiting, dizziness, muscle and joint pain, and a rash.

Bees and Wasps

The familiar symptoms of bee and wasp stings include pain, redness, swelling, and itchiness in the area of the sting. Multiple stings can have much more severe consequences, such as anaphylaxis, a life-threatening allergic reaction that occurs in hypersensitive persons.

Snakes

Venomous pit viper bites usually begin to swell within 10 minutes and sometimes are painful. Other symptoms include skin blisters and discoloration, weakness, sweating, nausea, faintness, dizziness, bruising, and tender lymph nodes. Severe poisoning can also lead to tingling in the scalp, fingers, and toes, muscle contractions, an elevated heart rate, rapid breathing, large drops in body temperature and blood pressure, vomiting of blood, and coma.

Many pit viper and coral snakes (20%-60%) fail to poison (envenomate) their victim, or introduce only a small amount of venom into the victim's body. The wounds, however, can still become infected by the harmful microorganisms that snakes carry in their mouths.

Coral snake bites are painful but may be hard to see. One to seven hours after being bitten, a person begins to experience the effects of the venom, which include tingling at the wound site, weakness, nausea, vomiting, excessive salivation, and irrational behavior. Major nerves of the body can become paralyzed for 6 to 14 days, causing double vision, difficulty swallowing and speaking, respiratory failure, and other problems. Six to eight weeks may be needed before normal muscular strength is regained.

Jellyfish

Jellyfish venom is delivered by barbs called nematocysts, which are located on the creature's tentacles and penetrate the skin of people who brush up against them. Instant painful and itchy red lesions usually result. The pain can continue up to 48 hours. Severe cases may lead to skin necrosis, muscle spasms and cramps, vomiting, nausea, diarrhea, headaches, excessive sweating, and other symptoms. In rare instances, cardio respiratory failure may also occur.

Sting Rays

Tail spines are the delivery mechanism for stingray venom. Deep puncture wounds result that can cause an infection if pieces of spine become embedded in the wound. A typical stingray injury scenario involves a person who inadvertently steps on a resting stingray and is lashed in the ankle by its tail. Stingray venom produces immediate, excruciating pain that lasts several hours. Sometimes the victim suffers a severe reaction, including vomiting, diarrhea, hemorrhage (bleeding), a drop in blood pressure, and cardiac arrhythmia (disordered heart beat).

Emergency Management

- If stinger is present, remove it.
  - Scrape stinger out, that is, with the edge of a credit card.
  - Avoid using tweezers or forceps as these can squeeze venom from the venom sac into the wound.
- Wash area gently.
- Remove jewelry from injured area before swelling begins, if possible.
- Place injection site slightly below the level of the patient's heart.
- Do not apply cold to snakebites.
- Consult medical direction regarding constricting band for snakebite.
- Observe for development of signs and symptoms of an allergic reaction, treat as needed.

? CHAPTER QUESTIONS

1. Hypothermia occurs when:
   a. The body loses more heat than it produces.
   b. Cold food or drink is ingested.
   c. The body produces more heat than it loses.
   d. Specific parts of the body are exposed to cold temperatures.

2. Emergency care for local cold injuries includes:
   a. packing the affected area with snow or a cold pack
   b. encouraging the patient to walk on an injured extremity to restore circulation
   c. rubbing the affected area to restore circulation as soon as possible
   d. immersing the affected area in warm (tepid) water, just above body temperature (100°F-110°F)

3. All of the following are heat-related emergencies except:

    a. heat cramps

    b. heat exhaustion

    c. heat stroke

    d. heat index

Reference

US Department of Transportation, National Highway Traffic Safety Administration. *EMT-Basic National Standard Curriculum*. Washington, DC: US Department of Transportation, National Highway Traffic Safety Administration; 1994.

Chapter 25
Submersion, Drowning, and Diving Emergencies

It is 8:30 PM on a beautiful summer night when a frantic call comes into the 911 system for a 12-year-old child drowning. Dispatch calls your unit for a high-priority assignment, "Child Unconscious from a Pool Accident." Upon arrival, you see a crowd of people waiting in the street for your arrival. They point to the backyard. You see the sense of urgency in their request.

You grab your technician bag, oxygen bag, bag-valve-mask (BVM), and defibrillator, and begin to go into the backyard. Upon arrival you see a man attempting to remove what appears to be a limp child from the backyard swimming pool.

What is your next step?

WATER-RELATED EMERGENCIES

Near Drowning/Drowning

- In the United States, drowning deaths number more than 8000 per year, with 1500 of these deaths occurring in children.
- Drowning is defined as death secondary to asphyxia while immersed in a liquid, usually water, or within 24 hours of submersion.
- An additional 1200 reported immersion deaths are boating related (90% of boating deaths), 500 are motor vehicle associated, and 1000 reported drownings are of undetermined etiology. Scuba diving accounts for an estimated 700 to 800 deaths per year (etiologies include inadequate experience/training, exhaustion, panic, carelessness, and barotrauma).

Pathophysiology

- Submersion injury occurs when a person is submerged in water, attempts to breathe, and either aspirates water (wet drowning) or has laryngospasm without aspiration (dry drowning).
- The most important contributory factors to morbidity and mortality from near drowning are hypoxemia and a decrease in oxygen delivery to vital tissues. The pathophysiology of near drowning is intimately related to the multiorgan effects of hypoxemia.

Response to Submersion, Drowning, and Diving Emergencies

- Ensure the safety of the rescue personnel.
- Suspect possible spine injury if diving accident is involved or unknown (maintain high index of suspicion).
- Consider length of time in cold-water drowning. Any pulseless, non-breathing patient who has been submerged in cold water should be resuscitated.

Emergency Management

- In-line immobilization and removal from water with backboard if spine injury is suspected.
- If there is no suspected spine injury, place patient on left side to allow water, vomitus, and secretions to drain from upper airway.
- Suction as needed.
- Administer oxygen if not already done during the initial assessment.
- If gastric distention interferes with artificial ventilation, the patient should be placed on his left side. With suction immediately available, the EMT should place his hand over the epigastric area of the abdomen and apply firm pressure to relieve the distention. This procedure should only be done if the gastric distention interferes with the ability of the EMT to artificially ventilate the patient effectively.

Specific Assessment and Management—Near Drowning

- Submersion episode with at least transient recovery

Pathophysiology

WET VERSUS DRY DROWNING

- Fluid in posterior oropharynx stimulates laryngospasm.
- Aspiration occurs after muscular relaxation.
- Suffocation occurs with or without aspiration.
- Aspiration presents as airway obstruction.

FRESH VERSUS SALTWATER CONSIDERATIONS

- Despite mechanism differences, there is no difference in metabolic result.
- Hypothermic considerations in near drowning:
  - Common concomitant syndrome.
  - May be organ protective in cold-water near drowning.
  - Always treat hypoxia first.
  - Treat all near-drowning patients for hypothermia.

Emergency Management

- Establish patent airway, suction as needed.
- Ventilate as necessary.
- High-concentration oxygen should be administered.

Trauma Considerations

- Immersion episode of unknown etiology warrants trauma management.
- Postresuscitation complications:

- Adult respiratory distress syndrome (ARDS) or renal failure often occurs postresuscitation.
    - Symptoms may not appear for 24 hours or more, postresuscitation.
    - All near-drowning patients should be transported for evaluation.
- Specific pathology—Diving emergencies:
    - Application of gas laws
        — Boyle's law—At a constant temperature, the volume of a gas varies inversely with the pressure.
        — Dalton's law—In a mixture of gases, the total pressure is equal to the sum of the partial pressures of each gas.
        — Henry's law—The weight of a gas dissolved by a given volume of liquid at a constant temperature is directly proportional to the pressure.

Pathophysiology

- Increased pressure dissolves gases into blood.
- Oxygen metabolizes.
- Nitrogen dissolves.

Primary etiology is too rapid an ascent from depth.

Classification of Diving Emergencies

- Decompression illnesses
    - Excess nitrogen bubbles out of solution on depressurization.
    - Occurs in joints, tendons, spinal cord, skin, brain, inner ear.
    - Occludes circulation.

Principal Signs and Symptoms

- Joint pain
- Fatigue
- Paresthesias
- CNS disturbances

Emergency Management

- High-concentration oxygen
- Treat for shock
- Place patient in supine position
- Transport to emergency department
- Definitive care is typically hyperbaric oxygen therapy (HBO)

Pulmonary Overpressure Accidents

Air trapped in lungs by:

- Breath holding.
- Bronchospasm.
- Mucous plug.
- Shallow depths (<6 in) most dangerous.
- Pressure decreases and volume increases on ascent.
- Lung tissue ruptures in severe cases, producing a pneumothorax.

Principal Signs and Symptoms

- Respiratory distress
- Substernal chest pain
- Diminished breath sounds

Specific Treatment

- Rest.
- Supplemental oxygen.
- Hyperbaric oxygen not usually required.
- Treatment is the same as for pneumothorax of any etiology.

Arterial Gas Embolism (AGE)

- Air in bloodstream secondary to pulmonary overpressure
- Access to pulmonary circulation from ruptured alveoli
- Entrance to central circulation via left atrium
- Occlusion of small vessels occurs
- Cardiac compromise
- Pulmonary compromise
- Cerebral compromise

Principal Signs and Symptoms

- Usually appear within 10 minutes of surfacing (most commonly within 2 minutes).
- Varies according to organ system that is primarily affected.
- Most common presentation is similar to cerebral vascular accident (CVA).
- Hemispheric presentations are rare.
- Vertigo.
- Confusion.
- Loss of consciousness.
- Visual disturbances.

Emergency Management

- High flow oxygen.
- Transport supine, not in Trendelenburg position.
- Best treatment may be immediate hyperbaric oxygen.
- Treat as for near drowning.
- Treat according to other symptoms.
- Attempt to keep the patient at or below the altitude of the injury during transport.

Nitrogen Narcosis

- Excess nitrogen is dissolved in bloodstream under pressure.
- Most common appearance is at depths of 70 to 100 ft.
- Gas anesthetic effect is due to lipid solubility.
- Result is intoxication.
- Accidents at depth often result from impaired judgment.

Principal Signs and Symptoms

- Intoxication, impaired judgment
- Altered level of consciousness

Specific Treatment

- Self-resolving upon ascent
- Return to shallow depths

Other Diving-Related Illnesses

- Oxygen toxicity
  - ○ Usually seen only with prolonged exposure or excess concentration
- Contaminated gases
- Hypercapnia
- Hyperventilation

DIVERS ALERT NETWORK (DAN)

- Nonprofit organization affiliated with Duke University Medical Center
- Specializes in diving-related illnesses
- Available for consultation and referral
- (919) 684-9111 for emergencies
- (919) 684-2948 for non-emergency consultation and referral

? CHAPTER QUESTIONS

1. You respond to a call from a scuba diver who ascended from the depths rapidly following his dive a few hours ago. He is complaining of deep pain in his shoulders and elbows, made worse with any movement. You suspect:

   a. arterial gas embolism

   b. decompression illness

   c. recompression injury

   d. nitrogen narcosis

2. After a rapid ascent, a scuba diver developed a sudden onset of severe chest pain followed by a loss of consciousness. Your care during transport to the emergency department should be to protect the airway and:

   a. place the patient in the Trendelenburg position

   b. perform a needle thoracentesis

   c. administer 100% oxygen

   d. administer nitrous oxide

Reference

US Department of Transportation, National Highway Traffic Safety Administration. *EMT-Basic National Standard Curriculum*. Washington, DC: US Department of Transportation, National Highway Traffic Safety Administration; 1994.

Chapter 26
Behavioral Emergencies

You and your partner are dispatched to the scene of major highway overpass where a 30-year-old man has just jumped from the bridge. He is lying supine on the ground below the bridge. The fall is approximately 50 ft. The patient appears to be conscious and is attempting to move. What is your next step in evaluating the scene?

Behavior is a manner in which a person acts or performs any or all activities including physical and mental activity.

BEHAVIORAL EMERGENCY

A situation where the patient exhibits abnormal behavior within a given situation that is unacceptable or intolerable to the patient, family, or community. This behavior can be due to extremes of emotion leading to violence or other inappropriate behavior or due to a psychological or physical condition such as lack of oxygen or low blood sugar in diabetics.

BEHAVIORAL CHANGE

General factors that may alter a patient's behavior—The number of factors which may alter a patient's behavior include situational stresses, medical illnesses, psychiatric problems, and alcohol or drugs. Below is a list of common causes for behavior alteration:

- Low blood sugar
- Lack of oxygen
- Inadequate blood flow to the brain
- Head trauma
- Mind-altering substances
- Psychogenic—Resulting in psychotic thinking, depression, or panic
- Excessive cold
- Excessive heat

PSYCHOLOGICAL CRISES

- Panic
- Agitation
- Bizarre thinking and behavior
- Danger to self—Self-destructive behavior, suicide
- Danger to others—Threatening behavior, violence

ASSESSMENT FOR SUICIDE RISK

Depression

- Sad, tearful
- Thoughts of death or taking one's life

Suicidal Gestures

- The EMT must recognize and intervene in self-destructive behavior before the patient commits the act of suicide. Risk factors may include:
  - Individuals over 40, single, widowed or divorced, alcoholic, depressed
  - A defined lethal plan of action which has been verbalized
  - Unusual gathering of articles which can cause death such as purchase of a gun, large volumes of pills, and the like
  - Previous history of self-destructive behavior
  - Recent diagnosis of serious illness
  - Recent loss of significant loved one
  - Arrest, imprisonment, loss of job

Assessment

- Patient in an unsafe environment or with unsafe objects in hands
- Display of self-destructive behavior during initial assessment or prior to emergency response
- Important questions to be considered:
  - How does the patient feel?
  - Are there suicidal tendencies?
  - Is patient a threat to self or others?
  - Is there an underlying medical problem?
  - Any interventions?

Emergency Management

- Scene size-up, personal safety.
- Patient assessment.
- Calm the patient—Do not leave patient alone.
- Restrain if necessary. Consider need for law enforcement.
- Transport, if overdose is suspected, bring medications or drugs found to medical facility.

COMMON PSYCHIATRIC DISORDERS

Affective Disorders

Affective disorders are a group of mental disorders characterized by mood disturbances such as depression, bipolar, and dysrhythmic disorders.

Alcohol Intoxication

Patients with emergencies related to alcohol are common. An intoxicated patient often gives an inaccurate medical history, abnormal response to physical problems, and has the potential for violent and disruptive behavior.

Amnesic Psychogenic Dissociative Disorder

An amnesic psychogenic dissociative disorder is an inability to remember personal information after a severe psychological stress. The patient is usually calm and other memories are intact.

Conversion Disorder

A conversion disorder is the loss of a physical function with no physical cause. The cause of a conversion disorder is often found to be a psychological conflict, such as a need to avoid an unpleasant task or a need to be removed from an unpleasant situation. The conversion places the patient in a situation where he can receive support. Symptoms are a loss of some bodily function.

Depersonalization

Depersonalization is an altered perception of the body or a sense of being outside of the body, characterized by feelings that one's actions and speech cannot be controlled. Depersonalization is usually a protecting mechanism to protect the self.

Drug Intoxication

In most instances, patients with acute drug intoxication present with physical symptoms or are brought in unresponsive by friends.

Dystonia

Haldol, Thorazine, and Compazine may cause dystonia, which is a reaction to medications that causes muscle spasm or contractions that usually involve the tongue, neck, and jaw. Treatment is Cogentin (benztropine mesylate).

Fugue Disorder

A fugue disorder is an abrupt, massive amnesic event with alteration of consciousness that presents as a new personality. A fugue disorder is often precipitated by extreme stress and is associated with drug and alcohol abuse.

Hypochondriasis

Hypochondriasis is a condition where the person has an abnormal preoccupation with the belief that they have a serious illness.

Panic Attacks

Panic attacks are acute, recurrent attacks of panic having no tangible cause. Symptoms include shortness of breath, chest pain, tachycardia, sweating, nausea, vomiting, diarrhea, and a feeling of approaching death.

Phobias

A phobia is a persistent and irrational fear of a specific activity or object that results in a compelling desire to avoid the situation. Phobias are classified into three types:

- Agoraphobias (a variety of everyday situations)
- Social phobias (embarrassment in public)
- Simple phobias (specific situations, eg, tunnels, flying, elevators)

Symptoms may include fear, shortness of breath, chest pain, tachycardia, sweating, nausea, vomiting, diarrhea, and a feeling that something terrible is about to happen.

Posttraumatic Stress Disorder

Posttraumatic stress disorder (PTSD) is a condition where a patient experiences recurrent dreams or thoughts about a traumatic event with feelings of detachment and estrangement from the environment. The disorder is associated with sleep disorders, hyperalertness, difficulty concentrating, and memory impairment.

The cause of PTSD is commonly military combat, rape, or a disaster. Symptoms may include fear, shortness of breath, chest pain, tachycardia, sweating, nausea, vomiting, diarrhea, and a feeling that something terrible is about to happen.

Organic Disorders

Organic disorders encompass a large group of acute and chronic mental disorders associated with brain damage or cerebral dysfunction. The patient may present with impaired consciousness, orientation, intellect, judgment, thought processing, or with hallucination and mood changes.

Paranoid Disorder

Paranoia disorder is a condition where the patient shows persistent delusions of persecution. Behavior can be consistent with the delusion, or bizarre and incoherent. The disorder usually occurs in mid or late adult life and may include anger that leads to violent behavior.

Schizophrenia

Schizophrenia is a group of mental disorders with disordered thinking and bizarre behaviors. Clinically, patients show disturbances of thought with delusions. Speech may be coherent but unassociated with the situation, mute, completely incoherent, or catatonic. Effect may be flat or inappropriate. Perception is disordered with visual and auditory hallucinations.

SOMATOFORM DISORDERS

Somatoform disorders are physical symptoms with no detectable organic physical cause; they are not under conscious control of the patient.

Somatization

Somatization is a condition where a person has multiple somatic complaints with 15 or more symptoms lasting over several years. The cause of somatization is unknown. Symptoms include multiple physical complaints, numerous surgeries, and many medical consults. The condition is frequently associated with alcohol abuse.

- 18 months to 3 years—Autonomy versus shame and doubt, self-control without loss of self-esteem, the ability to cooperate and express oneself.

- 3 to 5 years—Initiative versus guilt, realistic sense of purpose and ability to evaluate one's own behavior versus self-denial and self-restriction.

- 6 to 12 years—Industry versus inferiority, realization of competence, preservation, versus feeling that one will never be "any good" and withdrawal from school and peers.

- 12 to 20 years—Identity versus role diffusion, coherent sense of self; plans to actualize one's abilities versus feelings of confusion, indecisiveness, and the possibility of antisocial behavior.
- 18 to 25 years—Intimacy versus isolation, capacity for love as mutual devotion, commitment to work and relationships versus impersonal relationships and prejudice.
- 25 to 65 years—Generatively versus stagnation, creativity, production, concern for others versus self-indulgence, and impoverishment of self.
- 65 years to death—Integrity versus despair, acceptance of the worth and uniqueness of one's life versus a sense of loss and contempt for others.

PHYSICAL CHANGES DURING STRESS

Alarm Stage

The alarm state is a condition where an increase in epinephrine and norepinephrine release occurs. The fight-or-flight reaction is activated. Blood pressure, pulse, respiratory rate, blood sugar, and alertness are increased.

Resistance Stage

The resistance stage is a stage where hormonal levels adjust and the patient uses coping and defensive behavior.

Exhaustion

When exhaustion occurs, the immune response decreases, the defense mechanisms are exaggerated, thinking is disorganized, sensory input is misperceived (auditory and visual illusions), reality concepts are distorted, and violent behavior can occur. Physical system failure and death can occur.

SUICIDOLOGY

The science of suicide includes causes, prediction of susceptibility, and prevention. In the United States, over 31,000 people intentionally kill themselves annually, which is equivalent to 1 every 20 minute. In recent years, suicides have doubled in children aged 10 through 19 years. Suicide is the ninth leading cause of death in the United States. More people die from suicide (11.9 per 100,000) than from homicide (8.5 per 100,000). Nearly 60% of all suicides are caused from firearms. Most suicide victims have consulted a physician within 6 months of the suicide and 10% have seen a physician within 1 week of the suicide. Health-care workers can prevent a suicide if they recognize the individual is at risk and intervene.

Warning Signs of Suicidal Ideation

- Specific lethal plan that does not include the possibility for rescue
- Depression (65% of suicides have a history of depression)
- History of suicide attempts (65% of suicides have a history of attempts)
- Limited psychological and social resources
- Taking actions to put their lives in order
- Giving away possessions
- Failure at work or school
- Recent loss and dealing with grief
- Poor work or school performance

- History of alcohol abuse
- History of drug abuse

Medical/Legal Considerations

- An emotionally disturbed patient who consents to care and transport significantly reduces legal problems.
- How to handle the patient who resists treatment:
  - Emotionally disturbed patient will often resist treatment.
  - May threaten EMTs and other responders.
  - To provide care against patient's will, you must show a reasonable belief the patient would harm himself or others.
  - If a threat to self or others, patient may be transported without consent after contacting medical direction. This action is performed by law enforcement.
- Avoiding unreasonable force.
  - Reasonable force depends on what force was necessary to keep patient from injuring himself or others.
  - Reasonable force is determined by looking at all circumstances involved.
    — Patient's size and strength
    — Type of abnormal behavior
    — Sex of patient
    — Mental state of patient and method of restraint
  - Be aware; after a period of combativeness and aggression, some calm patients may cause unexpected and sudden injury to self and others.
  - Avoid acts or physical force that may cause injury to the patient.
  - EMS personnel may use reasonable force to defend against an attack by emotionally disturbed patients.

Police and Medical Direction Involvement

- Seek medical direction when considering restraining a patient.
- Ask for police assistance if during scene size-up the patient appears or acts aggressive, or combative.

Protection Against False Accusations

- Documentation of abnormal behavior exhibited by the patient is very important.
- Have witnesses in attendance especially during transport, if possible.
- Accusing EMTs of sexual misconduct is common by emotionally disturbed patients—Have help, same-sex attendants, and third-party witnesses.

PRINCIPLES FOR ASSESSING BEHAVIORAL EMERGENCY PATIENTS

- Identify yourself and let the person know you are there to help.
- Inform him/her of what you are doing.
- Ask questions in a calm, reassuring voice.
- Allow the patient to tell what happened without being judgmental.

- Show you are listening by rephrasing or repeating part of what is said.
- Acknowledge the patient's feelings.
- Assess the patient's mental status.
  - Appearance
  - Activity
  - Speech
  - Orientation for time, person, and place

ASSESSMENT OF POTENTIAL VIOLENCE

- Scene size-up.
- History—The EMT should check with family and bystanders to determine if the patient has a known history of aggression or combativeness.
- Posture—Stands or sits in a position which threatens self or others. May have fists clenched or lethal objects in hands.
- Vocal activity—Yells or verbally threatens harm to self or others.
- Physical activity—Moves toward caregiver, carries heavy or threatening objects, has quick irregular movements, muscles tense.

METHODS TO CALM BEHAVIORAL EMERGENCY PATIENTS

- Acknowledge that the person seems upset, and restate that you are there to help.
- Inform him of what you are doing.
- Ask questions in a calm, reassuring voice.
- Maintain a comfortable distance.
- Encourage the patient to state what is troubling him.
- Do not make quick moves.
- Respond honestly to patient's questions.
- Do not threaten, challenge, or argue with disturbed patients.
- Tell the truth, do not lie to the patient.
- Do not "play along" with visual or auditory disturbances of the patient.
- Involve trusted family members or friends.
- Be prepared to stay at scene for a long time. Always remain with the patient.
- Avoid unnecessary physical contact. Call additional help if needed.
- Use good eye contact.

Restraining Patients

Restraint should be avoided unless patient is a danger to self and others. When using restraints, have police present, if possible, and get approval from medical direction. If restraints must be used, do the following:

- Be sure to have adequate help.
- Plan your activities.
- Use only the force necessary for restraint.
- Estimate range of motion of patient's arms and legs and stay beyond range until ready.

- Once decision has been made—Act quickly.
- Have one EMT talk to patient throughout restraining.
- Approach with four persons, one assigned to each limb all at the same time.
- Secure limbs together with equipment approved by medical direction.
- Turn patient face down on stretcher.
- Secure to stretcher with multiple straps.
- Cover face with surgical mask if patient is spitting on EMTs.
- Reassess circulation frequently.
- Document indication for restraining patients and technique of restraint.
- Avoid unnecessary force.

MANAGING OTHER BEHAVIORAL ISSUES

- Always try to talk patient into cooperation.
- Do not belittle or threaten patients.
- Be calm and patient in your attitude.
- Do not agree with disturbed thinking.
- Be reassuring and avoid arguing with irrational patients.
- Suggest appropriate steps to take.
- Lower distressing stimuli.
- Avoid restraints unless necessary.
- Treat with respect.

? CHAPTER QUESTIONS

1. Which of the following is most likely at low risk for suicide?

   a. Older man without a spouse, unemployed, and in poor health

   b. People who are depressed

   c. Persons with a serious debilitating illness

   d. Married men, living spouse, employed

2. In which stage of the stress response does it become more likely that the person might react with violent behavior?

   a. Alarm stage

   b. Resistance stage

   c. Exhaustion stage

   d. Fight or flight stage

Reference

US Department of Transportation, National Highway Traffic Safety Administration. *EMT-Basic National Standard Curriculum*. Washington, DC: US Department of Transportation, National Highway Traffic Safety Administration; 1994.

Chapter 27
Obstetric and Gynecological Emergencies

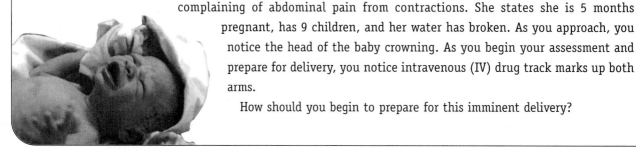

You are the first arriving EMS unit on-scene. As you enter the apartment, you find a 27-year-old woman complaining of abdominal pain from contractions. She states she is 5 months pregnant, has 9 children, and her water has broken. As you approach, you notice the head of the baby crowning. As you begin your assessment and prepare for delivery, you notice intravenous (IV) drug track marks up both arms.

How should you begin to prepare for this imminent delivery?

REPRODUCTIVE ANATOMY AND PHYSIOLOGY

(Fig. 27-1)

- Fetus—Developing unborn baby
- Uterus—Organ in which a fetus grows, responsible for labor and expulsion of infant
- Birth canal—Vagina and lower part of the uterus
- Placenta—Fetal organ through which fetus exchanges nourishment and waste products during pregnancy
- Umbilical cord—Cord that is an extension of the placenta through which fetus receives nourishment while in the uterus
- Amniotic sac (bag of water)—The sac that surrounds the fetus inside the uterus
- Vagina—Lower part of the birth canal
- Perineum—Skin area between vagina and anus, commonly torn during delivery
- Crowning—The bulging-out of the vagina which is opening as the fetus' head or presenting part presses against it
- "Bloody show"—Mucus and blood that may come out of the vagina as labor begins
- Labor—The time and process (defined in three or four stages) beginning with the first uterine muscle contraction until delivery of the placenta
  - Delivery is imminent.
  - Crowning.
  - In the process of delivering.

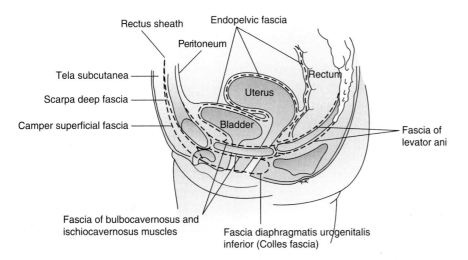

Figure 27-1 OB anatomy. *(Reprinted with permission from DeCherney AH, Nathan L. Current Diagnosis & Treatment Obstetrics and Gynecology. 10th ed. New York: McGraw-Hill; 2007:8.)*

- Presenting part—The part of the infant/fetus that comes first (usually the head)
- Abortion/miscarriage—Delivery of products of conception early in pregnancy

ASSESSMENT OF THE PREGNANT PATIENT

- Your primary goal is to focus on whether you will need to deliver in the pre-hospital setting or whether you have time to transport.
- A complete assessment should include an extensive history. Questions to ask include:
  - Age of the patient?
  - Is there a possibility of the patient being pregnant?
  - Did the patient miss her period and when was the last menstrual period?
  - Any abdominal pain (location/quality)?
  - Any nausea or vomiting?
  - EDC—Expected date of confinement (due date)?
  - Gravida—Number of pregnancies?
  - Para—Number of pregnancies that made it far enough that a fetus would have been expected to be viable?
  - Ab—Abortions, spontaneous or elective?
  - Prenatal care?
  - ROM—Any rupture of membranes?
  - Vaginal bleeding present?
  - Expulsion of the mucous plug?
  - Contractions, and what is the frequency?
  - Are there any preexisting medical conditions or illnesses that are a consequence of pregnancy?
  - Medications, including prenatal vitamins?
  - Last oral intake?

GYNECOLOGICAL EMERGENCIES

Ectopic Pregnancy

- Zygote implants in a location other than the uterine cavity.
- About 95% are in the fallopian tube.
- This is a life-threatening emergency!

Signs and Symptoms

- Abdominal pain may be absent.
- Some patients do not miss their period.
- Some patients have negative pregnancy tests.
- Lower abdominal pain or unexplained hypovolemia in a woman of child-bearing age is an ectopic pregnancy until proven otherwise!

Emergency Management

- High-concentration oxygen.
- Treatment for hypovolemia.
- Transport immediately.

Pelvic Inflammatory Disease

- Acute or chronic infection that involves the fallopian tubes, ovaries, uterus, and peritoneum.
- Most commonly caused by gonorrhea.
- Staphylococcus, streptococcus, coliform bacteria also cause infections.

Signs and Symptoms

- Lower abdominal pain.
- Gradual onset over 2 to 3 days, beginning 1 to 2 weeks after last period.
- Fever, chills, nausea, and vomiting.
- Yellow-green vaginal discharge.
- The patient walks bent forward, holding abdomen.

Emergency Management

- High-concentration oxygen
- Transport

Spontaneous Abortion

- Miscarriage
- Pregnancy terminating before the 20th week
- Usually occurs in the first trimester

Signs and Symptoms

- Vaginal bleeding
- Cramping, lower abdominal pain, or pain in the back
- Passage of fetal tissue
- Complications include:
  - Incomplete abortion
  - Hypovolemia
  - Infection leading to sepsis

Emergency Management

- High-concentration oxygen
- Transport in the Trendelenburg position
- Transport any tissue to the hospital
- Provide emotional support

Preeclampsia

- Acute hypertension after the 24th week of gestation
- 5% to 7% of all pregnancies
- Most often occurs with first pregnancies
- Other risk factors include young mothers, no prenatal care, multiple gestations, lower socioeconomic status
- Triad—Hypertension, proteinuria, edema

Signs and Symptoms

- Hypertension
  - Systolic greater than 140 mm Hg
  - Diastolic greater than 90 mm Hg
  - Or either reading greater than 30 mm Hg above patient's normal blood pressure
- Edema, particularly of the hands, face, and is present early in the day
- Rapid weight gain
  - 3 lb/wk in the second trimester
  - Greater than 1 lb/wk in the third trimester
- Decreased urine output
- Headache and blurred vision
- Nausea and vomiting
- Epigastric pain
- Pulmonary edema
- Complications:
  - Eclampsia
  - Premature separation of the placenta
  - Cerebral hemorrhage
  - Retinal damage
  - Pulmonary edema
  - Lower birth weight infants

Emergency Management

- High-concentration oxygen
- Transport left lateral recumbent
- Avoid excessive stimulation
- Reduce light in patient compartment

Eclampsia

- Most severe form of pregnancy-induced hypertension
- Occurs in less than 1% of all pregnancies

Signs and Symptoms

- Include signs and symptoms of preeclampsia
- Seizures
- Coma
- Complications:
  - 10% maternal mortality rate
  - 25% fetal mortality rate

Emergency Management

- High-concentration oxygen, assist ventilations as needed.
- Transport left lateral recumbent.
- Reduce light.
- Transport immediately.
- Consider advanced life support (ALS) intercept.

Abruptio Placenta

- Premature separation of the placenta
- High-risk groups include:
  - Older patients
  - Hypertensive patients
  - Multigravidas

Signs and Symptoms

- Mild to moderate vaginal bleeding.
- Sharp abdominal pain.
- Rigid tender uterus.
- Hypovolemia.
- Remember: Third trimester abdominal pain equals abruptio placenta until proven otherwise.

Management

- High-concentration oxygen.
- Transport left lateral recumbent.
- Treat hypovolemia.
- Transport rapidly.

Placenta Previa

- Implantation of the placenta over the cervical opening

Signs and Symptoms

- Painless, bright red vaginal bleeding
- Soft nontender uterus
- Hypovolemia

Management

- High-concentration oxygen.
- Transport left lateral recumbent.

- Treat hypovolemia.
- Transport rapidly.

Uterine Rupture

- Blunt trauma to the pregnant uterus
- Prolonged labor against an obstruction
- Weaken uterine wall from old cesarean scar

Signs and Symptoms

- Tearing abdominal pain.
- Hypovolemic shock.
- Firm rigid abdomen.
- Vaginal bleeding may or may not be present.

Emergency Management

- High-concentration oxygen administration.
- Anticipate shock.
- Consider ALS intercept.

EMERGENCY CHILDBIRTH—NORMAL DELIVERY

- Predelivery considerations—*Remember* BSI/PPE!
  - Have the OB kit open and begin setup.
  - Have oxygen and resuscitation equipment available for both mother and baby.
- It is best to transport an expecting mother, unless delivery is expected within a few minutes based on assessment of:
  - How long have you been pregnant?
  - Are there contractions or pain?
  - Any bleeding or discharge?
  - Is crowning occurring with contractions?
  - What is the frequency and duration of contractions?
  - Does she feel as if she is having a bowel movement with increasing pressure in the vaginal area?
  - Does she feel the need to push?
  - Rock hard abdomen?

Precautions

- Use body substance isolation.
- Do not touch vaginal areas except during delivery and when your partner is present.
- Do not let the mother go to bathroom.
- Do not hold mother's legs together.
- Recognize your own limitations and transport even if delivery must occur during transport.
- If delivery is eminent with crowning, contact medical direction for decision to commit to delivery on site. If delivery does not occur within 10 minutes, contact medical direction for permission to transport.

Delivery Procedures

(Fig. 27-2)

- Apply gloves, mask, gown, eye protection for infection control precautions.
- Have mother lie with knees drawn up and spread apart.
- Elevate buttocks with blankets or pillow.
- Create sterile field around vaginal opening with sterile towels or paper barriers.
- When the infant's head appears during crowning, place fingers on bony part of skull (not fontanels or face) and exert very gentle pressure to prevent explosive delivery. Use caution to avoid fontanels.
- If the amniotic sac does not break, or has not broken, use a clamp to puncture the sac and push it away from the infant's head and mouth as they appear.
- As the infant's head is being born, determine if the umbilical cord is around the infant's neck; slip over the shoulder or clamp, cut and unwrap.
- After the infant's head is born, support the head; suction the mouth two or three times and the nostrils. Use caution to avoid contact with the back of the mouth.
- As the torso and full body are born, support the infant with both hands.
- As the feet are born, grasp the feet.
- Wipe blood and mucus from mouth and nose with sterile gauze, suction mouth and nose again.
- Wrap infant in a warm blanket and place on its side, head slightly lower than trunk.
- Keep infant level with vagina until the cord is cut.
- Assign partner to monitor infant and complete initial care of the newborn.
- Clamp, tie, and cut umbilical cord (between the clamps) as pulsations cease, approximately four fingers' width from infant.
- Observe for delivery of placenta while preparing mother and infant for transport.
- When delivered, wrap placenta in towel and put in plastic bag, transport placenta to hospital with mother.

Figure 27-2   Delivery. **A.** Anterior rotation of the head. **B.** Extension of the head. **C.** External rotation of the head. *(Reprinted with permission from DeCherney AH, Nathan L. Current Diagnosis & Treatment Obstetrics and Gynecology. 10th ed. New York: McGraw-Hill; 2007:208.)*

- Place sterile pad over vaginal opening, lower mother's legs, help her hold them together.
- Record time of delivery and transport mother, infant, and placenta to hospital.

APGAR SCORING

The APGAR score is a quick way to assess a newborn infant (see Table 27-1). It is composed of five separate components. Each of the parts is assigned a score from 0 to 2. The composite score is computed at 1 and 5 minutes. Scores of 7 or above are considered normal. Scores of 4 to 6 are intermediate. Lower scores suggest the baby was subject to birth stress.

TABLE 27-1: APGAR Scoring Chart

Signs	0	1	2	1 Min	5 Min
Heart rate	Absent	<100	>100		
Respiratory effort	Absent	Slow, irregular	Good, crying		
Muscle tone	Limp	Some flexion	Active motion		
Reflex irritability	No response	Grimace	Cough, sneeze, cry		
Color	Blue, pale	Body pink	Completely pink		
	Blue	extremities blue			
			Total Score:		

Vaginal bleeding following delivery—Up to 500 cc of blood loss is normal following delivery. A 500-cc blood loss is well tolerated by the mother following delivery. The EMT must be aware of this loss so as not to cause undue psychological stress on him/herself or the new mother.

With excessive blood loss, massage the uterus.

- Hand with fingers fully extended.
- Place on lower abdomen above pubis.
- Massage (knead) over area.
- Bleeding continues—Check massage technique and transport immediately, providing oxygen and ongoing assessment.

Regardless of estimated blood loss, if mother appears in shock (hypoperfusion), treat as such and transport prior to uterine massage. Massage en route.

INITIAL CARE OF THE NEWBORN

(Fig. 27-3 and 27-4)

Abnormal Deliveries

Prolapsed Cord

- Condition where the cord presents through the birth canal before delivery of the head; presents a serious emergency which endangers the life of the unborn fetus.

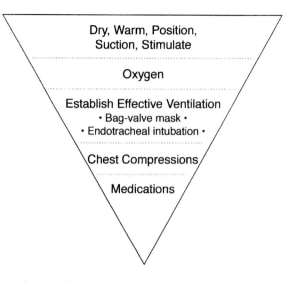

Figure 27-3   Inverted pyramid. *(From http://www.health. state.ny.us/nysdoh/ems/ppcctoc.htm.)*

- ○ Size-up.
- ○ Initial assessment.
- ○ Mother should have high-flow oxygen.
- ○ History and physical examination.
- ○ Assess baseline vitals.
- ○ Treatment based on signs and symptoms.
- ○ Position mother with head down or buttocks raised using gravity to lessen pressure in birth canal.
- ○ Insert sterile gloved hand into vagina pushing the presenting part of the fetus away from the pulsating cord.
- ○ Transport rapidly, keeping pressure on presenting part and monitoring pulsations in the cord.

Breech Birth Presentation

- Breech presentation occurs when the buttocks or lower extremities are low in the uterus and will be the first part of the fetus delivered.
- Newborn at great risk for delivery trauma, prolapsed cord more common, transport immediately upon recognition of breech presentation.
- Delivery does not occur within 10 minutes.
- Emergency medical care.
- Immediate rapid transportation upon recognition.
- Place mother on oxygen.
- Place mother in head down position with pelvis elevated.

Limb Presentation

- Occurs when a limb of the infant protrudes from the birth canal. Is more commonly a foot when infant is in breech presentation.
  - ○ Immediate rapid transportation upon recognition.
  - ○ Place mother on oxygen.
  - ○ Place mother in head down position with pelvis elevated.

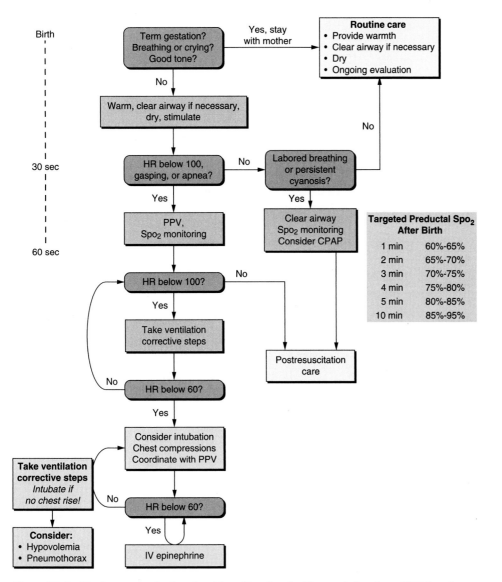

Figure 27-4 Newborn resuscitation algorithm. (Reprinted with permission from *2010 American Heart Association Guidelines for Cardiopulmonary Resuscitation and Emergency Cardiovascular Care. Part 15: Neonatal Resuscitation. Circulation.* 2010;122(suppl 3): S909-S919. © 2010 American Heart Association, Inc.

Multiple Births

- Be prepared for more than one resuscitation.
- Call for additional assistance.

Meconium

Amniotic fluid that is greenish or brownish-yellow rather than clear; an indication of possible fetal distress during labor.

- Do not stimulate before suctioning oropharynx.
- Suction.

- Maintain airway.
- Transport as soon as possible.

Premature Birth

- Always at risk for hypothermia
- Usually requires resuscitation, should be done unless physically impossible

? CHAPTER QUESTIONS

1. Which of the following conditions indicates a predelivery emergency for a pregnant patient?

   a. Swelling of the face and/or extremities

   b. A fever

   c. Flulike symptoms

   d. Nausea

2. Vaginal bleeding is discovered during your physical examination. You should:

   a. Place a sanitary napkin over the vaginal opening.

   b. Massage the uterus to control internal bleeding.

   c. Pack the vagina with sterile gauze or a dressing.

   d. Apply direct pressure to the vaginal area until bleeding is controlled.

3. Which of the following is true regarding trauma to a pregnant woman?

   a. Keep spine boards absolutely flat to facilitate blood flow to the fetus.

   b. Even minor trauma to the abdomen can cause serious fetal injuries.

   c. Early signs of shock are very obvious in pregnant women.

   d. If a pregnant woman dies as a result of an accident, CPR may save the life of the unborn infant.

4. Expect delivery of the infant within a few minutes if:

   a. The patient's "water breaks."

   b. The patient's abdomen gets very soft.

   c. The patient has the sensation of a bowel movement.

   d. Contractions are 5 minutes apart, and last 15 to 30 seconds.

5. Emergency care of the patient in active labor for a normal delivery includes:

   a. immediately clamping and cutting the umbilical cord if wrapped around the infant's neck

   b. suctioning the infant's nose first, as newborns are obligate nose-breathers

   c. exerting gentle pressure against the infant's skull to prevent explosive delivery

   d. having the patient lay on her left side during the delivery

6. As your patient delivers the infant, your emergency medical care should include:

    a. holding the infant upside down by the feet to help drain fluid

    b. cutting, then clamping, the umbilical cord

    c. massaging the uterus to decrease vaginal bleeding after delivery

    d. yanking on the umbilical cord after delivery to assist with placental expulsion

7. Which of the following is not a correct treatment for a cord presentation?

    a. Cover the cord with a saline-moist, sterile towel.

    b. With a sterile gloved hand, place the cord back into the vagina.

    c. Position the mother with her head down in the "knee-chest" position.

    d. Insert a sterile gloved hand into the vagina and push the presenting part of the fetus back and away from the cord.

8. Meconium staining is:

    a. the passing of a bowel movement by the infant in the amniotic fluid

    b. urine expelled by the infant during delivery

    c. a yellowish bubbly fluid caused by the infant's lungs being compressed during delivery

    d. blood that has leaked out of the umbilical cord during delivery

9. Additional care that you should provide to a premature infant includes:

    a. not suctioning the infant's mouth, as you may cause trauma

    b. placing a surgical mask on the infant's face to prevent contamination

    c. drying the infant thoroughly and wrapping in warm blankets, covering the head

    d. applying high-concentration oxygen by a pediatric nonrebreather mask

10. The signs of a severely depressed newborn include:

    a. poor or absent skeletal muscle tone

    b. an APGAR score of under 6

    c. a heart rate over 140 or under 100 beats per minute

    d. a respiratory rate under 60 beats per minute

11. An abnormally low placenta may tear or separate from the uterus, causing painless hemorrhaging. This condition is known as:

    a. ectopic pregnancy

    b. ruptured uterus

    c. placenta previa

    d. abruptio placenta

12. Eclampsia most frequently occurs during the last trimester and most often affects women in their 20s who are pregnant for the first time. Signs and symptoms of toxemia, or eclampsia, include:

    a. vaginal bleeding without pain

    b. increased urinary output

    c. seizures

    d. history of severe allergic reactions

13. An ectopic pregnancy means:

   a. The egg has implanted outside the uterus.

   b. A naturally aborted fetus due to any number of reasons.

   c. A pregnancy that continues past the expected due date.

   d. The fetus is developing in an abnormal position in the uterus.

14. The fetus, or unborn infant, develops in the:

   a. vagina

   b. placenta

   c. cervix

   d. uterus

15. The organ through which the fetus receives oxygen and nourishment from the mother is the:

   a. placenta

   b. umbilical cord

   c. amniotic sac

   d. uterus

16. The fluid-filled bag in which the infant floats is called the:

   a. placenta

   b. uterus

   c. amniotic sac

   d. vagina

17. During the first stage of labor, which of the following occurs?

   a. The placenta separates from the uterine wall.

   b. The cervix becomes fully dilated.

   c. The infant's head appears at the opening of the birth canal.

   d. All of the above.

18. Indications that delivery is imminent include:

   a. the onset of contractions

   b. bulging of the perineum

   c. the "bloody show"

   d. the breaking of the amniotic sac

19. During the third stage of labor:

   a. The infant is actually delivered.

   b. The amniotic sac ruptures.

   c. The placenta is expelled from the uterus.

   d. The head of the infant appears at the opening of the birth canal.

20. Questions that should be asked regarding due date include:

   a. How many previous pregnancies are there?

   b. How many children does the patient have?

   c. Has the patient had any prenatal care?

   d. All of the above.

CROSSWORD

Across

1. The medical term used for listening to lung sounds.
4. _____ medical history.
5. To check for a pulse on an unconscious adult patient, the EMT should palpate the _____ pulse.
8. During evaluation of a patient who is exhibiting signs of a stroke, the EMT should use the Cincinnati Prehospital Stroke Scale. Using this scale includes evaluating _____ droop, arm lift, and speech.
11. Another name for a cerebral vascular accident.
12. The medical term "renal calculus" is known as a kidney _____.
13. The "L" in SAMPLE stands for _____ meal or oral intake.
14. The medication used most frequently in an EMS system.
15. The heart has four _____ that prevent blood from flowing back into a specific chamber.

Down

2. Situations in which a drug should not be used because it may harm the patient.
3. A medication that is given to patients who are experiencing signs/symptoms of a myocardial infarction.
5. The mnemonic used to describe various respiratory distress syndromes.
6. How much of a drug should be administered.
7. An abnormal curvature of the spine.
9. The mnemonic used for the defibrillator.
10. The medication diabetic patients administer to themselves to lower blood sugar.

Section 5

Trauma

Chapter 28
Mechanism of Injury, Kinematics of Trauma

Your volunteer ambulance company is toned out for a forthwith pedestrian auto accident with the patient still pinned under the motor vehicle. The first responder arrives on-scene and confirms the incident. She states the patient is an 8-year-old girl pinned under a sport-utility vehicle (SUV), she is alert to voice, and she is complaining of severe abdominal pain. You arrive moments after that report; the fire department is operating on-scene removing the patient from under the vehicle with airbags to lift the vehicle off the patient. You approach the scene, determine scene safety, and establish there is one patient, and the firefighters are removing the victim as you arrive at the vehicle's side.

Your initial assessment reveals an 8-year-old girl with multiple grotesque deformities to both upper and lower extremities, no obvious life-threatening hemorrhaging, and obvious abrasion to the right upper quadrant of her abdomen.

Does this patient have a significant mechanism of injury (MOI)?

Figure 28-1 shows the interior of a vehicle following a high-speed lateral impact motor vehicle collision. Notice the seat and steering column displacement. This car struck a tree on the driver's side at a high rate of speed. What type of injuries would you expect to see with this type of mechanism of injury (MOI)?

KINEMATICS OF TRAUMA

- Trauma is the leading cause of death and disability in the United States among children and young adults (ages 1-44).
- Trauma is the third leading cause of death in all age groups.
- Annually, one in four Americans is injured severely enough to seek medical attention. An estimated 23 to 28 million people are treated in the ED annually for injury, of which 90% are not admitted to the hospital.
- Traumatic injury occurs to the body when the body tissues are exposed to energy levels beyond their tolerance. Work is defined as force acting over a distance. Forces that bend, pull, or compress tissues beyond their inherent limits result in the work that causes injury.

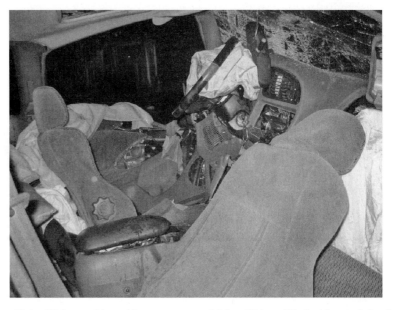

Figure 28-1 High-speed lateral impact motor vehicle collision. *(Used with permission from Peter DiPrima.)*

- Kinetic energy (KE) is the energy of a moving object (motion).
  - The formula for determining kinetic energy is:

$$KE = \frac{\text{mass (weight)} \times \text{velocity (speed)}^2}{2}$$

- In the case of a motor vehicle crash, the kinetic energy of the speeding car is converted into the work of stopping the car (crushing the car). Similarly, the passengers have kinetic energy, and this is converted to the work of stopping them (injury).
- The energy that is available to cause injury doubles when an object's weight doubles, but quadruples when its speed doubles.
- Velocity has a greater influence than mass.
- Increasing a car's speed from 50 mph to 70 mph doubles the energy that is available to cause injury.
- Potential energy—The product of mass (weight), force of gravity, and height.
- A child in a tree has potential energy. When the child falls, the potential energy is converted into kinetic energy. As the child hits the ground, the kinetic energy is converted into work, that is, the work of bringing the child's body to a stop and thereby damaging tissues, bones, and so on.

BLUNT TRAUMA: "LEADING CAUSE OF TRAUMATIC DEATH IN THE UNITED STATES"

- Motor vehicle crashes (MVC)—One of the most common sources of blunt trauma.
  - Each MVC typically consists of three collisions:

Figure 28-2   Significant mechanism of injury; car versus tree. *(Used with permission from Peter DiPrima.)*

— First—Vehicle against a hard object—MOI

— Second—Passenger against the interior of the car

— Third—Passenger's internal organs against the solid structures of the body

With new automotive technology (ie, air bags, energy-absorbing structural components, restraint systems), the severity of injuries to passengers in a motor vehicle collision is reduced. Air bags, which were introduced in the automotive community in the 80s and 90s, deploy very aggressively at speeds of 140 to 200 mph. This rapid deployment increased the potential of significant injury to unrestrained passengers, as well as children under 12 years old.

It is important to understand the effects of seating position, restraint type, restraint use, and vehicle type in assessing an patient from an MVC.

• Types of crashes (Figs. 28-2 through 28-7):

  ○ Frontal collisions—Is there intrusion into patient compartment? Were restraints used? Did the air bag deploy?

Figure 28-3   High-speed motor vehicle collision. *(Used with permission from Peter DiPrima.)*

Figure 28-4 A. Van versus tree. **B.** Photo of inside the van. Notice the seat displacement and steering column displacement. (*Used with permission from Peter DiPrima.*)

- ○ Rear-end collisions—High potential for whiplash injuries. Were restraints used?
- ○ Lateral collisions—T-bone, were restraints used? Twenty-five percent of severe aortic injuries result from lateral MVCs.
- ○ Rollover collisions—Ejection or partial ejection. Were restraints used?
- ○ Rotational impacts.

PENETRATING TRAUMA

- Second largest cause of traumatic death in United States.
- Low-velocity penetrating injuries, that is, knives, ice picks, and the like. Injury closely follows path of penetrating object.

Figure 28-5 Lateral impact motor vehicle collision with a rollover. *(Used with permission from Peter DiPrima.)*

- Medium-velocity and high-velocity penetrating injuries—Bullet, pressure waves emanating from path of bullet can cause remote damage (cavitation). If the mass of a bullet is doubled, the energy that can cause injury is doubled. If the velocity (speed) of the bullet is doubled, the energy that can cause damage is quadrupled.

FALLS

- Considered to be the most common cause of trauma.
- The severity of an injury from a fall is directly related to the height of the fall and the surface the patient lands on.
- A fall from more than 12 to 15 ft, or three times the victim's height, is considered to be a significant mechanism of injury.

Figure 28-6 Lateral impact car versus tree. *(Used with permission from Peter DiPrima.)*

Figure 28-7   High-speed rollover motor vehicle collision with passenger ejection. *(Used with permission from Captain Richard Mancuso, Station 2, Lakeland FD.)*

- Always consider internal injuries in a patient who has fallen from a significant height.
- Factors involving mechanism of injury from a fall include:
  - Height of the fall
  - Type of surface struck
  - The part of body that hit first
- Always consider syncope or other underlying medical causes of the fall.

BLAST INJURIES

- Three mechanisms of injury involving a blast injury:
  - Primary phase—Injuries occur from the pressure wave of the blast. (Injuries are seen to gas-containing or hollow organs.)

- Secondary phase—Injuries occur by flying debris.
- Tertiary phase—Injuries occur when the victim is thrown against an object.

TRAUMA PATIENT ASSESSMENT

- Three key decision points in trauma assessment process:
  - MOI determination
  - General impression of the patient
  - Priority determination—At end of initial assessment, is this a load-and-go situation?

Distinction Between Rapid Trauma Examination and Focused Assessment

- Rapid trauma examination is quick and covers key areas of body with patients that have a significant MOI.
- Focused examination on patients without a significant MOI focuses only on an injured area.

Distinction Between Rapid Trauma Examination and the Detailed Examination

- Rapid examination is quick and looks for "major" life-threatening injuries.
- Detailed examination is slower, more complete, and checks the "nooks and crannies." It is performed en route to hospital in most cases.

General Idea

- Care for serious patients occurs at hospitals/operating rooms
- Trauma care for serious patients is a balance of care for life-threatening injuries and transport.
- Early identification of serious patients is the key!

MOI determination is as important in initial assessment decisions as actual patient care.

? CHAPTER QUESTIONS

1. The type of crash predicts the injury pattern associated with vehicular trauma.

   a. True

   b. False

2. MVCs cause three points of impact that produce injury. They include collision with the object, body impact with the vehicle, and:

   a. organ impact on the body

   b. side impact crashes

   c. both a and b

   d. none of the above

Chapter 29
Bleeding and Shock

Your unit is dispatched to University Avenue and West 190th Street for a victim of a stabbing. Upon arriving at the scene, you notice police frantically waving you down in front of the local bodega.

The scene is safe to operate. As you survey the scene, you notice a very large pool of blood surrounding what appears to be a female patient. The patient is found lying prone in front of the location, unconscious and unresponsive. As you log roll the patient using c-spine precautions, your partner notices a very large knife impaled in the patients sternum. You estimate blood loss to be significant and the patient is pale, cool, and diaphoretic. The patient has agonal breathing, and rescue breathing is started by another responder on-scene. Your partner tells you she cannot palpate a radial or femoral pulse, but she has a weak and thready carotipulse.

With this assessment, what type of shock is this patient presenting?

PATHOPHYSIOLOGY OF SHOCK

- Shock is defined as "inadequate tissue perfusion."
- Shock can result from trauma, fluid loss, heart attack, infection, spinal cord injury, and the like.
- Occurs first at the cellular level, and if allowed, can progress to organ failure and death.

PHYSIOLOGY OF PERFUSION

- Cells of the body require a constant supply of oxygen and nutrients (glucose) along with the elimination of carbon dioxide and waste products.
- The needs of the cells are fulfilled by the circulatory system in conjunction with our respiratory and gastrointestinal systems.
- Perfusion is dependent on three components of the circulatory system:
  - Pump (heart) (rate)
  - Fluid volume (blood)
  - Container (blood vessels)

Any derangement of any of these components can affect perfusion.

- The following organs require the most oxygen, and in the pecking order during decreased perfusion receive oxygenated blood over other organs and tissues:
  - The heart (circulatory system)
  - The brain (nervous system)

- ○ The lungs (respiratory system)
- ○ The kidneys

THE PUMP "HEART"

- The pump of the circulatory system receives blood from venous system.
- Pumps blood to the lungs to receive oxygen.
- Pumps blood to the peripheral tissues.

Stroke Volume

The amount of blood pumped by the heart in one contraction. Stroke volume is effected by preload, contractile force, and afterload.

Preload

- The amount of blood delivered to the heart during diastole.
- It is dependent on venous return.
- Variable venous capacitance can increase or reduce blood return to the heart.
- Increased preload = increased stroke volume.

Contractile Force

The force generated by the heart during each contraction.

Frank-Starling Mechanism

- The greater the preload, the more the ventricles are stretched.
- The greater the stretch, the greater the contractile force.

Afterload

- Resistance against which the heart must pump
- When resistance is overcome, blood can be ejected
- Determined by the degree of arterial peripheral vasoconstriction
- Vasoconstriction = increased resistance = increased afterload = decreased stroke volume

Cardiac Output

- Amount of blood pumped by the heart in 1 minute or stroke volume × heart rate = cardiac output
- Expressed in liters per minute
- An increase in stroke volume or heart rate = increased cardiac output
- A decrease in stroke volume or heart rate = decreased cardiac output

$$\text{Cardiac Output} = (\text{Stroke Volume}) \times (\text{Heart Rate})$$

Blood Pressure

Defined as cardiac output × peripheral vascular resistance (afterload)

- Increased afterload = increased blood pressure
- Decreased afterload = decreased blood pressure

Baroreceptors

- Sensory fibers located in the aortic and carotid bodies.
- They monitor changes in blood pressure.
- If blood pressure increases, baroreceptors tell the brain to decrease heart rate, preload, and afterload.
- If blood pressure falls, baroreceptors signal the brain to activate the sympathetic nervous system to increase heart rate, preload, contractile force, afterload, and cardiac output.

THE FLUID "BLOOD"

- Blood is the fluid of the cardiovascular system.
- Blood is more viscous, thicker, and more adhesive than water.
- Because the cardiovascular system is closed, an adequate volume of blood must be present to fill system.
- Blood transports oxygen, carbon dioxide, nutrients, hormones, metabolic waste products, and heat.

THE CONTAINER "BLOOD VESSELS"

- The blood vessels serve as the container of the cardiovascular system.
- They are a continuous, closed, pressurized pipeline that moves blood throughout the cardiovascular system.
- The blood vessels of the body include arteries, arterioles, capillaries, venules, and veins.
- Under the control of the autonomic nervous system, they regulate blood flow to different areas of the body by adjusting their size and rerouting blood flow through microcirculation.

Microcirculation

- Responsive to local tissue needs.
- Capillary beds can adjust size to supply undernourished tissue and bypass tissue with no immediate need.
- Precapillary sphincters and postcapillary sphincters open and close to feed or bypass tissues.

Blood Flow

- Occurs because of peripheral resistance and pressure within the system.
- Peripheral resistance is dependent on inner diameter and length of the vessel, and blood viscosity.
- Very little resistance in the aorta and arteries.
- Significant changes are seen in arterioles, which can change size fivefold.

System Pressures

- Contraction of the venous side increases preload and stroke volume.
- Contraction of the arteriole side increases afterload and blood pressure.

Oxygen Transport

- In addition to perfusion, oxygenation of peripheral tissues is essential.
- Oxygen diffuses across the alveolar-capillary membrane.

- Oxygen binds to the hemoglobin molecule of the red blood cells.
- Ideally, 97% to 100% of hemoglobin is saturated with oxygen.

Fick Principle

- Conditions for effective movement and utilization of oxygen in the body
- Adequate FiO_2 (concentration of O_2 in inspired air)
- Appropriate oxygen diffusion from alveoli into bloodstream
- Adequate number of red blood cells
- Proper tissue perfusion
- Efficient off-loading at the tissue level

Tissue Perfusion

- Tissue perfusion is dependent on the circulatory system and oxygenation by the respiratory system.
- Inadequate tissue perfusion can be caused by:
  - Inadequate pumping
  - Inadequate preload
  - Inadequate cardiac contractile strength
- Excessive afterload:
  - Inadequate heart rate
  - Inadequate fluid volume
  - Hypovolemia
  - Inadequate container
  - Excessive dilation without change in fluid volume
  - Excessive systemic vascular resistance

PHYSIOLOGICAL RESPONSE TO SHOCK

- Normally the body can compensate for decreased tissue perfusion through a variety of mechanisms.
- When composition fails, shock develops, and if uncorrected becomes irreversible.
- Systemic response occurs:
  - Progressive vasoconstriction
  - Increased blood flow to major organs
  - Shunted from skin, GI, and the like
  - Increased cardiac output
  - Increased respiratory rate and volume
  - Decreased urine output
  - Decreased gastric activity

SHOCK AT THE CELLULAR LEVEL

Metabolism in Normal Conditions (Aerobic)

- Cell energy comes from glucose broken down through glycolysis into pyruvic acid.
- Pyruvic acid is further broken down in the Krebs cycle into CO_2, water, and energy.

Metabolism Poor Perfusion States (Anaerobic)

- Glucose breaks down into pyruvic acid, but not enough oxygen is present to enter into the Krebs cycle.
- Pyruvic acid accumulates, degrades into lactic acid, which also accumulates along with other metabolic acids.
- Cells die; tissues die; organs fail; organ systems fail; death ultimately ensues.
- Not enough O_2 in the cell for aerobic metabolism.
- Shifts to anaerobic metabolism using glycogen and fat (until stores depleted).
- Increased cell permeability.
- Na^+ and H_2O enter cell causing cellular swelling.
- K^+ leaks out of cell.
- Then Ca^{2+} enters cell.
- Buildup of lactic acid and CO_2 in cell.
- Cell eventually ruptures.

STAGES OF SHOCK

Compensated Shock

The body's defense mechanism in an attempt to preserve major organs.

- Precapillary sphincters close, blood is shunted to the core organs.
- Increased heart rate and strength of contractions.
- Increased respiratory function, bronchodilation.
- Will continue until problem is solved or shock progresses to next stage.
- Can be difficult to detect with subtle indicators.
- Tachycardia.
- Decreased skin perfusion.
- Alterations in mental status.
- Some medications such as propranolol can hide signs and symptoms (beta-blockers).

Decompensated Shock

- Precapillary sphincters open, blood pressure falls.
- *Cardiac output falls.*
- Blood surges into tissue beds, blood flow stagnates.
- Red cells stack up in rouleaux.
- Easier to detect than compensated shock.
- Prolonged capillary refill time.
- Marked increase in heart rate.
- Rapid, thready pulse.
- Agitation, restlessness, confusion.
- *Decreased BP.*

Irreversible Shock

- Compensatory mechanisms fail, cell death begins, vital organs falter.
- Cannot be differentiated in the field.

- Patient may be resuscitated but will die later (ARDS, renal and liver failure, sepsis).
- Organs have been deprived of O_2 for too long and cells have died causing organ failure.
- Brain, lungs, heart, kidneys.
- Development of DIC (disseminating intravascular coagulopathy).

Disseminating Intravascular Coagulopathy (DIC)

- Presence of injured or lysed cells results in the release of phospholipids into the blood, triggering the intrinsic pathway.
- Prolonged states of low CO result in injury to the vascular endothelium, which also triggers the intrinsic pathway.
- Systemic coagulation.
- Diffuse fibrin formation.
- Clotting factors are exhausted.
- Activation of coagulation causes activation of fibrinolytic system.

TYPES OF SHOCK

Hypovolemic Shock

- Shock due to loss of intravascular fluid volume.

Possible Causes

- Internal or external hemorrhage
- Traumatic hemorrhage
- Long bone or open fractures
- Severe dehydration from GI losses
- Plasma losses from burns
- Diabetic ketoacidosis
- Excessive sweating
- Can result from internal third-space loss, possible causes include:
  - Bowel obstruction
  - Peritonitis
  - Pancreatitis
  - Liver failure resulting in ascites

Internal Bleeding

- Hematemesis—Blood in vomit
- Melena—Black, tarry stool
- Hemoptysis—Coughing up blood
- Pain, tenderness, bruising, or swelling
- Broken ribs, bruises over the chest, distended abdomen

Characteristics of Bleeding

- Arterial—Blood is bright red and spurts.
- Venous—Blood is dark red and does not spurt.
- Capillary—Blood oozes out and is controlled easily.

External Bleeding

- Hemorrhage = bleeding.
- Body cannot tolerate greater than 20% blood loss.
- The average adult male has approximately 6 L of blood.
- Blood loss of 1 L can be dangerous in adults; in pediatrics, loss of 100 to 200 mL is serious.
- Hypovolemic shock is a volume problem.

What signs and symptoms would you expect to see and how would you treat the patient in the opening scenario in this chapter?

Controlling External Bleeding

DIRECT PRESSURE AND ELEVATION

- Direct pressure is the most common and effective way to control bleeding.
- Elevation controls bleeding.
- Wrap a pressure dressing around the wound once bleeding is controlled.
- If bleeding continues, apply additional dressings on top.

Pressure points

- If bleeding continues, apply pressure on pressure point.
- Pressure at *proximal* pulse point greatly slows down circulation to extremity.
- The brachial artery and femoral artery are the two most common pressure points used.

Applying a tourniquet

- Fold a triangular bandage into four in cravat.
- Wrap the bandage.
- Use a stick as a handle to twist and secure.
- Write "TK" on the patient's forehead, time it was placed, and what location on the body.

> **Clinical Significance**
>
> Stages of hypovolemia:
> Stage-1: 10%-15% blood loss
> Stage-2: 15%-30% blood loss
> Stage-3: 30%-45% blood loss
> Stage-4: >45% blood loss

Cardiogenic Shock

- Inability to pump enough blood to supply all body parts.
- Primary cause is severe left ventricular failure (AMI, CHF).
- Accompanying hypotension decreases coronary artery perfusion, worsening the situation.
- Other compensatory mechanisms—Increased peripheral resistance, increased myocardial O_2 demand (both worsen the situation).

Other Causes

- Chronic progressive heart disease.
- Rupture of papillary heart muscles or intraventricular septum.
- End-stage valvular disease.
- Patients may be normovolemic or hypovolemic.
- Usually have pulmonary edema.
- Pump failure (cardiogenic shock).
- Inadequate function of the heart.

- The heart muscle can no longer generate enough pressure to circulate blood to all organs.
- Causes a backup of blood into the lungs.
- Results in pulmonary edema.

A major difference between cardiogenic shock and other types of shock is the presence of pulmonary edema and dyspnea. Cardiogenic shock is a pump failure problem!

- What signs and symptoms would you expect to see?
- How would you manage a patient exhibiting signs and symptoms of cardiogenic shock?

Neurogenic Shock

- Shock resulting from inadequate peripheral resistance due to widespread vasodilatation (hypotension associated with c-spine or a high thoracic spinal cord injury).

Common Causes

- Spinal cord injury
- Central nervous system injuries

Neurogenic shock is a loss of vasomotor tone below the injury.

- What signs and symptoms would you expect to see?
  - Skin warm and dry below injury
  - Loss of sympathetic tone to the heart (bradycardia)

How would you treat a neurogenic shock patient?

Septic Shock

- Shock resulting from systemic vasodilatation.
- Systemic increased vascular permeability.
- Usually a result of gram (–) bacterial infection.
- Development of bacteremia septic shock.
- Vessel and content failure.
- Caused by severe bacterial infections, *toxins,* or infected tissues.
- Toxins damage vessel walls, causing them to *leak* and become unable to contract well.
- Leads to *dilation* of vessels and loss of plasma, causing shock.

How do you want to treat a septic shock patient?

Anaphylactic Shock

Anaphylactic shock is defined as a widespread hypersensitivity reaction to a specific antigen resulting in vasodilatation, peripheral pooling, relative hypovolemia leading to decreased perfusion, and impaired cellular metabolism.

- Provokes an extensive immune and inflammatory response
- Vasodilation
- Increased permeability
- Peripheral pooling
- Tissue edema
- Sudden onset and death can occur in minutes
- Anxiety

- Difficulty breathing
- GI cramps
- Edema
- Urticaria
- Pruritis
- Allergic reactions
- Vasodilation = produces drop in *BP*
- Bronchoconstriction = dyspnea

How would you treat a patient in anaphylactic shock?

- Psychogenic shock is caused by a sudden reaction of the nervous system that produces a temporary, generalized, vascular dilation.
- Commonly referred to as fainting or syncope.
- Causes range from fear or bad news to unpleasant sights.

EVALUATION OF THE SHOCK PATIENT

- Initial approach, approach with caution.
- What is the patient's mental status?
- Respiratory effort?
- Skin color?

Initial Assessment

- Check for airway patency; correct problems as needed.
- Assess breathing rate, quality; correct any life-threatening problems by administering high-concentration oxygen.
- Correct any obvious external bleeding.
- Location of palpable pulse as indicator of circulatory status.
  - Radial pulse—BP at least 80 mm Hg
  - Femoral pulse—BP at least 70 mm Hg
  - Carotid pulse—BP at least 60 mm Hg
- Assess skin color, temperature, and moisture.
  - Pale = decreased diffusion
  - Cyanotic = inadequate oxygenation
  - Mottled = late sign of shock
  - Cool = indicates vasoconstriction
- Assess capillary refill time in pediatric patients (less than 2 seconds is a normal finding).
- Level of consciousness is very early sign of impending circulatory collapse.
- Manifestations of reduction in cerebral flow include:
  - Agitation
  - Disorientation
  - Confusion
  - Inappropriateness of response
  - Unresponsiveness
- While altered mental status may result from drug/alcohol intake, assume the cause is decreased cerebral perfusion.

Secondary Assessment

- Rapid transport for life-threatening conditions
- Ideally, expose the head, neck, chest, and abdomen
- Reassess vital signs
- Gather a patient history when appropriate

GENERAL SHOCK MANAGEMENT

- *Ensure patent airway.*
- Maintain cervical spine support.
- Maintain airflow through the use of airway adjuncts or intubation, preferred in unresponsive shock patients.
- Provide suctioning as necessary.
- *Maintain adequate respiratory function.*
- Assist ventilations with BVM or other appropriate adjunct.
- Perform other interventions as needed to correct shock-related conditions leading to respiratory compromise.
- *Control major bleeding and treat hypotension.*
- Positioning of patient (supine with legs elevated 10-12 in).
- Upright if cardiogenic shock with pulmonary edema (check respirations and assist as needed).

? CHAPTER QUESTIONS

1. Which of the following forms of shock is most commonly seen in the trauma patient?

   a. hypovolemic shock
   b. cardiogenic shock
   c. septic shock
   d. none of the above

2. A patient has lost 15% to 30% of their total blood volume, what class of shock would they be in?

   a. Class I
   b. Class II
   c. Class III
   d. Class IV

3. What is the most common cause of cardiogenic shock?

   a. dysrhythmias
   b. myocardial infarction
   c. chest trauma
   d. congenital valve disorders

Reference

US Department of Transportation, National Highway Traffic Safety Administration. *EMT-Basic National Standard Curriculum.* Washington, DC: US Department of Transportation, National Highway Traffic Safety Administration; 1994.

Chapter 30
Soft Tissue Injuries

Upon arrival at the scene, you find a huge crowd standing around a patient who is lying on the floor. As you approach, a police officer tells you that witnesses state that the patient was at the bar about 1 hour ago and had a couple of drinks before a woman, who said she was his ex-girlfriend, walked into the bar and shot him. He is now supine on the street corner with an obvious gunshot wound to the chest. His mental status is alert, and he is sweating profusely.

What is your first step in assessing this patient?

FUNCTION OF THE SKIN

- Skin protects the body.
- Skin is watertight and not penetrable by bacteria.
- Skin regulates body temperature. Water evaporates from the skin surface in hot weather, and surface blood vessels constrict in cold weather.

LAYERS OF THE SKIN

(Fig. 30-1)

- Epidermis—Outermost layer consists of dead cells constantly being rubbed off and replaced.
  - Deeper part of the epidermis contains cells which contain some pigment granules.
- Dermis—Contains many special structures of the skin:
  - Sweat glands
  - Sebaceous glands
  - Hair follicles
  - Blood vessels
  - Specialized nerve endings
- Subcutaneous tissue—Beneath the skin is a layer composed largely of fat that serves as a body insulator.

TYPES OF SOFT TISSUE INJURIES (STI)

Closed Soft Tissue Injuries

Contusion (Bruise)

- Epidermis remains intact.
- Cells are damaged and blood vessels torn in the dermis.

Figure 30-1 Layers of the skin. *(Reprinted with permission from Bruncardi FC, Andersen DK, Billiar TR, et al. (eds). Schwartz's Principles of Surgery. 8th ed. New York: McGraw-Hill; 2005:430.)*

- Swelling and pain are typically present.
- Blood accumulation causes discoloration.

Hematoma

- Collection of blood beneath the skin.
- Larger amount of tissue damage as compared to contusion.
- Larger vessels are damaged.
- May lose one or more liters of blood.

Crush Injuries

- Crushing force applied to the body
- Can cause internal organ rupture
- Internal bleeding may be severe with shock (hypoperfusion)

Emergency Management

- Body substance isolation
- Proper airway/artificial ventilation/oxygenation
- If shock (hypoperfusion) or internal bleeding is suspected
  - Treat for shock (hypoperfusion)
  - Splint a painful, swollen, deformed extremity
  - Transport
  - Complete the pre-hospital care report. Document all pertinent findings of the patient assessment, treatment, and transport decisions.

Open Soft Tissue Injuries

Abrasion

- Outermost layer of skin is damaged by shearing forces.
- Painful injury, even though superficial.
- Very little or no oozing of blood.

Laceration

- Break in skin of varying depth.
- May be linear (regular) or stellate (irregular) and occur in isolation or together with other types of soft tissue injury.
- Caused by forceful impact with sharp object.
- Bleeding may be severe.

Avulsion

Flaps of skin or tissue are torn loose or pulled completely off.

Penetration/Puncture

- Caused by sharp pointed object.
- May be no external bleeding.
- Internal bleeding may be severe.
- Exit wound may be present.
- Examples:
  - Gunshot wound
  - Stab wound

Amputations

- Involves the extremities and other body parts.
- Massive bleeding may be present or bleeding may be limited.

Crush Injuries

- Damage to soft tissue and internal organs.
- May cause painful, swollen, deformed extremities.
- External bleeding may be minimal or absent.
- Internal bleeding may be severe.

Emergency Management

- Body substance isolation.
- Maintain proper airway/artificial ventilation/oxygenation.
- Management of open soft tissue injuries.
- Expose the wound.
- Control the bleeding.
- Prevent further contamination.
- Apply dry sterile dressing to the wound and bandage securely in place.
- Keep the patient calm and quiet.
- Treat for shock (hypoperfusion), if signs and symptoms are present.

Special Considerations

- *Chest injuries*—Occlusive dressing to open wound
  - Administer high-concentration oxygen.
  - Position of comfort if no spinal injury suspected.
- *Abdominal injuries*—Evisceration (organs protruding through the wound)
  - Do not touch or try to replace the exposed organ.
  - Cover exposed organs and wound with a sterile dressing, moistened with sterile water or saline, and secure in place.
  - Flex the patient's hips and knees, if uninjured.
- *Impaled objects*—Do not remove the impaled object, unless it is through the cheek and obstructing the airway, if it would interfere with chest compressions, or if interferes with transport.
  - Manually secure the object.
  - Expose the wound area.
  - Control bleeding.
  - Utilize a bulky dressing to help stabilize the object.
- *Amputations*—Concerns for reattachment
  - Wrap the amputated part in a sterile dressing.
  - Wrap or bag the amputated part in plastic and keep cool.
  - Transport the amputated part with the patient.
  - Do not complete partial amputations.
  - Immobilize to prevent further injury.
- *Open neck injury*
  - May cause air embolism.
  - Cover with an occlusive dressing.

? CHAPTER QUESTIONS

1. A wound under the skin that involves a blood vessel, characterized by a large lump with bluish discoloration is called a:

   a. crush injury

   b. concussion

   c. hematoma

   d. contusion

2. When performing the initial assessment and focused history and physical examination on a trauma patient, which of the following should be kept in mind?

   a. Severe bleeding should be treated as soon as your initial assessment is completed.

   b. BSI (body substance isolation) precautions should be taken if there is any external bleeding.

   c. DCAP-BTLS (*d*eformities, *c*ontusions, *a*brasions, *p*unctures/*p*enetrations, *b*urns, *t*enderness, *l*acerations, *s*welling, *c*repitation) during your rapid trauma assessment.

   d. SAMPLE (*s*igns/*s*ymptoms, *a*llergies, *m*edications, *p*ast medical problems, *l*ast oral intake, *e*vents) history should be obtained prior to your physical examination.

3. When providing emergency medical care for a closed soft tissue injury, remember that:

a. large contusions, hematomas, and crush injuries usually heal themselves without treatment

b. modern protective gloves have made hand washing unnecessary

c. splinting painful, swollen, deformed extremities reduces the patient's pain

d. high-concentration oxygen is usually not appropriate for soft tissue injuries

4. All the types of open wounds have one thing in common. That is:

a. They all involve underlying soft tissue that is torn loose or pulled completely off.

b. The patient is at risk for contamination with dirt, bacteria, and infection.

c. They are all more serious internally than they appear externally.

d. The wounds are all linear.

5. Scraping, rubbing, or shearing away of the outermost layer of the skin is called a/an:

a. contusion

b. laceration

c. abrasion

d. avulsion

6. Which of the following statements is true regarding punctures and penetrations?

a. Powder burns around a gunshot wound are indicative of a small-caliber bullet.

b. They are often more serious internally than they appear externally.

c. The entrance wound of a gunshot is larger than the exit wound when shot at close range.

d. Stab wounds are always easily detected due to the external bleeding.

7. When caring for a patient with a large, open neck injury, remember:

a. Dark, oozing blood indicates the carotid artery has been damaged.

b. To apply a pressure dressing circumferentially around the neck to control bleeding.

c. To cover the wound with an occlusive dressing, taped on three sides.

d. To immediately place a gloved hand over the wound to prevent air embolism.

Reference

US Department of Transportation, National Highway Traffic Safety Administration. *EMT-Basic National Standard Curriculum*. Washington, DC: US Department of Transportation, National Highway Traffic Safety Administration; 1994.

Chapter 31
Burn Emergencies

Upon arriving at the scene, police officers meet you at the street and tell you that a group of children threw gasoline on a homeless man and then lit him on fire. The fire department is on-scene and tells you that the patient put the fire out himself prior to their arrival. The scene is determined to be safe.

Upon initiating the initial assessment, you determine the patient has an open airway, but the patient is coughing up carbonaceous sputum. He states he feels like his throat is closing and you notice singed nose and facial hair. He is dyspneic, and has partial-thickness burns to the anterior portion of his chest.

How should you begin to treat this patient?

BURN CLASSIFICATION

Classification is according to depth of burn injury (Fig. 31-1).

- Partial thickness (second degree) involves both the epidermis and the dermis, but does not involve underlying tissue.
- Superficial (first degree) involves only the epidermis.
- Reddened skin
  - Intense pain
- Pain at the site
  - White to red skin that is moist and mottled
  - Blisters
- Full thickness (third degree)—Burn extends through all the dermal layers and may involve subcutaneous layers, muscle, bone, or organs.
  - Skin becomes dry and leathery and may appear white, dark brown, or charred.
  - Loss of sensation—Little or no pain, hard to the touch, pain at periphery.

DETERMINING THE SEVERITY OF A BURN

Rule of Nines

- Adult (Fig. 31-2A)
  - Head and neck—9%
  - Each upper extremity—9%
  - Anterior trunk—18%
  - Posterior trunk—18%

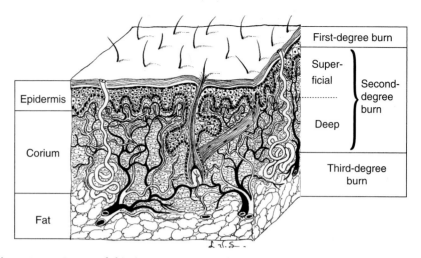

Figure 31-1   Layers of skin in comparison to thickness of burn. (*Reprinted with permission from Doherty GM, Way LW. Current Surgical Diagnosis and Treatment. 12th ed. McGraw-Hill;246.*)

- ○ Each lower extremity—18%
- ○ Genitalia—1%
- • Pediatric (Fig. 31-2B)
  - ○ Head and neck—18%
  - ○ Each upper extremity—9%
  - ○ Anterior trunk—18%
  - ○ Posterior trunk—18%
  - ○ Each lower extremity—13.5%
  - ○ Genitalia—1%

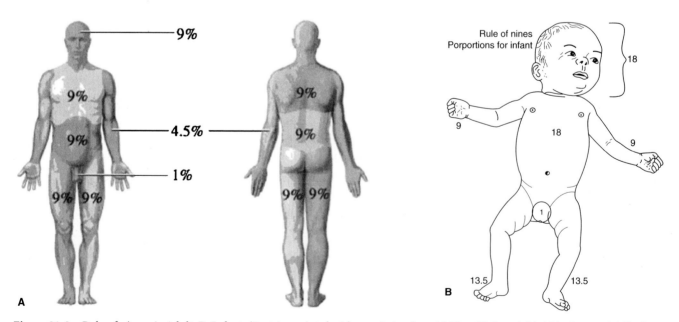

Figure 31-2   Rule of nines. **A.** Adult. **B.** Infant. (*Part A reprinted with permission from McPhee SJ, Papadakis MA. Current Medical Diagnosis & Treatment. 46th ed. New York: McGraw-Hill; 2007: 1627. Part B from http://www.health.state.ny.us/nysdoh/ems/ppcctoc.htm.*)

FACTORS INCLUDED DURING EVALUATION OF A BURN PATIENT

- Location of the burn
  - Face and upper airway
  - Hands
  - Feet
  - Genitalia
- Preexisting medical conditions
- Age of the patient
  - Less than 5 years of age
  - Greater than 55 years of age

Severity

- Critical burns
  - Full-thickness burns involving the hands, feet, face, or genitalia
  - Burns associated with respiratory injury
  - Full-thickness burns covering more than 10% of the body surface
  - Partial-thickness burns covering more than 30% of the body surface area (BSA)
  - Burns complicated by painful, swollen, deformed extremity
  - Moderate burns in young children or elderly patients
  - Burns encompassing any body part
- Moderate burns
  - Full-thickness burns of 2% to 10% of the BSA excluding hands, feet, face, genitalia, and upper airway
  - Partial-thickness burns of 15% to 30% of the BSA
  - Superficial burns of greater than 50% BSA
- Minor burns
  - Full-thickness burns of less than 2% of the BSA
  - Partial-thickness burns of less than 15% of the BSA

EMERGENCY MANAGEMENT

- Stop the burning process, initially with water or saline.
- Remove smoldering clothing and jewelry.
- Body substance isolation.
- Continually monitor the airway for evidence of closure.
- Prevent further contamination.
- Cover the burned area with a dry sterile dressing.
- Do not use any type of ointment, lotion, or antiseptic.
- Do not break blisters.

- Transport.
- Know local protocols for transport to appropriate burn center.

PEDIATRIC BURN PATIENT CONSIDERATIONS

- Greater surface area in relationship to the total body size.
- Results in greater fluid and heat loss.
- Any full-thickness burn or partial-thickness burn greater than 20%, or burn involving the hands, feet, face, airway, or genitalia, is considered to be a critical burn in a child.
- Any partial-thickness burn of 10% to 20% is considered a moderate burn in a child.
- Any partial-thickness burn less than 10% is considered a minor burn.
- Higher risk for shock (hypoperfusion), airway problem, or hypothermia.
- Consider possibility of child abuse.

TYPES OF BURNS

Chemical Burns

"Scene safety"

- Take the necessary scene safety precautions to protect yourself from exposure to hazardous materials.
- Wear gloves and eye protection.
- Emergency medical care
  - Dry powders should be brushed off prior to flushing.
  - Immediately begin to flush with large amounts of water.
  - Continue flushing the contaminated area when en route to the receiving facility.
  - Do not contaminate uninjured areas when flushing.

Electrical Burns

"Scene safety"

- Do not attempt to remove patient from the electrical source unless trained to do so.
- If the patient is still in contact with the electrical source or you are unsure, do not touch the patient.

EMERGENCY MANAGEMENT

- Administer high-concentration oxygen.
- Monitor the patient closely for respiratory and cardiac arrest.
- Often more severe than external indications. (Consider automated external defibrillator [AED].)
- Treat the soft tissue injuries associated with the burn. Look for both entrance and exit wounds.

? CHAPTER QUESTIONS

1. The layers of skin are:

   a. the epidermis, dermis, and subcutaneous layer
   b. the superficial layer, the partial-thickness layer, and the full-thickness layer
   c. the primary dermis, secondary dermis, and adjunct dermis
   d. the superior layer, medial layer, and inferior layer

2. Which of the following statements concerning degrees of burn is true?

   a. A first-degree burn is the most serious, and is the deepest.
   b. A full-thickness burn is also known as a third-degree burn.
   c. A second-degree burn is characterized by red, dry skin.
   d. A superficial burn is also called a second-degree burn.

3. According to the rule of nines, which of the following is equal to 9% of an adult's BSA?

   a. External genitalia
   b. The anterior trunk
   c. The head and neck
   d. Each lower extremity

4. A patient has sustained hot-liquid burns to the abdomen and anterior portion of each leg. What percentage of BSA has been burned, according to the rule of nines?

   a. 45%
   b. 27%
   c. 18%
   d. 36%

5. The difference in the rule of nines for a child as opposed to an adult is:

   a. Each lower extremity of the child is 9%.
   b. Each upper extremity of a child is 4.5%.
   c. The head and neck of a child is 18%.
   d. The entire back of a child is 9%.

Chapter 32
Muscoskeletal Injuries

You are responding to a report of a patient pinned between a tractor trailer and a loading dock. Upon arrival, the bystanders have already removed the truck from the patient. The patient is conscious and alert and is complaining of severe pain to his pelvic region. You begin your assessment and determine the patient has a possible fractured pelvis.
How would you begin your treatment of this patient?

BONE AND JOINT INJURIES

Mechanisms of injury resulting from:

- Direct force
- Indirect force
- Twisting force

Types of injuries:

- Open—Break in the continuity of the skin
- Closed—No break in the continuity of the skin

Signs and Symptoms

- Deformity or angulation
- Pain and tenderness
- Grating (crepitus)
- Swelling
- Bruising (discoloration)
- Exposed bone ends
- Joint locked into position

Emergency Management

- Body substance isolation.
- Administer oxygen if not already done and indicated.
- After life-threatening injuries have been treated, splint injuries in preparation for transport.
- Elevate the extremity.

Splinting Rationale

- Prevent movement of bone fragments, bone ends, or angulated joints.
- Minimize complications and damage to muscles, nerves, or blood vessels caused by broken bones.

- Reduce the risk of a closed, painful, swollen, deformed extremity to an open, painful, swollen, deformed extremity.
- Minimize the reduction of blood flow as a result of bone ends compressing blood vessels.
- Reduce excessive bleeding due to tissue damage caused by bone ends.
- Decrease pain associated with movement of bone ends.
- Reduce the possibility of paralysis of extremities due to a damaged spine.

Rules of Splinting

- Assess pulse, motor, and sensation distal to the injury prior to and following splint application, and record findings.
- Immobilize the joint above and below the injury.
- Remove or cut away clothing.
- Cover open wounds with a sterile dressing.
- If there is a severe deformity or the distal extremity is cyanotic or lacks pulses, align with gentle traction before splinting.
- Do not intentionally replace the protruding bones.
- Pad each splint to prevent pressure and discomfort to the patient.
- Splint the patient before moving when feasible and no life threats.
- When in doubt, splint the injury when feasible and no life threats.
- If patient has signs of shock (hypoperfusion), align in normal anatomical position and transport.

Complications of Splinting

- Compression of nerves, tissues, and blood vessels from the splint
- Delay in transport of a patient with life-threatening injury
- Splint applied too tight on the extremity reducing distal circulation
- Aggravation of the bone or joint injury
- Cause or aggravate tissue, nerve, vessel, or muscle damage from excessive bone or joint movement

Splinting a Joint Injury

- Body substance isolation.
- Apply manual stabilization.
- Assess pulse, motor, and sensory function.
- Align with gentle traction if distal extremity is cyanotic or lacks pulses and no resistance is met.
- Immobilize the site of injury.
- Immobilize bone above and below the site of injury.
- Reassess pulse, motor, and sensation after application of splint and record.

Traction Splinting

Indications for use is a painful, swollen, deformed midthigh with no joint or lower leg injury (midshaft femur fracture).

Contraindications of the Use of a Traction Splint

- Injury is close to the knee.
- Injury to the knee exists.
- Injury to the hip/pelvis.
- Partial amputation or avulsion with bone separation, distal limb is connected only by marginal tissue. Traction would risk separation.
- Lower leg or ankle injury.

Traction Splinting Procedure

- Assess pulse, motor, and sensation distal to the injury, and record.
- Body substance isolation.
- Perform manual stabilization of the injured leg.
- Apply manual traction—Required when using a bipolar traction splint.
- Prepare/adjust splint to proper length.
- Position splint under injured leg.
- Apply proximal securing device (ischial strap).
- Apply distal securing device (ankle hitch).
- Apply mechanical traction.
- Position/secure support straps.
- Reevaluate proximal/distal securing devices.
- Reassess pulses, motor, sensation distal to the injury after application of the splint, and record.
- Secure torso to the long board to immobilize hip.
- Secure splint to the long board to prevent movement of splint.

? CHAPTER QUESTIONS

1. The three kinds of muscles found in the body, each with a specific function, are called:

   a. voluntary, involuntary, and cardiac muscles
   b. controlled, autonomic, and contracting muscles
   c. long, flat, and specialized muscles
   d. flat, striated, and walled muscles

2. Injuries to the musculoskeletal system include:

   a. a dislocation, which is the displacement of a bone
   b. a strain, which is damage to, or tearing of, ligaments
   c. a sprain, which is the overextending or stretching of a muscle and/or tendon
   d. a comminuted injury, which is the detachment of a muscle from a bone

3. Bone and joint injuries may exhibit crepitus, which is:

   a. deformity or angulation of the injured extremity
   b. swelling of the injury site
   c. the discoloration of the skin at and around the injury site
   d. the sound or feeling of broken bone fragments grinding against each other

4. Emergency medical care of bone and joint injuries should include:

   a. splinting any painful extremity
   b. applying a heat pack to the injury to alleviate pain
   c. determining the injury, such as a fracture, dislocation, and the like
   d. realigning deformed extremities prior to splinting

5. The basic reasons for splinting a bone or joint injury include:

   a. preventing further movement to reduce the chance of further injury

   b. replacing exposed bone ends back into the extremity

   c. setting the bone ends back into their proper position

   d. preventing swelling which might complicate the emergency-room (ER) physician's examination

6. When caring for an extremity injury, the EMT-Basic should assess the distal pulse, motor function, and sensation:

   a. after application of a splint

   b. both before and after application of a splint

   c. prior to application of a splint

   d. every 5 minutes until arrival at the hospital

Reference

US Department of Transportation, National Highway Traffic Safety Administration. *EMT-Basic National Standard Curriculum.* Washington, DC: US Department of Transportation, National Highway Traffic Safety Administration; 1994.

Chapter 33
Head Injuries

A 911 call is received, and your ambulance is dispatched for a man with a head injury which occurred from a fall from a ladder. Upon arrival you find a 30-year-old man lying in a fetal position with what appears to be a head laceration.

As you approach and determine scene safety, you find the patient to be exhibiting what appears to be seizure activity.

What is your next step?

INJURIES TO THE BRAIN AND SKULL

- Traumatic brain injuries (TBI) are the leading cause of death and disability for children and adults ages 1 to 45 years of age.
- 1.6 million head injuries occur each year in the United States.
- Approximately 52,000 people die each year from TBI.
- 70,000 to 90,000 people are left with neurological disabilities.

THE IMPORTANCE OF AIRWAY, BREATHING, CIRCULATION (ABCs)

- Airway
  - Is the airway open?
    - — Use the modified jaw thrust maneuver for opening the airway of a suspected c-spine injury.
  - Is the airway patent?
- Breathing
  - Is the patient breathing?
  - Is the breathing pattern irregular?
  - Don't be shy; be aggressive with managing the breathing of a head-injured patient.
  - Rescue breathing (hyperventilation) should be limited to 20 breaths per minute.
- Circulation
  - Check for a radial, brachial, femoral, or carotid pulse.
  - No pulse, begin CPR according to AHA guidelines.
  - Treat for shock.
  - Is bleeding controlled?

HEAD INJURIES

(Fig. 33-1)

- Injuries to the scalp.
  - Very vascular, may bleed more than expected.
  - Control bleeding with direct pressure.
  - Injuries to the brain—Injury of brain tissue or bleeding into the skull will cause an increase of pressure in the skull.

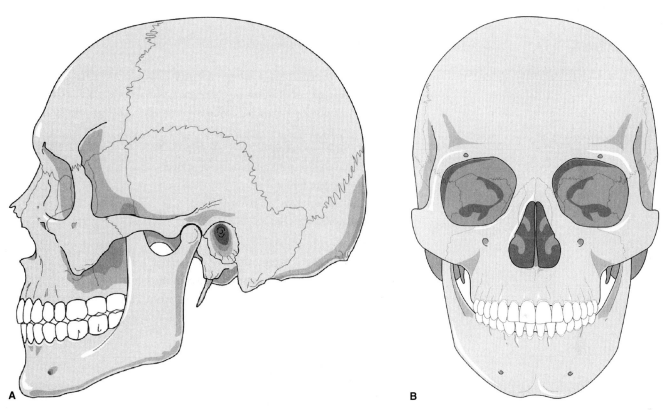

Figure 33-1 Image of the skull. **A.** Side view. **B.** Frontal view. *(LifeART image copyright 2011 Wolters Kluwer Health, Ltd./Lippincott Williams & Wilkins. All rights reserved.)*

Related Nontraumatic Conditions

- Nontraumatic injuries to the brain may occur due to clots or hemorrhaging.
- Nontraumatic brain injuries can be a cause of altered mental status.
- Signs and symptoms parallel that of traumatic injuries with the exception of evidence of trauma and a lack of mechanism of injury.

Skull Injury—Signs and Symptoms

- Mechanism of injury
- Contusions, lacerations, hematomas to the scalp
- Deformity to the skull
- Blood or fluid (cerebrospinal fluid [CSF]) leakage from the ears or nose
- Bruising (discoloration) around the eyes
- Bruising (discoloration) behind the ears (mastoid process)

Traumatic Brain Injury (TBI)—Signs and Symptoms

- Altered or decreasing mental status is the best indicator of a brain injury (GCS <9).
  - Confusion, disorientation, or repetitive questioning
  - Conscious—Deteriorating mental status
  - Unresponsive
- Irregular breathing pattern
- Consideration of mechanism of injury
  - Deformity of windshield
  - Deformity of helmet
- Contusions, lacerations, hematomas to the scalp
- Deformity to the skull
- Blood or fluid (CSF) leakage from the ears and nose
- Bruising (discoloration) around the eyes (raccoon eyes)
- Bruising (discoloration) behind the ears (mastoid process) (Battle sign)
- Neurologic disability
- Nausea and/or vomiting
- Unequal pupil size with altered mental status
- Systolic blood pressure
- Seizure activity may be seen
- Oxygen saturation less than 90%

Open Head Injury—Signs and Symptoms

- Consideration of mechanism of injury.
  - Deformity of windshield
  - Deformity of helmet
- Contusions, lacerations, hematomas to the scalp.
- Deformity to the skull.
- Penetrating injury—Do not remove impaled objects in the skull.
- Soft area or depression upon palpation.
- Exposed brain tissue if open.
- Bleeding from the open bone injury.
- Blood or fluid (CSF) leakage from the ears and nose.
- Bruising (discoloration) around the eyes.
- Bruising (discoloration) behind the ears (mastoid process).
- Nausea and/or vomiting.
- Possible signs and symptoms of a closed head injury may exist if brain injury has occurred.

Signs of Cerebral Herniation

- Unconscious and unresponsive
- Dilated pupils with no reaction to light
- Asymmetric pupils
- Nonresponsive to painful stimulus
- Posturing
  - Decorticate
  - Decerebrate
- Cushing reflex
  - ↑ in blood pressure, ↓ in pulse, and an irregular respiratory pattern.

Emergency Management

- Body substance isolation.
- Maintain airway/artificial ventilation/oxygenation. Maintain an oxygen saturation of greater than 90%.
- Initial assessment with spinal immobilization should be done on-scene with a complete detailed physical examination en route.
- With any head injury, the emergency medical technician (EMT) must suspect spinal injury. Immobilize the spine.
- Closely monitor the airway, breathing, pulse, and mental status for deterioration.
- Control bleeding.
- Do not apply pressure to an open or depressed skull injury.
- Dress and bandage open wound as indicated in the treatment of soft tissue injuries.
- If a medical injury or nontraumatic injury exists, place patient on the left side.
- Be prepared for changes in patient condition.
- Immediately transport the patient.

? CHAPTER QUESTIONS

1. The outermost layer of the three meninges is called the:

   a. pia mater
   b. dura mater
   c. alma mater
   d. arachnoid

2. Signs and symptoms of a brain injury may include:

   a. discoloration behind the ears (Battle sign)
   b. a ketone odor to the breath, which indicates the presence of CSF
   c. neck vein distention
   d. total or partial paralysis

3. When assessing the vital signs of a head injury patient, keep in mind that:

   a. Head injury alone will not result in signs and symptoms of shock.
   b. Sudden hypotension indicates increased intracranial pressure.
   c. A rapid or rising pulse indicates rising intracranial pressure.
   d. Hypotension in a head injury patient is due to bleeding elsewhere.

4. Cushing reflex is a sign of severe head injury, and causes:

   a. seizure-like activity and apnea
   b. increased BP, decreased pulse, and respiratory pattern changes
   c. decorticate posturing and abnormal breathing patterns
   d. unconsciousness, decerebrate posturing, and vomiting

Chapter 34
Injuries to the Spine

Your unit is dispatched to the scene of a motor vehicle collision. The scene is safe to operate and you approach the vehicle. You note major damage to the driver's side of the car with major intrusion into the passenger compartment. The driver of vehicle is unconscious and appears to be the only patient. How are you going to treat this patient?

SPINAL CORD INJURIES

- Mis-management of spinal injuries can result in paralysis.
- Approximately 20,000 people suffer spinal cord injuries each year.
- The most common age group for spinal cord injuries is 16 to 35 years old.
- Most common cause of spinal injuries is motor vehicle collisions.

THE NERVOUS SYSTEM REVIEW

Spinal Cord

- Consists of 31 segments; each gives rise to a pair of spinal nerves.
- Provides conduction pathways to and from the brain.
- Functions as a center for reflex action.

Peripheral Nervous System

- Cranial nerves—12 pairs are numbered according to order in which they arise; conducts impulses between brain and structures in head, neck, thoracic, and abdominal cavities.
- Spinal nerves—31 pairs; each nerve consists of a dorsal (sensory) root and a ventral (motor) root.

Autonomic Nervous System

- Involves involuntary or autonomic function.
- Impulses are conveyed to smooth muscle, cardiac muscle, and glandular epithelium.
- Center is located in the hypothalamus.
- Two parts—Sympathetic and parasympathetic.

Function of the Sympathetic Nervous System

- Increases cardiovascular response
- Pupil dilation

- Decreases peristalsis
- Regulates temperature
- Increases blood sugar
- Increases secretion of sweat glands
- Adrenal medulla—Epinephrine

Function of the Parasympathetic Nervous System

- Third, seventh, and tenth cranial nerves
- Pupillary constriction
- Decreases heart rate
- Stimulates watery secretions
- Relaxes bladder and rectal sphincters

Function of the Skeletal System in Relation to the Spine

The skeletal system provides protection and support to the spinal cord. Components of the skeletal system in relation to the spine include:

- Skull (Fig. 34-1)
- Spinal column (Fig. 34-2)
    ◦ Thirty-three bones
    ◦ Surrounds and protects the spinal cord

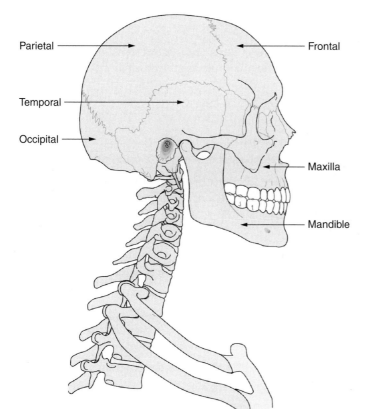

Figure 34-1 Skeletal system of the skull. (*LifeART image copyright 2011 Wolters Kluwer Health, Ltd./Lippincott Williams & Wilkins. All rights reserved.*)

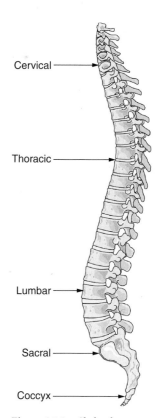

Figure 34-2 Skeletal system of the spine. (*LifeART image copyright 2011 Wolters Kluwer Health, Ltd./Lippincott Williams & Wilkins. All rights reserved.*)

INJURIES TO THE SPINE—MECHANISM OF INJURY

- Compression injuries can occur from falls, diving accidents, or motor vehicle accidents.
- Excessive flexion, extension, rotation can cause serious injury to the spine.
- Lateral bending can cause serious injury to the spine.
- Distraction injuries occur from:
    - Pulling apart the spine
    - Hangings

The EMT must maintain a high index of suspicion for the following mechanisms of injury:

- Motor vehicle crashes
- Pedestrian/vehicle collisions
- Falls
- Blunt trauma
- Penetrating trauma to head, neck, or torso
- Motorcycle crashes
- Hangings
- Diving accidents
- Any unknown mechanism of injury that involves an unconscious trauma victim

Signs and Symptoms

- Ability to walk, move extremities, or feel sensation (or lack of pain to spinal column) does not rule out the possibility of spinal column or cord damage.
- Tenderness in the area of injury.
- Pain associated with moving.
    - Do not ask the patient to move to try to elicit a pain response.
    - Do not move the patient to test for a pain response.
- Tell the patient not to move while asking questions.
- Pain independent of movement or palpation.
    - Along spinal column
    - Lower legs
    - May be intermittent
- Obvious deformity of the spine upon palpation.
- Soft tissue injuries associated with trauma.
    - Head and neck to cervical spine
    - Shoulders, back, or abdomen—Thoracic, lumbar
    - Lower extremities—Lumbar, sacral
- Numbness, weakness, or tingling in the extremities.
- Loss of sensation or paralysis below the suspected level of injury.
- Loss of sensation or paralysis in the upper or lower extremities.
- Incontinence.

Assessing the Potential Responsive Spine Injury Patient

- What is the mechanism of injury?
- Questions to ask:
  - Does your neck or back hurt?
  - What happened?
  - Where does it hurt?
  - Can you move your hands and feet?
  - Can you feel me touching your fingers?
  - Can you feel me touching your toes?
- Inspect for contusions, deformities, lacerations, punctures, penetrations, swelling.
- Palpate for areas of tenderness or deformity.
- Assess equality of strength of extremities:
  - Hand grip
  - Gently push feet against hands

Unresponsive Patient

- Mechanism of injury.
- Initial assessment.
- Inspect for:
  - DCAP-BTLS
- Palpate for areas of tenderness or deformity.
- Obtain information from others at the scene to determine information relevant to mechanism of injury or patient mental status prior to the EMTs' arrival.

Complications of Spinal Injuries

- Inadequate breathing effort
- Paralysis

Emergency Management

- Body substance isolation.
- Establish and maintain in-line immobilization.
  - Place the head in a neutral in-line position unless the patient complains of pain or the head is not easily moved into position.
  - Place head in alignment with spine.
  - Maintain constant manual in-line immobilization until the patient is properly secured to a backboard with the head immobilized.
- Perform initial assessment.
- Airway control must be done with in-line immobilization.
- Artificial ventilation must be done with in-line stabilization.
- Assess pulse, motor and sensory, in all extremities.
- Assess the cervical region and neck.
- Apply a rigid, cervical immobilization device.

- Properly size the cervical immobilization device. If it doesn't fit, use a rolled towel and tape to the board and have rescuer hold the head manually.
- An improperly fit immobilization device will do more harm than good.
- If found in a lying position, immobilize the patient to a long spine board.
- Position the device.
- Move the patient onto the device by log rolling.
- One EMT must maintain in-line immobilization of the head and spine.
- EMT at the head directs the movement of the patient.
- One to three other EMTs control the movement of the rest of the body.
- Quickly assess posterior body if not already done in focused history and physical examination.
- Position the long spine board under the patient.
- Place patient onto the board at the command of the EMT holding in-line immobilization using a slide, proper lift, and log roll or scoop stretcher so as to limit movement to the minimum amount possible. Which method to use must be decided based upon the situation, scene, and available resources.
- Pad voids between the patient and the board.
- Adult
  - Under the head.
  - Voids under torso. Be careful of extra movement.
- Infant and child—Pad under the shoulders to the toes to establish a neutral position.
- Immobilize torso to the board.
- Immobilize the patient's head to the board.
- Secure the legs to the board.
- Reassess pulses, motor and sensory, and record.
- If the patient is found in a sitting position in a chair, immobilize with a short spine immobilization device. Exception: If the patient must be removed urgently because of his injuries, the need to gain access to others, or dangers at the scene, he must then be lowered directly onto a long board and removed with manual immobilization provided.
- Position device behind the patient.
- Secure the device to the patient's torso.
- Evaluate torso fixation and adjust as necessary without excessive movement of the patient.
- Evaluate and pad behind the patient's head as necessary to maintain neutral in-line immobilization.
- Secure the patient's head to the device.
- Insert a long board under the patient's buttocks and rotate and lower him to it. If not possible, lower him to the long spine board.
- Reassess pulses, motor and sensory, in all extremities, and record.
- If the patient is found in a standing position, immobilize the patient to a long spine board.
  - Position the device behind patient.
  - Move the patient onto the device.
  - One rescuer on each side of the patient, one additional rescuer at the foot facing the patient.

- The rescuers on both sides of the patient reach with the hand closest to the patient under the arm to grasp the board, and use the hand farthest from the patient to secure the head.
- Once the position is guaranteed, place the leg closest to the board behind the board and begin to move the top of the board toward the ground. The rescuer at the foot of the board secures the board and the patient to prevent them from sliding, and the board is brought into a level horizontal position.
- If the patient is critically injured, perform a rapid extrication.
- Transport the patient immediately.
- Bring body into alignment.
- Transfer to long board without short spine board.

SPINAL IMMOBILIZATION

Indications for Use of Cervical Spine Immobilization Devices (CSID)

- Any suspected injury to the spine based on mechanism of injury, history, or signs and symptoms.
- Use in conjunction with short and long backboards.

Sizing

- Various types of rigid cervical immobilization devices exist; therefore, sizing is based on the specific design of the device.
- An improperly sized immobilization device has a potential for further injury.
- Do not obstruct the airway with the placement of a cervical immobilization device.
- If it doesn't fit, use a rolled towel and tape to the board and manually support the head. An improperly fitting device will do more harm than good.

Precautions

- Cervical immobilization devices alone do not provide adequate in-line immobilization.
- Manual immobilization must always be used with a cervical immobilization device until the head is secured to a board.

Short Backboards

Several different types of short board immobilization devices exist:

- Vest-type devices
- Rigid short board
  - Provides stabilization and immobilization to the head, neck, and torso.
  - Used to immobilize noncritical sitting patients with suspected spinal injuries.

Long Backboards (Full-Body Spinal Immobilization Devices)

Several different types of long board immobilization devices exist:

- Provide stabilization and immobilization to the head, neck, torso, pelvis, and extremities.
- Used to immobilize patients found in a lying, standing, or sitting position.
- Sometimes used in conjunction with short backboards.

Special Considerations

Indications for Rapid Extrication

- Unsafe scene.
- Unstable patient condition warrants immediate movement and transport.
- Patient blocks the EMTs' access to another, more seriously injured, patient.
- Rapid extrication is based on time and the patient, and not the preference of the EMTs.

Helmet Removal

Special assessment needs for patients wearing helmets:

- The helmet is removed to assure a properly maintained airway, or to adequately suction the patient, or to facilitate bag-valve-mask ventilation when necessary.

Indications for Leaving the Helmet in Place

- Good fit with little or no movement of the patient's head within the helmet.
- No impending airway or breathing problems.
- Removal would cause further injury to the patient.
- Proper spinal immobilization could be performed with helmet in place.
- No interference with the EMTs' ability to assess and reassess airway and breathing.

Indications for Removing the Helmet

- Inability to assess and/or reassess airway and breathing.
- Restriction of adequate management of the airway or breathing.
- Improperly fitted helmet allowing for excessive patient head movement within the helmet.
- Proper spinal immobilization cannot be performed due to helmet.
- Cardiac arrest.

Infants and Children

- Immobilize the infant or child on a rigid board appropriate for size (short, long, or padded splint), according to the procedure outlined in the "Spinal Immobilization" section.

Special considerations:

- Pad from the shoulders to the heels of the infant or child, if necessary, to maintain neutral immobilization.
- Properly size the cervical immobilization device. If it doesn't fit, use a rolled towel and tape to the board and manually support head. An improperly fitted immobilization device will do more harm than good.

? CHAPTER QUESTIONS

1. The 12 vertebrae that comprise the upper back are the:

   a. sacral spine

   b. coccyx

   c. lumbar spine

   d. thoracic spine

2. During the initial assessment of a trauma patient:

   a. Initiate immediate manual in-line spinal stabilization based on mechanism of injury.

   b. Open the airway of the unconscious patient using the head-tilt chin-lift method.

   c. The patient's skin may be cool, pale, and moist below the site of spinal injury, and warm and dry above the site of injury.

   d. Inadequate breathing will result from spinal cord damage involving the lumbar spine.

3. The three major complications of spinal injury include which of the following?

   a. systemic vasodilatation, resulting in reduced tissue perfusion

   b. paralysis of the respiratory muscles, occurring with injury to the lumbar spine

   c. paralysis to only one side of the body that does not resolve

   d. inadequate circulation indicated by tachycardia and cool, clammy skin

4. The steps in immobilizing a supine patient to a long backboard include:

   a. securing the patient's torso to the board prior to securing the head

   b. removing the C-collar once the patient is immobilized on the board

   c. not placing padding on the board, as it might move the spine out of alignment

   d. using the log roll, a move ideally performed by two rescuers, one at the head, the other at the hips

Reference

US Department of Transportation, National Highway Traffic Safety Administration. *EMT-Basic National Standard Curriculum.* Washington, DC: US Department of Transportation, National Highway Traffic Safety Administration; 1994.

Chapter 35

Injuries to the Eyes, Face, and Neck

It is after midnight on a summer night and you have been dispatched to the scene of a motor vehicle collision (MVC). Upon arrival, you establish the scene as being safe. You notice the patient walking around at the scene and he appears to be in his mid-twenties. You note the patient's car struck a light pole and there is significant damage to the front end of the car. The patient appears upset as you approach him. His right eye is swollen and you notice he has a laceration above both of his eyes. He states, "I had too much to drink!" He is concerned about the damage he did to his mother's car, and is complaining of neck pain.

How would you manage this patient?

Eye, face, and neck injuries are significant because of the associated loss of function that may occur secondary to the injury. The emergency medical technician (EMT) must not only deal with the seriousness of the injury, but also the emotional distress the patient may have when fearing loss of vision, scarring, or even significant hemorrhage.

THE EYE

(Fig. 35-1)

- The eyeball is a sphere about 1 in. in diameter.
- Its outer covering is the sclera (white portion).
- The cornea is the transparent region overlying the center.
- The pupil is the dark center, which is surrounded by the colored iris.
- The lens of the eye allows for the focusing of images on the retina, which is located to the back of the eye.
- Another structure of the eye is the conjunctiva, which lines the inner surface of the eyelids.
- Each side of the lens is a chamber. The anterior chamber contains aqueous humor, and posterior to the lens is the vitreous body that houses vitreous humor (gives the eye its shape).
- The eye is housed in the orbit socket of the skull.

THE FACE

- The face has 14 bones, 13 of which are immovable, with the only moveable one being the mandible.

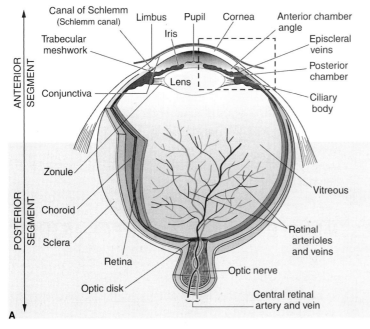

Figure 35-1A   Anatomy of the eye.

Figure 35-1B   Surrounding structures of the eye. (*Reprinted with permission from Brunton LL, Lazo JS, Parker KL. Goodman & Gilman's The Pharmacological Basis of Therapeutics. 11th ed. New York: McGraw-Hill; 2006:1710, 1708.*)

- The face is also extremely vascular, and bleeds readily to even minor trauma. Trauma to the face can not only distort these bony structures, but it may also cause hemorrhage and airway occlusion.
- Any trauma of sufficient force to injure the face can easily result in head or neck trauma as well.

THE NECK

- The neck contains major structures of the body:
  - Carotid arteries
  - Jugular veins
  - Larynx and trachea

- Damage to these vascular and airway structures can cause life-threatening bleeding and airway compromise.
- Injuries to the neck can easily cause life-threatening conditions.
- While injuries to these locations can vary, they do create some common findings:
  - They all tend to hemorrhage profusely.
  - Many times, these types of injuries are the result of an assault.
  - You may deal with not only physical trauma, but emotional trauma also.
  - These types of injuries should not be taken lightly by the EMT-B, as they can rapidly deteriorate as well.

ASSESSMENT: EYE, FACE, AND NECK INJURIES

- Scene size-up.
- Consider the MOI.
- It may be difficult to gather information from the patient because often they are in extreme pain and emotional distress.
- Determine the number of patients injured and the need for additional resources early.
- Finally, remember that since many of these types of injuries come by way of an assault, consider having a law enforcement officer there, should that be the cause of the injury.
- Initial assessment.
- Be aware of the alteration in the patient's mental status.
- Establish in-line manual stabilization of the head.
- Open the airway with a jaw-thrust if needed and suction out any blood or vomitus.
- Determine quality and adequacy of breathing.
- Typically bleeding is profuse and easy to assess. Be sure, however, that you are properly managing bleeds to the head.
- Determine the priority status of the patient.

Initial Assessment Findings that Demonstrate a Critical or High-Priority Patient

- Chemical burns to the eye
- Impaled object in the eye
- An extruded eyeball
- Respiratory distress
- Severe injuries to the face and neck
- Major bleeding
- Alteration in mental status

FOCUSED HISTORY AND PHYSICAL EXAMINATION

- Consistent with other traumatically injured patients, your completion of the physical examination, vitals, and SAMPLE (*s*igns/*s*ymptoms, *a*llergies, *m*edications, *p*ast medical problems, *l*ast oral intake, *e*vents) history are determined by your priority status.

- Often, injuries to the eye, face, and neck are critical, so commonly you'll complete a rapid trauma assessment followed by vitals and the SAMPLE history.
- Use the OPQRST (*o*nset, *p*rovokes, *q*uality, *r*adiates, *s*everity, *t*ime) mnemonic to assess any other complaints of pain.
- If the patient is critical, deliver only necessary treatment and initiate transport following the history and physical examination.

DETAILED PHYSICAL EXAMINATION AND ONGOING ASSESSMENT

- Detailed physical examination will be completed when the patient's condition is stable.
- If the patient is unstable, or if you are too close to the hospital, then skip the detailed examination and start the ongoing assessment.
- Repeat the ongoing assessment for the unstable patient every 5 minutes, and every 15 minutes for the stable patient.
- Notify the receiving facility of the patient's condition, response to your treatment, and estimated time of arrival.

ASSESSING THE EYE INJURED PATIENT

- Asses the orbits for bruising, swelling, lacerations, or tenderness.
- Assess the lids for bruising, swelling, and lacerations.
- Assess the conjunctiva for redness, pus, and foreign bodies.
- Assess the globes for redness, abnormal coloring, and lacerations.
- Assess the pupils for size, shape, equality, and reactivity.
- Evaluate eye muscle movement in all directions.
- Assess the eye for any abnormality.
- Assess motor function of the eyes by having patient follow your finger movement in a large "H" pattern.
- If the eye is swollen shut, avoid excessive manipulation.
- Do not force eyelid open unless you're flushing it.
- Consult medical direction prior to irrigating the eye.
- Do not add medicine to the eye.
- Sponge or wipe blood away that exits the eye; do not remove blood from the eye itself.
- Keep patient supine and quiet.
- Give the patient nothing by mouth.
- If you're going to cover the injured eye, just cover both at the same time to limit motion.

Foreign Object in the Eye

Methods in removing a foreign object include:

- Flushing foreign particle from the eye.
- Inverting the eyelid and removing the object.
- Removing object from the upper lid.
- Grasping eyelid and telling the patient to look down.
- Placing applicator swab along center of upper eyelid.

- Pulling eyelid up and over applicator swab.
- Once you expose the undersurface of the eye, the foreign material can be removed.

Orbit Injury

- Management includes placing a dressing and a cold pack over the eye to reduce swelling.
- Do not, however, use a cold pack if you suspect a globe injury.

Lid Injury

- Stop any bleeding with light pressure.
- Preserve any avulsed tissue.
- Cover with a moist sterile dressing.
- Also cover opposite eye.

Globe Injury

- Due to the various injuries possible, it is best to just apply patches lightly to both eyes.
- Apply a shield to the injured eye to avoid any pressure being exerted on it.

Chemical Burn Injury

- The burning mechanism can cause rapid and permanent injury.
- Start irrigation with large amounts of water immediately.

Extruded Eyeball

- Cover the eye carefully so that no additional pressure is applied to the eyeball.
- Cover the other eye as well to limit motion and rapidly transport.

Impaled Object in the Eye

- Like an extruded eyeball, care should be taken to rapidly treat it and provide transport.
- Place padding around the object.
- Impaled object in the eye.
- Stabilize the impaled object with a cup.
- Bandage the cup in place and provide transport.

Removing Contact Lenses

- Eye injuries may be further complicated by the presence of contact lenses.
- Examine with a penlight to assess for shadowing over the outer portion of the eye (soft lens), or shadowing over the iris (hard lens).
- Some people only wear one contact lens, so don't dismiss them until you look in both eyes.
- Seek medical direction for permission to remove the lens.
- The type of lens typically determines how it should be removed.

INJURIES TO THE FACE

- Injuries to the face occur often due to common mechanisms of injury (ie, MVC), and their location.
- About 75% of MVC victims sustain some type of facial trauma.
- Some injuries can be life threatening due to their imposition on airway maintenance.
- Don't forget to consider cervical injuries with any type of facial trauma.

Emergency Management

- Establish cervical stabilization.
- Carefully assess the oral cavity, and retrieve any broken-off teeth, torn-away tissue, or other foreign material.
- Suction blood from the mouth (may need to be constantly repeated).
- Provide oxygen via NRB (nonrebreather) or PPV (positive pressure ventilation), depending on breathing.
- Control any severe bleeding.
- Treat any avulsed teeth by wrapping in saline gauze.
- Treat for hypoperfusion (shock), and transport.

Impaled Object to the Cheek

- Generally, pack each side if the patient is stable.
- If the impalement compromises the airway, remove it in the direction of entry and pack both sides.

Injuries to the Nose

- Never pack the internal nares; however, external bleeds should be controlled.
- Try not to position the patient supine as any bleeding may compromise the airway.
- Treat nasal fractures with cold compresses.

Injuries to the Ear

- Apply direct pressure to external bleeding.
- Preserve any tissue avulsions.
- Never pack the ear, but rather allow a sterile dressing to collect the blood.

Injuries to the Neck

- Can be caused by blunt or penetrating trauma.
- Basic care includes:
  - Immobilization
  - Control of the airway, oxygen, and ventilation as needed
  - Cover neck wounds with occlusive dressing
  - Rapid transport

Severed Blood Vessel in the Neck

- Use a gloved hand to cover the wound initially.
- Use digital pressure on carotid artery only as a last resort.
- Apply an occlusive dressing.
- Cover with a regular bulky dressing.
- Only apply enough pressure to control the bleeding.
- Once bleeding is controlled, secure with roller gauze bandaging that is anchored around the shoulder and axillary region.
- Transport the patient on their left side with the head tilted down.
- If the patient is immobilized, then simply tilt the spinal board to the left.
- Continue oxygen therapy and treatment for shock.

? CHAPTER QUESTIONS

1. A patient that sustained a traumatic injury to the face must also be assessed for:

   a. brain injury

   b. airway obstruction

   c. spinal injury

   d. all of the above

2. Double vision, a marked decrease in vision, or a loss of sensation above the eyebrow, over the cheek, or in the upper lip may be caused by:

   a. detached retina

   b. orbital fracture

   c. cervical spine injury

   d. temporal bone fracture

Chapter 36
Chest, Abdomen, and Genitalia Injuries

You are dispatched to the state police station for a man with chest pain. Upon arrival you learn the patient was struck in the chest with an object during an attempted robbery. The patient's vital signs are as follows:

BP 124/72, RR 28 labored, HR 100; skin is pale, cool, and dry.

With this mechanism of injury (MOI), what type of injuries may this patient have?

- Unlike trauma to the extremities, thoracic and abdominal trauma rarely involve large visible injuries. In fact, an injury to these locations may be lethal, but have very minimal external signs of injury.
- Early recognition and treatment saves lives.
- Thoracic injuries can interfere with normal breathing and gas exchange, and abdominal injuries may result in significant abdominal bleeding.

ANATOMY OF THE CHEST

- Surrounded by ribs, with the sternum on the anterior thorax, and the spine in the posterior.
- Inferior border is diaphragm.
- Contains lungs, heart, trachea, esophagus, and major blood vessels.
- Lungs are surrounded by the visceral and parietal pleura, which plays a role in certain types of thoracic injuries (Fig. 36-1).

TYPES OF CHEST INJURIES

- Open chest injuries result from some type of penetrating mechanism.
- These injuries can allow the pleural space to fill with air that gets entrained from outside causing the collapse of the lung.
- At times, the hole in the chest may cause air to get pulled in and create an audible "sucking" sound. This is referred to as a "sucking chest wound."
- Open chest wounds can also cause vascular damage to blood vessels in the chest causing the hemothorax to fill with blood (collapsing the lung and causing hypoperfusion).
- Even small injuries are sufficient to cause life-threatening air or blood accumulation in the pleural space.

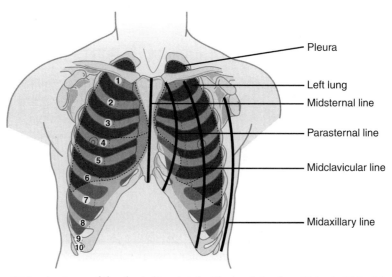

Figure 36-1   Anatomy of the chest. *(Reprinted with permission from Doherty GM, ed. Current Diagnosis & Treatment: Surgery, 13th ed. New York:McGraw-Hill; 2010:306.)*

Pneumothorax

- A pneumothorax is a type of chest injury that can occur with an open or closed chest injury. As mentioned previously, a hole in the chest wall can allow air to be sucked in during inhalation. The problem is, the air entering through the chest wound does not reach the alveoli for gas exchange. Rather, it accumulates in the "sub-atmospheric" space between the pleural linings until the lung collapses.
- The collapsing of the lung results in diminished ability to exchange oxygen and eliminate carbon dioxide.

Tension Pneumothorax

- This injury can progress from a pneumothorax when a large amount of air collects in the pleural cavity and causes significant disruption to the lungs.
- Another type of chest injury is referred to as a "closed" chest injury, and is the usual result of blunt forces applied to the chest wall.
- These injuries may be more challenging to discern because of the lack of external symptoms (other than some early signs of soft tissue trauma to the chest wall).
- Injuries that could result from closed chest wall injuries include both pneumothorax and tension pneumothorax, but also broken ribs, flail segments, and vascular trauma causing a hemothorax.

Signs and Symptoms

- Decreased or absent breath sounds on the affected side
- Jugular venous distension (late sign)
- Tracheal deviation toward unaffected side (late sign)
- Hyperesonance on percussion

- Unequal chest rise
- Dyspnea
- Tachypnea
- Tachycardia
- Hypotension
- Hypoxia
- Pale, cool, clammy skin
- Subcutaneous emphysema
- Cyanosis

Flail Segment

- A flail segment occurs when there are adjacent ribs that are fractured in numerous places.
- In effect, the flailed region becomes "detached" from the skeletal framework of the thoracic wall.
- As a result, the flailed segment moves opposite of the normal chest excursion during breathing because it is affected by the negative and positive pressure in the thorax created by breathing, rather than the muscular activity of the respiratory effort.
- This results in poor air exchange and hypoxemia.
- Paradoxical motion occurs when the flailed segment moves opposite of the normal chest wall.

Hemothorax

- A hemothorax could result from either a closed or open chest wall injury.
- The mechanism behind its occurrence is the hemorrhage of blood from a lacerated thoracic blood vessel, and the blood accumulates in the pleural space.
- As the blood accumulates, it forces the lung to collapse, which alters normal oxygenation, as well as promotes hypoperfusion as this is a type of internal bleeding which can make the patient hypovolemic.
- Hemothorax can result from either open or closed chest wall trauma. In either instance, its occurrence has a large effect on the patient's ability to oxygenate and maintain peripheral perfusion.

ASSESSMENT: CHEST INJURIES

- Scene size-up—As with other types of trauma, be certain that the scene is safe, making sure the injuries sustained are not from some type of violence or hazardous location.
- Take necessary BSI; consider eye and face protection.
- Analyze the MOI, and try to determine if the patient may have an open or closed thoracic injury.
  - Sport accidents usually cause closed chest injuries.
  - Falls could cause closed or open chest injuries.
  - Was there a fight or shooting (common with open injuries)?
  - Crushing mechanism usually causes closed chest injuries.
  - An explosion could cause an open or closed chest injury.

Initial Assessment

- Determine your general impression. As you approach, does the patient seem to be in significant respiratory distress?
- Remember to take in-line manual stabilization when needed.
- Assess the airway for patency. Be certain there is no blood, vomitus, or secretions causing occlusion.
- Closely assess the respiratory effort. If you note inadequate breathing, immediately start artificial ventilation. You will determine the cause of the poor breathing during the rapid trauma assessment.
- During your assessment of the circulatory status, the presence of tachycardia, poor capillary refill, poor peripheral perfusion, and weak/absent peripheral pulses are all indications of hypoperfusion, possibly from an internal (or even external) bleeding.
- The patient should be considered a priority if any of the following are present:
  - Loss of function or impairment to the airway, breathing, or circulation.
  - An acute change in mental status.
  - Abnormal findings during focused history and physical examination.
  - Indications of significant chest injury.
  - Subtle clues or findings that may indicate chest wall injuries.

Emergency Management

- When dealing with chest trauma, remember that the following conditions must be supported immediately:
  - Airway inadequacy (blood, vomitus, foreign bodies, etc.)
  - Breathing insufficiency (poor minute ventilation)
  - Circulatory compromise (hemorrhage, hypoperfusion)
- Maintain an open airway and establish cervical immobilization.
- Use a jaw-thrust maneuver if cervical spine injury suspected.
- Use an OPA or NPA if the airway is still difficult to control.
- Provide oral suctioning as needed.
- Provide oxygen therapy at 15 L/min.
- Evaluate/assure breathing adequacy.
- Provide artificial ventilation if needed; however, avoid forceful ventilations as this may aggravate chest injuries.
- Provide stabilization to any impaled object found in the chest.
  - If found, do not remove the impaled object.
- Occlude any open soft tissue injuries noted.
  - First with your gloved hand, then with an occlusive dressing.
- Completely immobilize the patient.
  - As needed for spinal precautions.
- Treat the patient for shock, and provide rapid transport to the hospital.
  - Warmth, positioning, oxygen therapy, and the like.

> ▶**Note:**
>
> The following injuries are considered immediate life threats and should be treated immediately:
> - Open chest wound
> - Flail segment
> - Major hemorrhage

Specific Management of Chest Injuries

Open Chest Wound

- Place a nonporous dressing to the chest wall and tape it on three sides.
- This helps limit inward movement of air during breathing and relief of trapped air on exhalation.

Flail Segment

- Upon finding a flail segment, initially provide stabilization with your hand (to limit paradoxical motion). Continue stabilization by applying a bulky dressing or clean towel to the chest wall for splinting purposes.
- Secure the dressing. You can use the patient's arm to help splint the flail segment.

Detailed Physical Examination and Ongoing Assessment

- En route to the hospital, if time and the patient's condition permit, perform a detailed physical examination to assess for any problems that may have been overlooked during the rapid trauma assessment.
- During the ongoing assessment, reevaluate the effectiveness of your treatment and assess for further deterioration. Reassess and record the baseline vital signs.
- Contact the receiving hospital, and keep them advised of any further changes in the patient's status.

ANATOMY OF THE ABDOMEN

- The abdomen contains major organs of the digestive, urinary, and endocrine systems.
- Organs are enveloped by a visceral and parietal peritoneum.
- Organs within the abdomen can be characterized as:
  - Hollow
  - Solid
  - Vascular

ABDOMINAL INJURIES

- Injuries to the abdomen could be caused by either blunt or penetrating trauma.
- Like chest injuries, abdominal injuries are considered to be either open or closed in nature.
- Because of the number of organs within the abdominal cavity (including highly vascular ones), trauma to the abdomen can cause significant disturbances in homeostasis, as well as acute hemorrhage and death should a vascular structure become damaged.

TRAUMA ASSESSMENT: ABDOMINAL INJURIES

- Scene size-up
- The MOI can give you clues as to the nature of the injury to the abdomen (blunt or penetrating injury).
- Ensure your own safety, and search the scene for clues such as guns, knives, sharp metal, etc.
- If the mechanism of injury was a motor vehicle collision (MVC) (which is the most common cause of blunt trauma), try to determine particularities of the crash (type of vehicle, speed of travel, points of impact, etc.).
- Contact additional resources as necessary.
- Determine if any other victims (whether abdominally injured or not) are on-scene and in need of care.

Initial Assessment

- Form a general impression upon your approach to the patient.
- Note the position the patient is in; this may give you a clue as to the nature of the problem.
- Continue with your assessment of the patient's mental status by using the AVPU (*a*lert, *v*erbal, *p*ainful stimulus, *u*nresponsive) mnemonic.
- Ensure the patient's airway is open by assessing the oral cavity and listening for abnormal airway sounds.
- Breathing may be noted to be hypopneic as abdominal pain tends to make the patient's breathing shallow.
- Assess circulation by taking a core and peripheral pulse, evaluate the quality of peripheral perfusion, and determine the skin characteristics.
- Determine priority status of the patient.
- Focused history and physical examination are necessary.
- Consider the patient's complaints, MOI, and clinical status when determining whether to perform a rapid trauma assessment or focused physical examination.
- While performing the rapid trauma assessment or the focused abdominal physical examination, be sure to use good assessment skills to detect any rigidity, guarding, soft tissue trauma, masses, tenderness, or other abnormal finding.
- Follow this with your assessment of baseline vitals and determination of the SAMPLE (*s*igns/*s*ymptoms, *a*llergies, *m*edications, *p*ast medical problems, *l*ast oral intake, *e*vents) history.
- Maintain an open airway and appropriate spinal protection.
- Provide high-flow oxygen at 15 L/min via an appropriate oxygenation adjunct.
- Reassess the breathing status; if found to be inadequate, then begin positive pressure ventilation (PPV).
- Treat for shock (hypoperfusion) as appropriate.

Abdominal Evisceration

- This occurs when the trauma to the abdomen allows abdominal tissue to protrude out.
- Do not touch or replace the tissue.
- First, cut away any clothing.
- Place a premoistened dressing over the wound, and gently tape it in place.
- Do not try to replace intestines within the abdomen.
- Apply an occlusive dressing (such as plastic wrap) over the moistened dressing.
- Secure all the material in place with tape or other suitable material.

Emergency Management: Abdominal Evisceration

- Control any external bleeding with pressure and dressings.
- Eviscerations should be treated as recommended.
- Position the patient supine with legs flexed at the knees if not contraindicated for any other reason.
- Stabilize any impaled object.
- Transport as quickly as possible.

GENITALIA ANATOMY

Both male and female anatomy (Figs. 36-2 and 36-3) is comprised largely of soft tissue.

Injuries to the Male Genitalia

- Lacerations
- Abrasions
- Avulsions
- Penetrations
- Amputations
- Contusions
- Severe pain

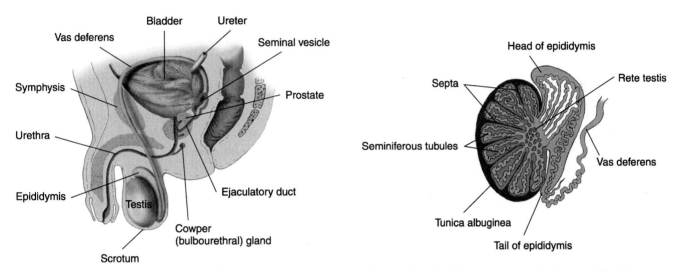

Figure 36-2 Male genitalia. *(Reprinted with permission from Ganong WF. Review of Medical Physiology. 22nd ed. McGraw-Hill; 2005.)*

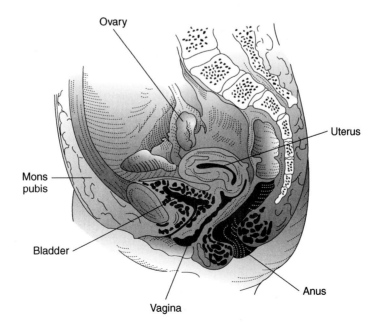

Figure 36-3 Female genitalia. *(Reprinted with permission from Benson RC. Handbook of Obstetrics & Gynecology. 8th ed. Lange/McGraw-Hill; 1983.)*

Injuries to the Female Genitalia

- Can occur from straddle injuries, sexual assault, blunt trauma, abortion attempts, traumatic childbirth, foreign body insertion
- Injury manifestation includes:
  - Soft tissue crush injuries
  - Amputation and avulsions
  - Lacerations
  - Contusions and hematoma
  - Severe pain

For Either Gender, Basic Assessment and Treatment

- Essentially, the injury will be managed consistent with other soft tissue injuries.
- Apply direct pressure to stop any bleeds (never pack the female's vagina).
- Save and transport any avulsed or amputated tissue.
- Consider the application of a cold compress to help with pain management and swelling.
- Try to have a same gender emergency medical technician (EMT) provide the care, and be empathetic to the fright, pain, and anxiety that typically accompany these types of injuries.

? CHAPTER QUESTIONS

1. Your patient has received an open chest wound from a screwdriver. Emergency management should include all the following except:

   a. high-concentration oxygen

   b. sealing the wound with an occlusive dressing

   c. placing in a position of comfort if there is no spinal injury

   d. cleaning the wound with saline

2. A 33-year-old male patient has been involved in a motor vehicle crash and has an open abdominal injury with a protruding bowel secondary to being partially ejected from the vehicle. Your treatment of the injury should include:

   a. replacing the exposed bowel

   b. keeping the patient's legs straight

   c. covering the exposed bowel with a sterile dressing moistened with saline

   d. covering the bowel with dry sterile gauze prior to transport

Chapter 37
Agricultural and Industrial Accidents

EMS and the fire department are dispatched to the scene of a construction accident on a river barge (Fig. 37-1). The only access to the incident is via boat. The responding fire department dispatched a marine unit to the dock where you and your partner will board with your equipment.

What are some safety issues you will need to perform during your scene size-up?

INTRODUCTION TO INDUSTRIAL ACCIDENTS

- According to the National Institute for Occupational Safety and Health (NIOSH), during the period from 1980 through 1995, at least 93,338 workers in the United States died as a result of trauma suffered on the job.
- That is an average of about 16 deaths per day. The Bureau of Labor Statistics (Department of Labor) Census of Fatal Occupational Injuries (CFOI) has identified 5915 workplace deaths from acute traumatic injury in 2000.
- The Bureau of Labor Statistics also estimates that 5.7 million injuries to workers occurred in 1997 alone, while NIOSH estimates that about 3.6 million occupational injuries were serious enough to be treated in hospital emergency rooms in 1998.
- With this staggering data presented from NIOSH, it is absolutely crucial for EMTs to evaluate scene safety during an industrial or agricultural accident. General industry safety standards can be found in the Code of Federal Regulations under Section 29 CFR 1910; this includes fire fighting and EMS safety regulations.

Causes of Injuries Associated with Machinery

- *Rotation* machinery causes injuries when a machine that uses circular motion draws a body part into the machinery.
- *Reciprocating* machinery causes injuries by having vertical or horizontal movement in a single plane which draws a body part in, or traps it between moving parts and a fixed object.
- *Transversing* machinery causes injuries in a line, such as a conveyer belt or clothing line at a cleaner. Moving elements can drag or trap a patient between the moving elements and a fixed object.
- *Cutting* machinery causes injuries from a band saw, or table saw. Injuries seen are usually amputations.

Figure 37-1   River barge. *(Used with permission from Peter DiPrima.)*

- *Punching* machinery causes injuries from a press that stamps or creates holes in a single stroke. The injuries that occur are usually crushing or puncture.
- *Shearing* machinery causes injuries when two pieces of machinery move parallel to each other. Injuries that occur include cuts, amputations, or crushing injuries.
- *Bending* machinery causes injuries when the material or machinery draws an extremity into the machine. Common injuries seen are fractures and crushing injuries.

Common Injuries Seen

- Fractures
- Crushing injuries
- Amputations
- Burns
- Poisonings and or asphyxiation
- Compartment syndrome (remember the five *P*s of compartment syndrome are *p*ain, *p*aresthesia, *p*assive stretch, *p*ressure, and *p*ulselessness)

INTRODUCTION TO AGRICULTURAL ACCIDENTS

- According to the National Institute for Occupational Safety and Health, agriculture ranks among the most hazardous industries. Farmers are at very high risk for fatal and nonfatal injuries. Farming is one of the few industries in which the families (who often share the work and live on the premises) are also at risk for fatal and nonfatal injuries.
- Approximately 1,859,000 full-time workers were employed in production agriculture in the United States in 2003.
- An estimated 1.08 million children and adolescents under 20 years of age resided on farms in 2001, with about 593,000 of these youth performing

work on the farms. On an average, 103 children are killed annually on farms (1990-1996). Approximately 40% of these deaths are work related. In 2001, an estimated 22,600 children and adolescents were injured on farms; 8,400 of these injuries were due to farm work.

- In an average year, 110 American farm workers are crushed to death by tractor rollovers (1992-2000).
- Every day, about 228 agricultural workers suffer lost-work-time injuries, and about 5% of these result in permanent impairment.

Types of Agricultural Equipment Used

- Tractors
- Combines
- Strippers/pickers
- Augers
- Power takeoffs (PTO)
- Agricultural chemicals

Silo Rescue

- Silos are used to hold grain.
- They are enclosed and are not made for human occupancy.
- At the top they a have a reduced oxygen atmosphere.
- Material located inside could entrap an individual or produce gases as it deteriorates.

Silo Dangers

- Asphyxiation
- Entrapment
- Dust explosion
- Falls
- Collapse of the walls supporting the silo

SCENE MANAGEMENT

- Industrial or agricultural incidents will most likely be chaotic and sometimes confusing.
- It is very important to stay focused and safe!
- Scene size-up is crucial when operating on an industrial accident. Gather all information prior to committing to a situation that may cause injury or death to you or your partner.
- Remember to call for the appropriate resources early and do not perform any rescue by entering an unsafe or hazardous scene.

SPECIALIZED EQUIPMENT USED FOR MACHINERY EXTRICATION OR DISENTANGLEMENT

Figure 37-2 shows some of the heavy rescue equipment used for disentanglement. Figure 37-3 shows a close-up view of the Holmatro "O" cutter and spreader and a windshield cutter. Figure 37-4 shows the valve assembly used to operate an airbag system. Figure 37-5 shows examples of the 1, 3, 5, 12, and 17 ton airbag systems that are used for various types of equipment lifting.

Figure 37-2 Heavy rescue equipment used for disentanglement. *(Used with permission from Peter DiPrima.)*

Figure 37-3 The Holmatro "O" cutter, spreader and a windshield cutter. *(Used with permission from Peter DiPrima.)*

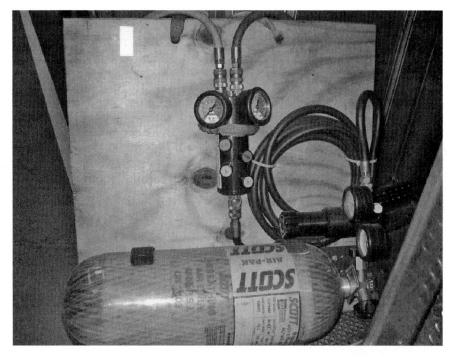

Figure 37-4 Valve assembly used to operate airbag system. *(Used with permission from Peter DiPrima.)*

Figure 37-5 Examples of the 1, 3, 5, 12, and 17 ton airbag system used for various types of equipment lifting. *(Used with permission from Peter DiPrima.)*

? CHAPTER QUESTIONS

Match the following terms with the appropriate definitions.

1. Transversing machinery
2. Cutting machinery
3. Punching machinery
4. Shearing machinery
5. Bending machinery

   a. Causes injury when the material or machinery draws an extremity into the machine; common injuries seen are fractures and crushing injuries

   b. Causes injury in a line, such as a conveyer belt or clothing line at a cleaner; moving elements can drag or trap a patient between the moving elements and a fixed object

   c. Causes injuries from a band saw, or table saw; injuries seen are usually amputations

   d. Causes injuries when two pieces of machinery move parallel to each other; injuries that occur include cuts, amputations, or crushing injuries

   e. Causes injuries from a press that stamps or creates holes in a single stroke; injuries that occur are usually crushing, or punctures

Reference

US Department of Transportation, National Highway Traffic Safety Administration. *EMT-Basic National Standard Curriculum.* Washington, DC: US Department of Transportation, National Highway Traffic Safety Administration; 1994.

CROSSWORD

Across

1. Movement of segments of the body without regard to the forces that caused the movement to occur.

8. A form of shock that presents with tachycardia, hypoperfusion, fever, tachypnea, and altered mental status.

10. The rule of _____ is used to estimate the total body surface area burned.

12. Superficial, partial, and full thickness _____.

13. _____ pressure.

14. _____ segment is two or more ribs broken in two or more places.

15. _____ shock is a form of shock that is defined by hypoperfusion from fluid or blood loss.

Down

2. _____ object is a foreign body that penetrates the skin and remains imbedded in body tissue.

3. The acronym for mechanism of injury.

4. The amount of blood discharged from the right and left ventricles per minute, or stroke volume multiplied by heart rate.

5. Another term used for shock.

6. _____ syndrome is when a muscle has prolonged pressure, for example, a leg stuck under collapsed building material.

7. Acronym for a traumatic brain injury.

9. A hole or wound made by a sharp object.

11. Innermost layer that surrounds the brain.

14. _____ thickness burns are burns that have blisters and redness with severe pain.

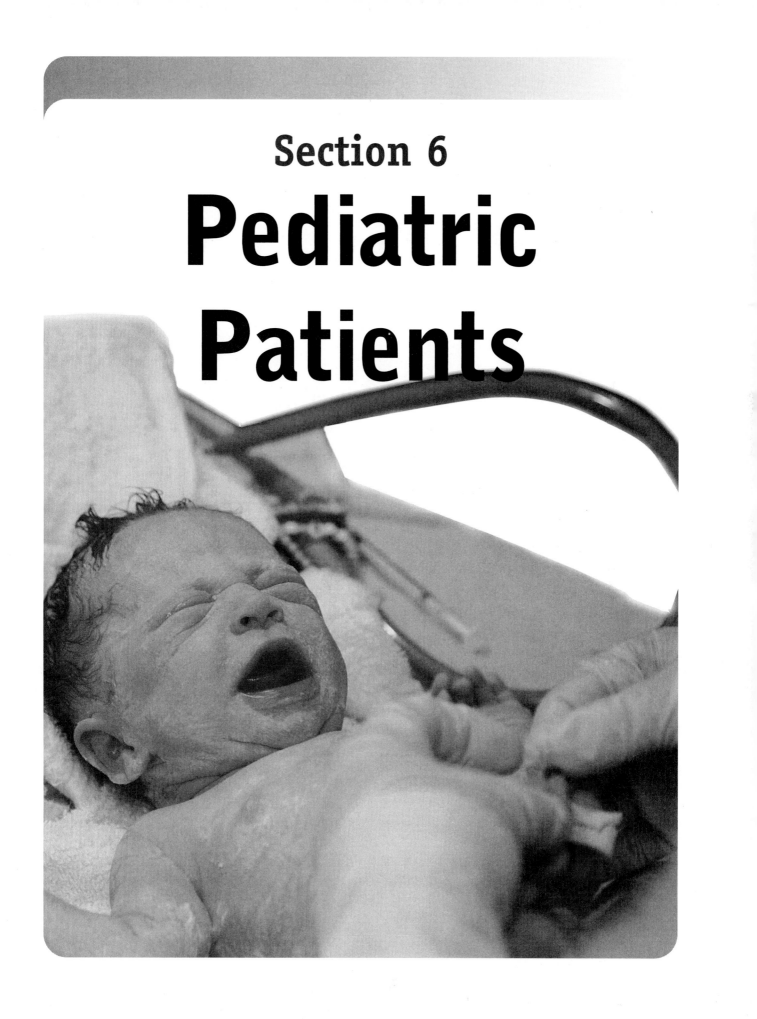

Section 6
Pediatric Patients

Chapter 38
Infants and Children

EMS is dispatched to a private house for an unconscious female child. Upon entering the house, from across the room you see a female child 2 years old listless in her mother's arms. As you approach, the patient's father urgently summons you to "help his daughter." The mother states the patient "stopped breathing and turned blue." You ask the mother if you can take the baby from her arms, and immediately begin assessing the patient's airway. What is your next step during your assessment?

THE HUMAN BODY (INFANTS AND CHILDREN)

Developmental Differences

Newborns (Birth to 1 Month) and Infants (1-12 Months)

- Minimal stranger anxiety.
- Separation anxiety from parents.
- Do not want to be suffocated by an oxygen mask.
- Need to be kept warm—Make sure hands and stethoscope are warmed before touching child.
- Breathing rate best obtained at a distance—Watch chest rise, note color, and level of activity.
- Examine heart and lungs first, head last. This is done to build confidence. It is best to obtain heart and lung sounds before the child becomes agitated.

Toddlers: 1-3 Years

- Do not like to be touched.
- Do not like being separated from parents.
- Do not like having clothing removed. Remove, examine, replace.
- Do not want to be suffocated by an oxygen mask.
- Assure child that he was not bad. Children think their illness/injury is punishment.
- Afraid of needles.
- Fear of pain.
- Should be examined trunk to head approach. This is done to build confidence. It should be done before child becomes agitated.

Preschool: 3-6 Years

- Do not like to be touched.
- Do not like being separated from parents.
- Do not like having clothing removed. Remove, examine, replace.
- Do not want to be suffocated by an oxygen mask.
- Assure child that he was not bad. Children think that the illness/injury is a punishment.
- Afraid of blood.
- Fear of pain.
- Fear of permanent injury.
- Modest.

School Age: 6-12 Years

- Afraid of blood.
- Fear of pain.
- Fear of permanent injury.
- Modest.
- Fear of disfigurement.

Adolescent: 12-18 Years

- Fear of permanent injury.
- Modest.
- Fear of disfigurement.
- Treat them as adults.
- These patients may desire to be assessed privately, away from parents or guardians.

Table 38-1 shows Pediatric Assessment Tools.

Anatomical and Physiological Concerns: The Pediatric Airway

- Small airways throughout the respiratory system are easily blocked by secretions and airway swelling.
- Tongue is large relative to small mandible and can block airway in an unconscious infant or child.
- Positioning the airway is different in infants and children, do not hyperextend the neck. Place the head in a neutral position.
- Infants are obligate nose breathers, so suctioning a secretion-filled nasopharynx can improve breathing problems in an infant.
- Children can compensate well for short periods of time.
  - Compensate by increasing breathing rate and increasing effort of breathing.
  - Compensation is followed rapidly by decompensation due to rapid respiratory muscle fatigue and general fatigue of the infant.

Airway

The most important component of pediatric care is airway, airway, airway!

- The pediatric airway is more anterior than the adult's.
- The diameter of the airway is smaller than the adult patient's.
- Large tongue in relation to the jaw.
- Infants favor breathing through the nose.

TABLE 38-1:   Pediatric Assessment Tools

Pediatric Pulse Rates		
Age	Low	High
Infant (birth-1 y)	100	160
Toddler (1-3 y)	90	150
Preschooler (3-6 y)	80	140
School-age (6-12 y)	70	120
Adolescent (12-18 y)	60	100

Pediatric Respiratory Rates	
Age	Rate (breaths per min)
Infant (birth-1 y)	30-60
Toddler (1-3 y)	24-40
Preschooler (3-6 y)	22-34
School-age (6-12 y)	18-30
Adolescent (12-18 y)	12-16

Low-Normal Pediatric Systolic Blood Pressure	
Age[*]	Low Normal
Infant (birth-1 y)	> 60[*]
Toddler (1-3 y)	>70[*]
Preschooler (3-6 y)	>75
School-age (6-12 y)	> 80
Adolescent (12-18 y)	> 90

[*]Normal vital sign ranges.

This curriculum was developed by the Fire Department of the City of New York under contract with the New York State Department of Health/Health Research Incorporated. Funding was provided through grant #6 H33 MC 00036 from the Emergency Medical Services for Children Program. The Emergency Medical Services for Children (EMSC) Program is administered by the Maternal and Child Health Bureau, Health Resources and Services Administration, Public Health Service, U.S. Department of Health and Human Services in cooperation with the National Highway Traffic Safety Administration.

Health Research Incorporated (HRI) retains title and copyright of this curriculum. This curriculum should not be published or duplicated without prior written consent of HRI, except as required by law. Any references to this curriculum should include the New York State Department of Health and the State of New York. Authors: Ann M. Fitton, EMT-P, Wilfredo Silvestry, EMT-P, John S. McFarland, EMT-P, Peter N. Andryuk, EMT-P, Contributors: Andres Rodriguez, EMT-P, John C. Clappin, Gustave Pappas, EMT-P.

Breathing

- Pediatric patients are dependent on the contraction of their diaphragm to breathe.
- Bradycardia is a late sign of low oxygenation in the pediatric patient.
- Pediatric patients compensate for respiratory distress by increasing their rate, but fatigue easily.

Circulation

- Compensate in shock effectively, but decompensate rapidly.
- Mental status change is a good indicator of hypoperfusion.
- Blood pressure is an unreliable indicator of perfusion in the pediatric patient.
- Hypovolemia can result from vomiting and diarrhea in children.
- Compare strength of central pulses with those of peripheral pulses.

Oxygen Therapy

- High concentration via pediatric nonrebreather mask
- Blow-by techniques such as
  - Holding oxygen tubing 2 in from the patient's face (and oxygen that is set at a liter flow of 1-6 L/min).
  - Insert tubing into a paper cup, and let the patient hold the cup by their face.

Artificial Ventilation

- Bag-valve-mask sizing is important.
- Mask seal:
  - Two-hand method (preferred method)
  - One-hand method
- Mouth-to-mask artificial ventilations with supplemental oxygen attached.
- Use of the bag-valve-mask requires skill and practice!
  - Squeeze bag slowly and evenly enough to make chest rise adequately.
  - Rates for child and infant are 20 breaths per minute.
  - Provide high-concentration oxygen by using an oxygen reservoir.

ASSESSMENT

General impression of a well versus sick child can be obtained from overall appearance. The emergency medical technician (EMT) should assess the following:

- Mental status
- Effort of breathing
- Color
- Quality of cry/speech
- Interaction with environment and parents
  - Normal behavior for child of this age
  - Playing
  - Moving around
  - Attentive versus nonattentive
  - Eye contact
  - Recognizes parents
  - Responds to parents' calling
- Emotional state
- Response to the EMT
- Tone/body position

General Approach to the Pediatric Patient Should Begin from Across the Room

- Mechanism of injury
- Assessment of surroundings
- General impression of well versus sick
- Respiratory assessment:
  - Note chest expansion/symmetry
  - Effort of breathing

- ○ Nasal flaring
- ○ Stridor, crowing, or noisy
- ○ Retractions
- ○ Grunting
- ○ Respiratory rate
- Perfusion assessment—Skin color

Hands-On Approach to Infant or Child Patient Assessment

- Assess breath sounds
- Assess circulation

Detailed Physical Examination

Begin with a trunk-to-head approach.

COMMON PROBLEMS ENCOUNTERED WITH PEDIATRIC PATIENTS

Airway Obstructions

Mild Airway Obstruction: Signs and Symptoms in the Pediatric Patient

- Good air exchange.
- Responsive and can forcefully cough.
- Wheezing may be present.

Severe Airway Obstruction: Signs and Symptoms in the Pediatric Patient

- Poor air exchange
- No air exchange
- High-pitched noise while inhaling (stridor)
- Increased difficulty breathing
- Cyanosis
- Unable to speak or cry
- May exhibit the "universal choking sign"
- Inability to move air

Emergency Management

1 YEAR TO ADOLESCENT (CONSCIOUS)

- Ask, "Are you choking?"
- Give abdominal thrusts/Heimlich maneuver.
- Repeat until foreign body is dislodged or the child goes unconscious.
- Summon advanced life support.

1 YEAR TO ADOLESCENT (UNCONSCIOUS)

- Begin cardiopulmonary resuscitation (CPR).
- Look into the mouth while opening the airway; use a finger sweep only if a foreign body is visible.
- Continue CPR for five cycles or 2 minutes, continue cycles until foreign object is dislodged and prepare for transport.

LESS THAN 1 YEAR OF AGE (CONSCIOUS)

- Confirm severe airway obstruction.
- Evaluate for sudden onset of severe difficulty breathing, ineffective or silent cough, weak or silent cry.
- Give five back slaps and five chest thrusts.
- Repeat until effective or the patient becomes unconscious.
- Summon advanced life support.

LESS THAN 1 YEAR OF AGE (UNCONSCIOUS)

- Begin CPR.
- Look into the mouth while opening the airway; use a finger sweep only if a foreign body is visible.
- Continue CPR for five cycles or 2 minutes, continue cycles until foreign object is dislodged and prepare for transport.

Respiratory Emergencies

- Recognize the difference between upper airway obstruction and lower airway disease.
  - Upper airway obstruction—Stridor on inspiration.
  - Lower airway disease:
    - — Wheezing and breathing effort on exhalation
    - — Rapid breathing (tachypnea) without stridor

Recognize Signs of Increased Effort of Breathing

Respiratory distress is indicated by any of the following:

- Nasal flaring
- Intercostal retraction (neck muscles), supraclavicular, subcostal retractions
- Stridor
- Neck and abdominal muscles—Retractions
- Audible wheezing
- Grunting

Respiratory Failure

Respiratory failure presents with the same signs and symptoms of respiratory distress, and any of the following:

- Breathing rate less than 10 per minute
- Heart rate greater than 60
- Cyanosis
- Decreased muscle tone

- Severe use of accessory muscles
- Poor peripheral perfusion
- Altered mental status
- Grunting

Respiratory Arrest

- Apneic
- Limp muscle tone
- Unconscious
- Slower, absent heart rate
- Weak or absent distal pulses

Emergency Management

- Provide high-concentration oxygen to all children with respiratory emergencies.
- Provide high-concentration oxygen and assist ventilation for severe respiratory distress.
  - Respiratory distress and altered mental status
  - Presence of cyanosis with oxygen
  - Respiratory distress with poor muscle tone

Childhood Respiratory Disease

Croup is a group of respiratory diseases that often affect infants and children under the age of 6. It is characterized by a barking cough; a whistling, obstructive sound (stridor) as the child breathes in; and hoarseness due to obstruction in the region of the larynx. It may be mild, moderate or severe, and severe cases, with breathing difficulty, can be fatal. Another type of croup is known as spasmodic croup. People with spasmodic croup first catch a cold, rarely with fever, and then the croupy cough begins. In some cases, spasmodic croup may begin suddenly without any preceding cold symptoms. Unlike viral croup, spasmodic croup usually recurs, and can occur in older children, and rarely even in adults. Spasmodic croup is thought to be related to allergies.

TABLE 38-2: The Westley Score: Classification of Croup Severity

Feature	Severity			
Chest wall retraction	None = 0	Mild = 1	Moderate = 2	Severe = 3
Stridor	None = 0	With agitation = 1	At rest = 2	
Cyanosis	None = 0	With agitation = 4		At rest = 5
Level of consciousness	Normal = 0 (including sleep)	Disoriented = 5		
Air entry	Normal = 0	Decreased = 1	Markedly decreased = 2	

Data from Muñiz A, Molodow RE, Defendi GL. Croup. Available on: http://emedicine.medscape.com/article/962972-overview.

- A Westley score of less than or equal to 2 designates mild croup (Table 38-2). The characteristic barking cough and hoarseness may be present but without resting stridor.
- A score of 3 to 7 is classified as moderate croup, and typically there will be signs of increased respiratory effort, including accessory muscle recruitment and sternal recession.
- A score of greater than or equal to 8 indicates severe croup, and these children are at the greatest risk of respiratory failure. There is marked in drawing of the sternum, and the child may become fatigued and distressed.

One alarming feature is the reduction of stridor in a child previously demonstrating severe obstructive signs. With worsening airway obstruction, air movement is so limited that the characteristic sound is lost.

Signs and Symptoms

Croup is characterized by a harsh "barking" cough and sneeze, inspiratory stridor (a high-pitched sound heard on inhalation), nausea/vomiting, and fever. Hoarseness is usually present. More severe cases will have respiratory distress.

The "barking" cough (often described as seal-like) of croup is diagnostic. Stridor will be provoked or worsened by agitation or crying. If stridor is also heard when the child is calm, critical narrowing of the airway may be imminent.

Epiglottitis

Epiglottitis is inflammation of the epiglottis the flap that sits at the base of the tongue, which keeps food from going into the trachea (windpipe). Due to its place in the airway, swelling of this structure can interfere with breathing and constitutes a medical emergency. The infection can cause the epiglottis to either obstruct or completely close off the windpipe.

- With the advent of the Hib vaccine, the incidence has been reduced, but the condition has not been eliminated.
- Epiglottitis involves bacterial infection of the epiglottis, most often caused by *Haemophilus influenzae* type B, although some cases are attributable to *Streptococcus pneumoniae* , *S. agalactiae*, *Staphylococcus aureus*, and *S. pyogenes*.

Epiglottitis typically affects children, and is associated with fever, difficulty in swallowing, drooling, hoarseness of voice, and stridor. However, it is important to note that since the introduction of the *H. infuenzae* vaccination in many Western countries (including the UK), the disease is becoming relatively more common in adults. The child often appears acutely ill, anxious, and has very quiet shallow breathing with the head held forward, insisting on sitting up in bed. The early symptoms are insidious but rapidly progressive, and swelling of the throat may lead to cyanosis and asphyxiation. Cases in adults are most typically seen among abusers of crack cocaine and have a more subacute presentation. George Washington is thought to have died of epiglottitis.

Seizures

- Seizures in children who have chronic seizures are rarely life threatening. However, seizures, including febrile, should be considered life threatening by the EMT.
- May be brief or prolonged.

- Assess for presence of injuries that may have occurred during seizures.
- Caused by fever, infections, poisoning, hypoglycemia, trauma, or decreased levels of oxygen, or could be idiopathic in children.
- History of seizures. Ask the following questions:
  - Has the child had prior seizure(s)?
  - If yes, is this the child's normal seizure pattern?
  - Has the child taken his antiseizure medications?

Emergency Management

- Ensure airway position and patency.
- Position patient on side if no possibility of cervical spine trauma.
- Have suction ready.
- Provide oxygen and, if in respiratory arrest or severe respiratory distress, ensure airway position and patency and ventilate with bag-valve-mask.
- Transport. Although brief seizures are not harmful, there may be a more dangerous underlying condition.

Altered Mental Status

Can be caused by a variety of conditions:

- Hypoglycemia
- Poisoning
- Postseizure
- Infection
- Head trauma
- Decreased oxygen levels
- Hypoperfusion (shock)

Emergency Management

- Ensure patency of airway.
- Be prepared to artificially ventilate/suction.
- Transport to the appropriate hospital.

Poisonings

Identify suspected container through adequate history. Bring container to receiving facility if possible.

Emergency Management

RESPONSIVE POISONING PATIENT

- Contact medical control.
- Consider need to administer activated charcoal.
- Provide oxygen.
- Transport.
- Continue to monitor patient—May become unresponsive.

UNRESPONSIVE ROISONING PATIENT

- Ensure patency of airway.
- Be prepared to artificially ventilate.

- Provide oxygen if indicated.
- Call medical control.
- Transport.
- Rule out trauma; trauma can cause altered mental status.

Fever

- Common reason for infant or child ambulance call.
- Many causes—Rarely life threatening. A severe cause is meningitis.
- Fever with a rash is a potentially serious consideration.

Emergency Management

- Transport.
- Be alert for seizures.

Shock (Hypoperfusion)

Rarely a primary cardiac event

Common Causes

- Diarrhea and dehydration
- Trauma
- Vomiting
- Blood loss
- Infection
- Abdominal injuries

Less Common Causes

- Allergic reactions
- Congenital cardiac disease

Signs and Symptoms

- Rapid respiratory rate
- Pale, cool, clammy skin
- Weak or absent peripheral pulses
- Delayed capillary refill
- Decreased urine output; measured by asking parents about diaper wetting and looking at the diaper
- Mental status changes
- Absence of tears, even when crying

Emergency Management

- Ensure airway/oxygen.
- Be prepared to artificially ventilate.
- Manage bleeding if present.
- Elevate legs.
- Keep warm.
- Transport. Note—need for rapid transport of infant and child patients, with secondary examination completed en route, if time permits.

Near Drowning

- Artificial ventilation is a top priority.
- Consider possibility of trauma.
- Consider possibility of hypothermia.
- Consider possible ingestion, especially alcohol.
- Protect airway, suction if necessary.
- Secondary drowning syndrome—Deterioration after breathing normally from minutes to hours after event. All near-drowning victims should be transported to the hospital.

Sudden Infant Death Syndrome (SIDS)

Signs and Symptoms

- Sudden death of infants in first year of life.
- Causes are many and not clearly understood.
- Baby most commonly discovered in the early morning.

Emergency Management

- Try to resuscitate unless rigor mortis.
- Parents will be in agony from emotional distress, remorse, and imagined guilt.
- Avoid any comments that might suggest blame to the parents.

Trauma

- Injuries are the number-one cause of death in infants and children.
- It is not uncommon for a child to be severely injured but display no early obvious signs.
- Blunt injury is most common.
- The pattern of injury will be different from adults.
  - Motor vehicle crashes
    - — Unrestrained passengers have head and neck injuries.
    - — Restrained passengers have abdominal and lower spine injuries.
  - Struck while riding bicycle—Head injury, spinal injury, abdominal injury
  - Pedestrian struck by vehicle—Abdominal injury with internal bleeding, possible painful, swollen, deformed thigh, head injury
  - Falls from height, diving into shallow water—Head and neck injuries
  - Burns
  - Sports injuries—Head and neck
  - Child abuse

REVIEW OF SPECIFIC BODY SYSTEMS

Head

- The single most important maneuver is to ensure an open airway by means of the modified jaw thrust.
- Children are likely to sustain head injury along with internal injuries. Signs and symptoms of shock (hypoperfusion) with a head injury should cause you to be suspicious of other possible injuries.

- Respiratory arrest is common secondary to head injuries and may occur during transport.
- Common signs and symptoms are nausea and vomiting.
- Most common cause of hypoxia in the unconscious head injury patient is the tongue obstructing the airway. Jaw thrust is critically important.
- Do not use sandbags to stabilize the head because the weight on child's head may cause injury if the board needs to be turned for emesis.

Chest

- Children have very soft pliable ribs.
- There may be significant injuries without external signs.

Abdomen

- More common site of injury in children than adults.
- Often a source of hidden injury.
- Always consider abdominal injury in the multiple trauma patients who is deteriorating without external signs.
- Gastric distention can distend abdomen and interfere with artificial ventilation efforts.

Extremities

Extremity injuries are managed in the same manner as adults.

CHILD ABUSE AND NEGLECT

- Child abuse encompasses the most serious harm committed against children. An abused child is one whose parent or legal guardian inflicts serious physical injury, creates a risk for serious injury, or commits a sex act against the child.
- Maltreatment including neglect means the child's physical, mental, or emotional condition has been impaired, or placed in imminent danger by the parent or legal guardian.
- The EMT must be aware of condition to be able to recognize the problem.
- Signs and symptoms of abuse:
  - Multiple bruises in various stages of healing.
  - Injury inconsistent with mechanism described.
  - Repeated calls to the same address.
  - Fresh burns.
  - Parents seem inappropriately unconcerned.
  - Conflicting stories.
  - Fear on the part of the child to discuss how the injury occurred.
  - Central nervous system (CNS) injuries are the most lethal—Shaken baby syndrome.
- Signs and symptoms of neglect:
  - Lack of adult supervision.
  - Malnourished appearing child.

- ○ Unsafe living environment.
- ○ Untreated chronic illness.
- • Do not accuse in the field.
  - ○ Accusation and confrontation delays transportation.
  - ○ Bring objective information to the receiving facility.
    - — Objective—What you see and what you hear—*not* what you think.

SPECIAL NEEDS PEDIATRIC PATIENTS

This can include many different types of situations.

- • Premature babies with lung disease
- • Babies and children with heart disease
- • Infants and children with neurologic disease
- • Children with chronic disease or altered function from birth

Often special needs children will be at home, technologically dependent.

Tracheotomy Tube

Common Complications
- • Obstruction
- • Bleeding
- • Air leak
- • Dislodged
- • Infection

Emergency Management
- • Maintain an open airway.
- • Suction as needed.
- • Maintain position of comfort.
- • Transport.

Home Ventilators

Usually the parent or guardian is familiar with operation of a home ventilator.

Emergency Management
- • Guarantee patent airway.
- • Artificially ventilate with high-concentration oxygen.
- • Transport.

Central Lines

- • Intravenous lines (IVs) that are placed near the heart for long-term use.
  - ○ Complications include cracked line, infection, clotting off, or bleeding.

Emergency Management

- If bleeding is present, apply pressure.
- Transport.

Gastrostomy tubes and gastric feeding are placed directly into stomach for feeding. These patients usually cannot be fed by mouth.

- Be alert for breathing problems.
- Ensure adequate airway.
- Have suction available.
- If a diabetic patient, be alert for altered mental status. Infant will become hypoglycemic quickly if they cannot be fed.
- Provide oxygen.
- Transport.

Shunts are devices running from the brain to the abdomen to drain excess cerebral spinal fluid. Will find reservoir on side of skull.

- Change in mental status
- Prone to respiratory arrest
  - Manage airway.
  - Ensure adequate artificial ventilation.
  - Transport.

FAMILY RESPONSE TO A CHILD'S ILLNESS OR INJURY

- A child cannot be cared for in isolation from the family; therefore, you have multiple patients.
- Striving for calm, supportive interaction with family will result in improved ability to deal with the child. Calm parents = calm child; agitated parents = agitated child.
- Anxiety arises from concern over child's pain; fear for child's well-being.
- Worsened by sense of helplessness.
- Parent may respond to EMT with anger or hysteria.
- Parents should remain part of the care unless child is not aware or medical conditions require separation.
- Parents should be instructed to calm child; can maintain position of comfort and/or hold oxygen.
- Parents may not have medical training, but they are experts on what is normal or abnormal for their children and what will have a calming effect.

Provider Response

- Anxiety from lack of experience with treating children as well as fear of failure.
- Skills can be learned and applied to children.
- Stress from identifying patient with their own children.
- Provider should realize that much of what they learned about adults applies to children; they need to remember the differences.
- Infrequent encounters with sick children; advance preparation is important (practice with equipment and examining children).

? CHAPTER QUESTIONS

1. Emotional and physical characteristics of adolescents include:

   a. believing that, generally, nothing bad can happen to them

   b. concerns about death and disability first emerge in this age group

   c. believing the illness or injury that they have is some form of punishment

   d. having vivid imaginations and being able to dramatize events

2. When examining and caring for an infant:

   a. Begin your assessment with the head, and end with the feet.

   b. Complete your scene size-up and initial assessment from across the room.

   c. Explain each procedure that you are going to do to the infant.

   d. Separate the infant from the caregiver during assessment.

3. An 8-year-old child:

   a. has no understanding of what EMS is about

   b. is preoccupied with his/her body and is extremely concerned about modesty

   c. is the most difficult to manage

   d. is able to rationalize, and may be curious about what you are doing

4. When treating a child, keep in mind that:

   a. The child's ribs are more rigid than an adult's.

   b. The tracheal diameter of a newborn is the same as that of an adult.

   c. The child's skin surface is small compared to body mass.

   d. Infants and children have a higher metabolic rate, so periods of poor oxygenation can be more dangerous.

5. Which of the following is correct regarding infants' and children's respiratory status?

   a. Compensatory mechanisms are the same as an adult's, and they will both gradually deteriorate.

   b. The leading cause of cardiac arrest in infants and children is failure of the respiratory system.

   c. It is not important to distinguish between an upper airway obstruction from a foreign body and an obstruction caused by a respiratory condition.

   d. Determining the origin of the child's respiratory dysfunction is essential in the pre-hospital setting to appropriately care for the patient.

6. A child is displaying nasal flaring and retractions, but is maintaining an adequate respiratory rate and depth. This child is in:

   a. decompensated respiratory failure

   b. compensated respiratory failure

   c. early decompensated failure

   d. late respiratory distress

7. Indications that a pediatric patient has a partial airway obstruction include:

a. crowing or other noisy respirations

b. ineffective or absent cough

c. no crying or talking

d. unresponsiveness

8. Important sounds to listen for include:

a. stridor, which sounds like rolling a few strands of hair near the ear

b. crackles, which are harsh, high-pitched sounds that occur during inspiration

c. rales, which are loud, gurgling sounds occurring during exhalation

d. wheezing, which is caused by air moving at a high rate through narrowed bronchioles

9. While assessing the circulation of a 2-year-old child, you should check all of the following except:

a. warmth and color of hands and feet

b. mental status

c. blood pressure

d. capillary refill

Reference

US Department of Transportation, National Highway Traffic Safety Administration. *EMT-Basic National Standard Curriculum.* Washington, DC: US Department of Transportation, National Highway Traffic Safety Administration; 1994.

Section 7
Operations

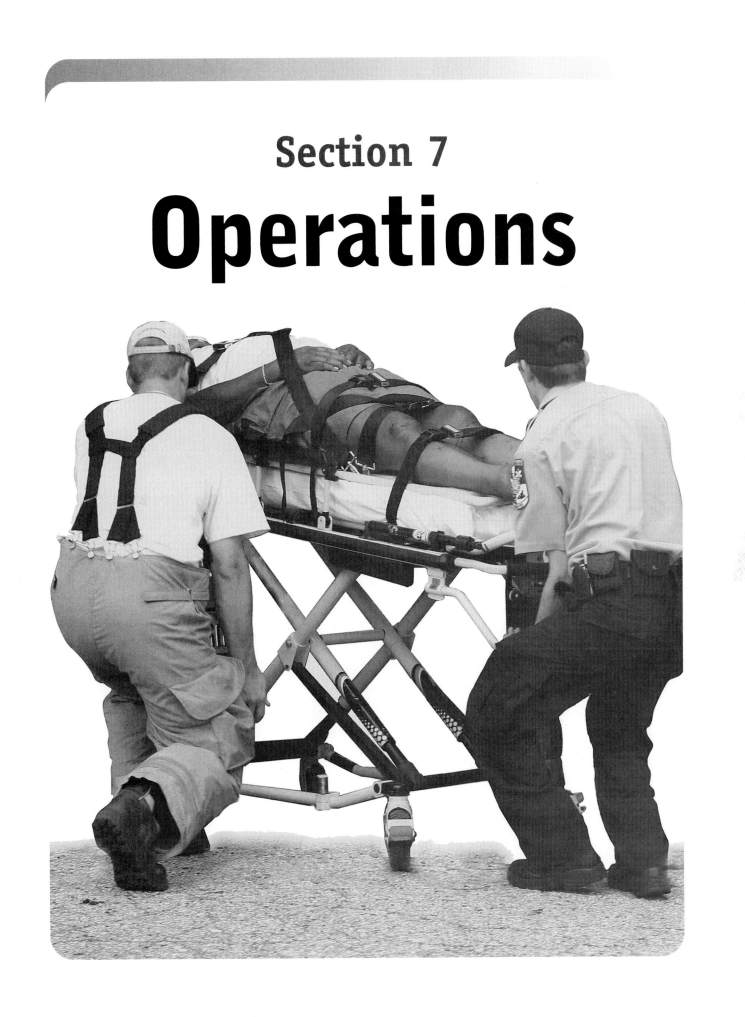

Chapter 39
Ambulance Operations

PHASES OF AN AMBULANCE CALL

Preassignment Operations and Check

- Preparation for the call
  - Necessary equipment needed for a medical assignment:
    — Basic supplies
    — Patient transfer equipment
    — Airways
    — Suction equipment
    — Artificial ventilation devices
    — Oxygen inhalation equipment
    — Cardiac compression equipment
    — Basic wound care supplies
    — Splinting supplies
    — Childbirth supplies
    — Medications
    — Automated external defibrillator
  - Essential nonmedical equipment needed:
    — Personal safety equipment per local, state, and federal standards
    — Preplanned routes or comprehensive street maps
- Personnel requirements:
  - At least one EMT in patient compartment is minimum staffing for an ambulance, two are preferred.
- Daily inspections of the vehicle systems include:
  - Fuel (Tank should be full.)
  - Oil (Level should be checked at the beginning of every tour/shift.) (Fig. 39-1)
  - Engine cooling system
  - Battery
  - Brakes (test)
  - Wheels and tires (Adequate tread should be on every tire for adequate traction.)
  - Headlights (working properly)
  - Stoplights (working properly)
  - Turn signals (working properly)
  - Emergency warning lights (working properly)

Transmission fluid dipstick

Engine oil dipstick

Figure 39-1   Under the hood of an ambulance.

- Wipers (working properly)
- Horn (working properly)
- Siren (working properly)
- Doors closing and latching (working properly)
- Communication system (working properly)
- Air conditioning/heating system/ventilation system (working properly)
- Equipment
  - Checked, maintained, restocked, and repaired as required.
  - Batteries for defibrillator, suction should be at full charge and ready for use.

Assignment Operations

Dispatch Center

- Central access
- 24 hour availability
- Trained dispatch personnel (emergency medical dispatch [EMD] certified)
- Dispatch information for responding units
  - Nature of call
  - Name, location, and callback number of caller
  - Location of patient
  - Number of patients and severity
  - Other special problems

En Route

- Seat belts should be worn.
- Notify dispatch (acknowledge assignment).
- Ascertain essential information.
  - Nature of the call
  - Location of the call
- Driving the ambulance with due regard for the public during emergency vehicle operations and nonemergency situations.

- Characteristics of good ambulance operators:
  - Physically fit
  - Mentally fit
  - Able to perform under stress
  - Positive attitude about abilities
  - Tolerant of other drivers
- Safe driving is as important as providing emergency medical care to the ill or injured patient (Fig. 39-2).
  - The driver and all passengers should wear safety belts.
  - Become familiar with the characteristics of your vehicle.
  - Be alert to changes in weather and road conditions.
  - Exercise caution in use of red lights and siren.
  - Select appropriate route.
  - Maintain safe following distance.
  - Drive with due regard for safety of all others.
  - Know appropriateness of using lights and sirens.
  - Headlights are the most visible warning device on an emergency vehicle.
- Obtain additional information from dispatch.
- Assign personnel to specific duties.
- Assess specific equipment needs.
- Positioning the unit:
  - For safety.
  - Uphill from leaking hazards.
  - 100 ft from wreckage.
  - In front of the wreckage or beyond the wreckage.
  - Set parking brake.

Figure 39-2 Ambulance accident. An ambulance on its way to a hospital swerved into an elevated train support attempting to avoid an oncoming vehicle. *(Used with permission from Peter DiPrima.)*

- ○ Utilize warning lights.
- ○ Shut off headlights unless there is a need to illuminate the scene.
- To exit the scene, avoid parking in a location that will hamper exit from the scene.
- Review state and local laws, regulations, or ordinances in the area relative to the operations of an emergency vehicle, including:
  - ○ Vehicle parking or standing
  - ○ Procedures at red lights, stop signs, and intersections
  - ○ Regulations regarding speed limits
  - ○ Direction of flow or specified turns
  - ○ Emergency or disaster routes
  - ○ Use of audible warning devices
  - ○ Use of visual warning devices
  - ○ Laws regarding a school bus

Escorts and Multiple Vehicle Response

- Extremely dangerous.
- Used only if unfamiliar with location of patient or receiving facility.
- No vehicle should use lights or siren.
- Provide a safe following distance.
- Recognize hazards of multiple vehicle response.

Intersection crashes (most common type of ambulance crash)

- Motorist arriving at intersection as light changes and does not stop.
- Multiple emergency vehicles following closely, and an awaiting motorist does not expect more than one, and vision is obstructed by vehicles.

Arrival at Scene

(Fig. 39-3)

- Notify dispatch.
- Size-up:
  - ○ Body substance isolation.
  - ○ Scene safety—Assess the scene for hazards.
  - ○ Mechanism of injury/nature of illness:
    — Medical
      - Mass casualty incident.
      - Determine the number of patients.
      - Obtain additional help as needed.
      - Begin triage.
      - Provide c-spine stabilization as necessary.
    — Trauma
      - Mass casualty incident.
      - Number of patients.
      - Obtain additional help.
      - Begin triage.
      - Spine stabilization if necessary.
      - Total number of patients.
      - Need for additional help or assistance.

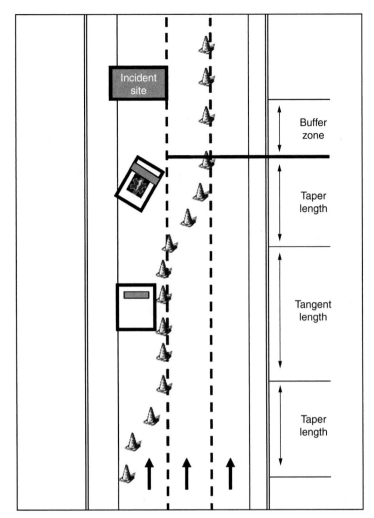

Figure 39-3 Proper rig placement at an accident scene. *(Used with permission from Peter DiPrima.)*

Actions at the Scene
- Be organized.
- Perform rapid/efficient treatment.
- Goal of transport in mind.

Transferring the Patient to the Ambulance
- Preparing the patient for transport.
- Completion of critical interventions.
- Check dressings and splints.
- Patient covered and secured to moving device.
- Lifting and moving is accomplished using the guidelines found in Chapter 6, section on preparing to lift and move patients.

En Route to the Receiving Facility
- Notify dispatch.
- On-going assessment should be continued.

- Additional vital sign measurements should be obtained.
- Notify receiving facility.
- Reassure patient.
- Complete pre-hospital care reports.

At Receiving Facility

- Notify dispatch.
- Transfer the patient at the facility.

Reports

- A complete verbal report is given at bedside.
- A complete written report is completed, and left prior to returning to service.

En Route to Station

- At station or receiving facility, notify dispatch.
- Prepare for the next call. Restock supplies that were used.
- Clean and disinfect the ambulance as needed.
- Clean and disinfect ambulance equipment.

Postrun

- Refuel unit.
- File reports.
- Complete cleaning and disinfection procedures.
- Notify dispatch.

AIR MEDICAL CONSIDERATION—UTILIZATION, LANDING ZONES, AND SAFETY

- When requesting a Medivac, provide:
  - Your agency
  - Location of incident (cross streets)
  - Landing zone (LZ) information
  - LZ sector name
  - Patient information
  - Radio frequency you are operating on

LZ PREPARATION

- The LZ should be 100′ × 100′, clear of overhead wires, free from debris, level flat, and clearly marked (Fig. 39-4).
- Turn off any lights that could blind the pilot during landing and takeoff.

During and After Landing

- Never approach the tail rotor.
- Protect the patient and yourself from rotor wash.

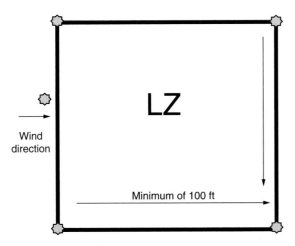

Figure 39-4 Landing zone.

? CHAPTER QUESTIONS

1. The phases of an ambulance call include all of the following except:

   a. daily vehicle and equipment inspection
   b. billing and collections
   c. en route to the receiving facility
   d. en route to the scene

2. Use of escort vehicles during an emergency response is often a:

   a. very quick way to respond
   b. more dangerous means of response and increases the chance for collision
   c. means of decreasing an ambulance collision
   d. way to make the driver's job easier

3. Emergency vehicle operators must drive with the safety of others in mind. This concept is known as driving:

   a. within the law
   b. with due regard
   c. in the emergency mode
   d. within intent

Chapter 40
Gaining Access and Extrication

FUNDAMENTALS OF EXTRICATION

- Role of the emergency medical technician (EMT) in nonrescue emergency medical services (EMS):
  - Administer necessary care to the patient before extrication and assure that the patient is removed in a way to minimize further injury.
  - Patient care precedes extrication unless delayed movement would endanger life of the patient or rescuer.
  - Working with others:
    — The nonrescue EMS provider will need to work together with the providers of rescue.
    — The nonrescue EMT should cooperate with the activities of the rescuers, and not allow their activities to interfere with patient care.
- Role of the EMT in rescue EMS:
  - In some instances, the EMS providers are also the rescue providers.
  - A chain of command should be established to assure patient care priorities.
    — Administer necessary care to the patient before extrication and assure that the patient is removed in a way to minimize further injury.
    — Patient care precedes extrication unless delayed movement would endanger life of the patient or rescuer.

EQUIPMENT

- Basic equipment should be on the ambulance at all times (Fig. 40-1)

PERSONAL SAFETY

- The number-one priority for all EMS personnel.
- Protective clothing that is appropriate for the situation should be utilized.

PATIENT SAFETY

Following the safety of the EMS responders, the next priority is the safety of the patient.

- The patient should be informed of the unique aspects of extrication.
- The patient should be protected from broken glass, sharp metal, and other hazards, including the environment.

Figure 40-1 Basic equipment carried on an ambulance. (*Used with permission from Peter DiPrima.*)

GETTING TO THE PATIENT

Simple access does not require equipment.

- Try opening each door.
- Roll down windows.
- Have patient unlock doors.

Complex access requires use of tools, special equipment. These are separate programs that should be taken (trench, high angle, and basic vehicle rescue).

REMOVING THE PATIENT

- Maintain cervical spine stabilization. Immobilize spine securely.
- Complete initial assessment, provide critical interventions.

? CHAPTER QUESTIONS

1. When gaining access to a patient, the EMT should:

   a. try opening each door
   b. roll down windows
   c. have patient unlock doors if capable
   d. all of the above are correct

2. The number-one priority at any EMS assignment is crew safety.

   a. True
   b. False

Chapter 41
Response to Hazardous Materials

It is a midsummer day; the temperature has peaked at 98°F, and the humidity is 58%. Dispatch summons your ambulance to an overturn on Interstate 1 involving a tanker tractor trailer. As information is gathered by the dispatcher, she relays the information to your unit. Reports are coming in to central dispatch of rollover motor vehicle collision with people trapped. Upon arrival, you find an overturned 18-wheel tanker truck. Your partner notices during your scene survey that a green haze is emanating from the tanker portion of the truck. You notify dispatch that you are relocating to a safe location, and set up a staging area about half-mile away. You let incoming units know of the staging area and request the response of the county hazardous materials unit. Bystanders are reporting the driver is trapped and is seriously injured. You use the binoculars to survey the scene from a distance and confirm the driver is pinned in the vehicle. You also notice a UN placard number on the side of the vehicle. The United Nations (UN) number is 3355.

Is this the appropriate response for this incident so far?

HAZARDOUS MATERIALS (HAZ-MAT)

Any substance or material capable of posing a risk to health, safety, and property. Traditionally, the fire service was called to manage these events. In 1986, emergency medical services (EMS) involvement was mandated by Congress when they passed the Superfund Amendments and Reauthorizations Act (SARA), Title III.

- In 1989, the Occupational Safety and Health Administration (OSHA) required specific training for all EMS personnel who might respond to haz-mat incidents.
- The Department of Transportation (DOT) regulates all aspects of transporting hazmat in the United States. This also includes design and type of container that must be used for transport.

EMT Response to Hazardous Materials

- Incident size-up (First priority is scene safety.)
- Recognition and/or confirmation that incident involves hazardous materials

Maintain a high index of suspicion when responding to incidents involving:

- Transportation
- Highway crashes

- Storage facilities
- Manufacturing plants
- Acts of terrorism

Use one of the following resources to identify the substance:

- Department of Transportation (DOT) North American Emergency Response Guide (NAERG)
- United Nations (UN) numbers
- National Fire Protection Agency (NFPA) 704 placard system
- DOT placards
- Shipping papers (found in the driver's compartment of tractor trailers, also known as the shipping manifest)
- Material safety data sheets (MSDS)

The above resources will assist the first responder in determining:

- Immediate need for evacuation
- Immediate action with ambulatory patients
- Zones, such as
  - Hot zone—Dangerous area
  - Warm zone—Entry/decontamination point
  - Cold zone—Safe area
- Assessment of toxicological risk
- Type of chemical
- Specific actions of a chemical and its reactivity to water
- Potential for secondary contamination
- Specific out-of-hospital medical treatment
- Appropriate techniques in decontamination of patients

Priority is to treat decontaminated patients and to transport patients that pose no risk of contaminating you or your equipment.

NFPA outlines levels of response, including what level of training is required by all personnel who may arrive first. All first responders must be trained to an awareness level.

- Emergency medical technicians (EMTs) who may transport "semidecontaminated patients" must be trained to the NFPA 473 Level-1.
- EMTs who may have to rapidly "decon" and assist in the decontamination corridor must be trained to the 473 Level-2.

Hazardous materials scene size-up includes a high degree of awareness. Responding to any one of the following could be a potential hazardous materials incident and should be approached with caution:

- Vehicle crashes
- Commercial vehicles
- Pest control vehicles
- Tankers
- Cars with alternative fuels
- Tractor-trailers
- Mass transportation
  - Railroads (Fig. 41-1)
  - Pipelines

Figure 41-1   Derailed train car carrying hazardous materials. The aftermath of Hurricane Katrina included one of many derailed train cars carrying hazardous materials (UN 3257).

- Mass storage facilities
  - Tanks/storage vessels
  - Warehouses
  - Hardware/agricultural stores
  - Agriculture
  - Manufacturing operations
  - Chemical plants
- Terrorism
- Shopping centers
- Other public environments
- Health-care facilities
- Laboratories

Recognizing Hazards

- Placarding of vehicles (required by law, some vehicles not placarded).
- Use of the NAERG could assist the paramedic in determining the specific chemical.

Common UN/DOT placard classifications are listed below:

- Explosives
- Gases
- Flammable liquids
- Flammable solids
- Oxidizers and organic peroxides
- Poisonous and etiologic agents
- Radioactive materials

- Corrosives
- Miscellaneous hazardous materials

NFPA 704 system for fixed facilities (Fig. 41-2a and b)

- Blue = health hazard
- Red = fire hazard
- Yellow = reactivity hazard

Health Hazard:
4—Deadly
3—Extreme danger
2—Hazardous
1—Slightly hazardous
0—Normal material

Fire Hazard:
Flash points
4—Below 73°F
3—Below 100°F
2—Below 200°F
1—Above 200°F
0—Will not burn

Special Hazards:
Oxidizer—OXY
Acid—ACID
Alkali—ALK
Corrosive—COR
Use no water—W
Radiation hazard—

Reactivity:
4—May detonate
3—Shock and heat may detonate
2—Violent chemical change
1—Unstable if heated
0—Stable

A

B

Figure 41-2 **A.** NFPA 704 placard. **B.** Example of the NFPA 704 on the entryway to a factory.

Identification of Substances

The origin of dealing with a hazardous material is often difficult—especially with unknown substances. Using resources such as the material safety data sheets (MSDS) may reveal detailed substance information. Shipping papers may also assist in revealing substance identification. Other resources used in responding to hazardous materials include:

- Poison control centers
- CAMEO (computer-aided management of emergency operations) computer database information
- Computer modeling for plumes
- CHEMTREC (Chemical Transportation Emergency Center) (1-800-424-9300; 24-hour toll-free hotline)
- Other reference sources
  - Textbooks
  - Handbooks
  - Technical specialists

Hazardous Material Response Teams utilize specialized recognition equipment to monitor and recognize unknown chemicals. This equipment includes:

- Air monitoring equipment
- Gas monitoring equipment
- Ph testing
- Chemical testing
- Colormetric tube testing

Hazardous Material Zones

(Fig. 41-3)

Hot Zone

- Contamination actually present
- Site of incident/release
- Entry with high-level personal protective equipment (PPE)
- Entry limited to trained hazardous materials team members

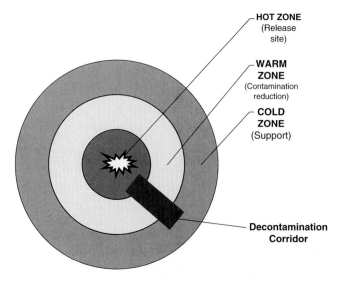

HOT ZONE
(Release site)

WARM ZONE
(Contamination reduction)

COLD ZONE
(Support)

Decontamination Corridor

Figure 41-3   Hazardous materials zones.

Warm Zone

- Buffer zone outside of hot zone
- Where decontamination corridor is located
- Corridor has "hot" and "cold" ends
- Authorized trained hazardous materials team members

Cold Zone

- Safe area
- Staging for personnel and equipment
- Where medical monitoring occurs
- One end of corridor
- Safe operation area for EMS personnel

Specific Terminology for Medical Hazardous Materials Operations

- Boiling point (BP)—The temperature at which the vapor pressure of the material being heated equals atmospheric pressure.
- Flammable/explosive limits—The highest and lowest concentrations of a substance that can explode or burn.
- Flash point (FP)—The lowest temperature at which the vapor given off by a substance forms an ignitable mixture with air.
- Ignition temperature—Minimum temperature to which a substance must be heated before it will spontaneously burn independently of the source of heat.
- Specific gravity—The ratio of the density of a solid or liquid to the density of water.
- Vapor density (VD)—The relative density of a vapor compared to air.
- Vapor pressure—A measure of how readily a solid or liquid mixes with air at its surface. Vapor pressure approaching 760 mm Hg indicates a volatile substance and suggests that there will be high concentration in the air.
- Water solubility—The degree to which a material or its vapors dissolve in water.
- Alpha radiation—Massive and travel only 3 to 4 in from their radioactive source.
- Beta radiation—More energetic and less massive than alpha particles. Beta particles can travel up to 100 ft from their source.
- Gamma radiation is not particles but forms of pure energy and can travel great distances from its source.

Specific Toxicological Terms

- Threshold limit value (TLV)—A TLV reflects the level of exposure that the typical worker can experience without an unreasonable risk of disease or injury. TLVs are not quantitative estimates of risk at different exposure levels or by different routes of exposure.
- Lethal concentration and doses (LD_{50})—An LD_{50} value is the amount of a solid or liquid material that it takes to kill 50% of test animals (eg, mice or rats) in one dose.
- Parts per million (PPM)—PPM is defined as the mass of the component in solution divided by the total mass of the solution multiplied by 10^6 (one million).

- Immediately dangerous to life and health (IDLH)—This concentration is considered to be the limit beyond which an individual will not be capable of escaping death or permanent injury without help in less than 30 minutes.
- Permissible exposure limit (PEL)—A permissible exposure limit (PEL) is the maximum amount or concentration of a chemical that a worker may be exposed to under OSHA regulations.
- Short-term exposure limit (TLV-STEL)—A short-term exposure limit (STEL) is defined as the concentration to which workers can be exposed continuously for a short period of time without suffering from:
  - Irritation
  - Chronic or irreversible tissue damage
  - Narcosis of sufficient degree to increase the likelihood of accidental injury, impair self-rescue, or materially reduce work efficiency
- Ceiling level (TLV-C)—At no time should this exposure limit be exceeded.

TYPES OF CONTAMINATION

- Primary contamination
  - Exposure to substance
  - Only harmful to individual
  - Little chance of exposure to others
- Secondary contamination
  - Exposure to substance.
  - Substance easily transferred.
  - Touching patient results in contamination.
  - Key concept in hazardous materials medical operations.
  - Gas exposure rarely results in secondary contamination.
  - Liquid and particulate matter more likely to result in secondary contamination.

HOW POISONS ARE ABSORBED

- Topical absorption
  - Skin and mucous membranes.
  - Not all skin absorbs at the same rate and not all poisons are easily absorbed.
- Respiratory inhalation
  - Absorption through bronchial tree
  - Oxygen-deficient atmospheres
- Gastrointestinal ingestion
  - Ingestion of substances
  - Factors affecting absorption
- Parenteral injection
  - Injection
  - Wound entry
  - Invasive medical procedures

CYCLE OF POISON ACTIONS

- Absorption
  - Time to delivery into blood stream
- Distribution
  - Distribution to target organs
  - Poison or drug binds to tissues/molecules
  - Actions
  - Deposits
- Biotransformation
  - Liver
- Elimination through
  - Gastrointestinal (GI)
  - Kidneys
  - Respiratory system
- Actions of poisons are determined by several factors including:
  - Acute toxicity
    — Immediate effect from substance
  - Delayed toxicity
    — No immediate effect
    — Symptoms appear later
    — Delayed pathology or disease
  - Local effects
    — Effect immediate at the contaminated site
    — Burn model
    — Progression of effects like burn
    — Topical or respiratory
    — Skin irritation—Acute bronchospasm
  - Systemic effects
    — Cardiovascular
    — Neurological
    — Hepatic
    — Renal
  - Dose response
    — Physiologic response to dosage.
    — How much to get an effect?
    — Essential concept for decontamination.
  - Synergistic effects
    — Combinations may react synergistically.
    — Standard pharmacologic approach.
    — Standard treatment can result in synergy.
    — Medical control/poison control reference.

COMMONLY ENCOUNTERED HAZARDOUS MATERIALS

- Corrosives (acids/alkalis)
- Pulmonary irritants (ammonia/chlorine)

- Pesticides (carbamates/organophosphates)
- Chemical asphyxiants (cyanide/CO)
- Hydrocarbon solvents (xylene/methylene chloride)

CONSIDERATIONS FOR PERFORMING INVASIVE PROCEDURES

Risk versus benefit (Will treating the patient contaminate you or further contaminate the patient?)

- The primary purpose of decontamination is to reduce the patient's dosage of material, decrease the threat of secondary contamination, and reduce the risk of rescuer injury and contamination.
- Environmental considerations are a consideration if there are no life threats. Trained hazardous materials response team members will prevent runoff of material. If there are life threats, patient comes first. Remember, only trained and fully protected haz-mat response team members should rescue victims of a hazardous materials incident.

Modes of Decontamination

- Dilution
  - Lavage with copious amounts of water
  - Water is universal decontamination solution
  - Dilution decreases dose and action
  - Reduction of topical absorption
- Absorption
  - Use of pads to "blot" up the material
  - Towels to dry the patient after lavage
  - Usually a secondary method to lavage
  - Common for environmental cleanup
- Neutralization
  - Almost never used in patient decontamination
  - Hazard of exothermic reactions
  - Time to determine neutralizing substance
  - Lavage usually dilutes and removes faster
- Disposal/isolation
  - Removal of clothing
  - Removal of substances

Decontamination Decision Making

- Field considerations include flight of walking contaminated victims to rescuers—"fast break" event—action required now.
- Conscious, contaminated people will "self-rescue" by walking out of hot zone.
- Immediate decontamination often not avoidable.
- Speed of hazardous material team response may hinder walking contaminated.

EMS Gross Decontamination and Treatment

- All EMS need gross decontamination capability.
- EMS should be prepared for quick decontamination.
- Need for rapid EMS PPE.
- Need quick transport isolation methods.

"Fast Break" Incident Decision Making

- Critical patient—Unknown/life-threatening material (remember patients who are contaminated are a risk to the EMS crew as well as equipment and the emergency department).
- Decontamination and treatment should be simultaneous.
- Remove clothing (80% of contamination is removed by having the patient remove their clothing).
- Treat life-threatening problems.
- Lavage—Water is universal decontamination solution.
- Contain/isolate patient.
- Transport.
- Noncritical—Unknown/life-threatening material
  - More contemplative approach
  - Decontamination and treatment simultaneous
  - Remove clothing
  - Treat life-threatening problems
  - Lavage—Water is universal decontamination solution
  - Contain/isolate patient
  - Transport
- Noncritical—Substance known
  - Slower approach
  - Environmental/privacy considerations
  - More thorough decontamination
  - Clothing removal
  - Thorough lavage/wash
  - Drying/reclothing PRN
  - Medical monitoring
  - Patient isolation PRN
  - Transport

Longer-Duration Event Decision Making

- Patients in hot zone—Nonambulatory
  - No rescue attempted
  - Wait for hazardous materials team
  - Team will set up decontamination corridor
- Haz-mat team will not make entry until:
  - Medical monitoring of entry team
  - Decontamination corridor established
  - Longer duration event
  - Often 60 minutes for team deployment

- ○ Set up time
- ○ Better opportunity for thorough decontamination
- ○ Better PPE
- ○ Less chance of secondary contamination
- ○ Better environmental protection

Decontamination Methods Used by Trained Personnel

- • Decontamination and PPE is driven by the substance encountered.
- • Decontamination solutions
  - ○ Do not attempt to neutralize.
  - ○ Lavage with copious amounts of water.
  - ○ Water is the universal solution.
  - ○ Tincture of green soap used to improve wash.
  - ○ Isopropyl alcohol is used for some isocyanates.
  - ○ Vegetable oil is used for some water-reactive substances.
- • Remove the clothing
  - ○ Also remove rings and jewelry.
  - ○ Shoes and socks.
  - ○ Cut off clothing PRN.
- • Thorough wash and rinse
  - ○ Allow fluid to drain away.
  - ○ Don't allow them to stay in the run-off.
- • Rewash and rinse
  - ○ Pay careful attention to difficult areas to decontaminate:
    — Scalp/hair
    — Ears/ear canals/nostrils
    — Axilla
    — Fingernails
    — Navel
    — Groin/buttocks/genitalia
    — Behind knees
    — Between toes, toenails

LEVELS OF TRAINED HAZARDOUS MATERIALS PERSONAL PROTECTION EQUIPMENT

There are four levels of protection (Fig. 41-4).

- • Level "A" protection
  - ○ Highest level of personal protection
  - ○ Highest degree of protection from chemical breakthrough
  - ○ Fully encapsulated suit
  - ○ Covers everything including SCBA
  - ○ Impermeable/sealed
  - ○ Typically used by hazardous materials team for entry into hot zone
- • Level "B" protection
  - ○ Level of protection typically worn by decontamination team
  - ○ Decontamination wears one level below entry
  - ○ Usually nonencapsulating protection

- ○ SCBA worn outside suit
- ○ Easier entry and SCBA bottle changes
- ○ Easier to work in
- ○ High degree of repellence
- Level "C" protection
  - ○ Nonpermeable clothing
  - ○ Eye, hand, and foot protection
  - ○ Used during transport of patients with potential of secondary contamination
- Level "D" protection
  - ○ Firefighter turnout clothing

A

B

Figure 41-4 Levels of protection. A. Level A protective haz-mat suit. B. Level B protective haz-mat suit. C. Level C protective haz-mat suit. D. Level C suit with personnel using powered air purifying respirators (PAPR) and CBRNE gas masks. *(A. Used with permission from the Georgia Institute of Technology. B. From http:// www.epa.gov/superfund/programs/er/ resource/d1_04.htm. C. Used with permission from the National Library of Medicine. D. Used with permission from Peter DiPrima.)*

Figure 41-4   *(Continued)*

Determining Appropriate PPE

- Depends on whether the chemical is known.
- A permeability chart is consulted to determine "breakthrough" time.
- Double or triple gloves or chemical-resistant gloves are used.
- Nitrile gloves have a high resistance to chemicals.
- If situation is emergent, take maximal barrier precautions—Full turnouts or Tyvek suit/gowns.
- Use high-efficiency particulate air (HEPA) filters and eye protection.
- Remove leather shoes, use rubber boots.
- Ideally, at least level "B" protection should be used.
- Ideally, use disposable protection.

PROCEDURES IN TRANSPORTING A SEMIDECONTAMINATED PATIENT (AS A LAST RESORT)

- Use as much disposable equipment as possible.
  - Reduces decontamination later
- Practicality of lining an ambulance interior with plastic:
  - Impractical
  - Time consuming

If airborne contaminants can permeate cabinets, it is unsafe for the driver to operate the ambulance. Patients who are "off-gassing" should not be placed in the patient compartment of the ambulance because of the risk of injuring the crew.

Medical Monitoring and Rehabilitation

Entry team/decontamination team readiness prior to entry:

- Assessment of vital signs and documentation.
- Team members should have normal values on file.
- Documentation flow sheet must be started.
  - Blood pressure
  - Pulse
  - Respiratory rate
  - Temperature
  - Body weight
  - Mental/neurological status
- Rescuer PPE can cause considerable heat stress.
- Prehydration prior to entry.
  - About 8 to 16 ounces of water or sport drink

After Exit, Personnel Should Return to the Medical Sector for "Rehab"

- Reassessment of vital signs and documentation.
- Documentation flow sheet must be started.
  - Blood pressure
  - Pulse
  - Respiratory rate
  - Temperature
  - Body weight
  - Mental/neurological status
- Rehydration at exit
  - About 8 to 16 ounces of water or sport drinks (such as Gatorade)
- Use weight to estimate fluid losses
  - Medical control/protocol determination
    — PO fluids

- No reentry until:
  - Vitals are back to normal
    — Nontachycardic
    — Alert
    — Normotensive
    — Body weight within percentage of normal

Heat stress factors include prehydration of the member, degree of physical fitness, ambient air temperature, degree of activity, and duration in the PPE.

? CHAPTER QUESTIONS

For questions 1 to 4, match the following definitions with the correct terms.

   a. Level "A" protection

   b. Level "B" protection

   c. Level "C" protection

   d. Level "D" protection

1. Nonpermeable clothing
2. Highest level of personal protection
3. Level of protection typically worn by decontamination team
4. Firefighters' gear
5. Through which of the following routes are poisons absorbed?

   a. topical

   b. respiratory

   c. gastrointestinal

   d. injection

   e. all of the above

6. Decontamination occurs in the cold zone.

   a. True

   b. False

Reference

US Department of Transportation, National Highway Traffic Safety Administration. *EMT-Basic National Standard Curriculum.* Washington, DC: US Department of Transportation, National Highway Traffic Safety Administration; 1994.

Chapter 42

Response to Mass Casualty Incidents/National Incident Management System

We are in the middle of a very busy hurricane season. The National Weather Service (NWS) has issued a hurricane warning for your response area, with probable landfall in the late evening of the following day. The NWS estimates the hurricane to hit your location with sustained winds of over 140 mph (category 4 storm).

Category 4 is classified as:

Winds: 131 to 155 mph.

Damage: extreme, almost total destruction of doors, windows. Some wall and roof failure. Major damage to lower floors of oceanfront buildings. Evacuations up to 6 miles inland. Pressure 27.17 to 27.90 in accompanied by a storm surge of 13 to 18 ft.

Local government is calling for a mandatory evacuation of all coastal areas. You are assigned through dispatch to respond to one of the local nursing homes and report to the southwest evacuation officer in charge of evacuating nonambulatory patients from this facility.

Upon arrival, you report to the command site of this facility and meet up with the south-west evacuation officer. She orders you and your partner to report to the 3rd floor with your stretcher and necessary equipment to operate. Upon arrival on the 3rd floor, you report what resources will be required for patient evacuation.

Who will you report your findings to, and who will be responsible for supplying the necessary equipment and staff to aid in the evacuation?

HOMELAND SECURITY PRESIDENTIAL DIRECTIVE 5

"To prevent, prepare for, respond to, and recover from terrorist attacks, major disasters, and other emergencies, the United States Government shall establish a single, comprehensive approach to domestic incident management. The objective of the United States Government is to ensure that all levels of government across the Nation have the capability to work efficiently and effectively together, using a national approach to domestic incident management."

WHAT IS THE NATIONAL INCIDENT MANAGEMENT SYSTEMS (NIMS)?

A core set of:

- Doctrine
- Concepts
- Principles
- Terminology
- Organizational processes that is applicable to all hazards

NIMS has six components:

- Command and management
- Preparedness
- Resource management
- Communications and information management
- Supporting technologies
- Ongoing management and maintenance

Command and Management

Standardizes incident management for all hazards across all levels of government. Based on three key constructs:

- Incident command system
- Multiagency coordination systems
- Public information systems

Preparedness

Establishes measures and capabilities that all agencies should develop.

Resource Management

Standardization in describing and tracking inventory before, during, and after an incident.

Communications and Information Management

Effective communications, information management, and intelligence sharing are paramount in operating at a domestic incident.

Supporting Technologies

Provide an architecture for science and technology support to incident management.

Ongoing Management

The Department of Homeland Security will establish a multijuristictional, multidisciplinary NIMS integration center.

MASS CASUALTY INCIDENTS

Disasters

Some people call these types of incidents disasters. It is important to remember that the term disaster has a specific legal meaning. States and localities declare "state of emergency." The President declares "major disasters."

Types of Disasters

Several events have the potential to cause mass casualty incidents (MCI):

- Natural disasters (floods, winter storms, hurricanes, tornados) (Figs. 42-1 and 42-2)
- Technical hazards (haz-mat incidents, building collapse)

Figure 42-1   Destruction left by Hurricane Katrina. *(Used with permission from Peter DiPrima.)*

Figure 42-2   The aftermath of Hurricane Katrina. *(Used with permission from Peter DiPrima.)*

Figure 42-3   A building explosion/collapse was caused by an individual who filled the four-story building with natural gas. *(Used with permission from Peter DiPrima.)*

- Transportation accidents (road, rail, aircraft, ship, etc.)
- Civil and political disorder (demonstrations, strikes, riots)
- Criminal or terrorist incidents (Fig. 42-3)

Mass Casualty Incidents

A mass casualty incident (or MCI) is any incident that injures or causes illness in enough people to overwhelm the resources usually available in a particular system or region.

Goals of MCI Management

- Do the greatest good for the greatest number.
- Manage scarce resources.
- Do not relocate the disaster.
- MCIs place great demands on resources, including equipment, rescuers, and facilities. Our goal as responders is not to relocate the disaster!
- Patient prioritization at the scene is important for effective patient distribution.
- Don't send all of the red tag patients to one hospital.

STAGES OF AN INCIDENT

- Initial notification
- Implementation

- Operations
- Escalation
- Stabilization
- De-escalation
- Termination

EMS INITIAL RESPONSE ROLES AND RESPONSIBILITIES

- *Initial response roles*—Emergency medical services (EMS) is a specific component of the overall incident management system. The first arriving unit should start the following actions:
- *First arriving unit*—The first emergency response unit to arrive at a mass casualty incident is by default "in charge" (the incident commander) until relieved. As a result, the individuals on the first emergency response unit must take immediate actions to begin to manage the entire incident. These actions may be the most important steps taken in the entire incident. The initial unit must resist the "temptation" to begin one-on-one patient care.
- *Assess scene for safety*—The object is to ensure no one else gets hurt. Assess the scene for safety much as you would for a normal response to any EMS incident, except that the scene is much bigger and requires a wider look. The following may pose a hazard: (1) fire, (2) electrical hazards, (3) spilled or contained flammable liquids, (4) hazardous materials, (5) nuclear, chemical, or biological agents, (6) other life threats, (7) debris that poses a threat to rescuers or their vehicles, and (8) secondary explosions.
- *Scene size-up*—How big is the incident and how bad is it?
  - Type of incident
  - Approximate number of patients
  - Severity of injuries
  - Area involved, including problems with scene access
- *Confirmation of incident*
  - Report situation—Contact dispatch with your size-up information.
  - Request assistance—Resources and mutual aid if needed.
  - Notify the Medical Command Center to insure rapid hospital notification.
- *Set up*—Set up the scene for the best management of mass casualties by on-scene and responding resources, including:
  - Staging.
  - Secure access and egress.
  - Secure adequate space for work areas.
    — Triage, treatment, transportation

SIMPLE TRIAGE AND RAPID TREATMENT (START)

Triage

Triage is a French word meaning "to sort."

Purpose of Triage

- Assigns treatment priorities.
- Separates MCI victims into easily identifiable groups.

- Determines required resources for treatment, transportation, and definitive care.
- Prioritizes patient distribution and transportation.

Benefits of Triage

- Identifies patients who require rapid medical care to save life and limb.
- Provides rational distribution of casualties.
- Separating the minor injuries reduces the urgent burden on each hospital—An average of 10% to 15% of MCI patients are serious enough to require extended hospitalization.

What Is START?

Start was developed by Hoag Hospital and the Newport Beach Fire Department to be used in the event of an MCI.

- START enables EMS providers to triage patients at an MCI in less than 60 seconds and is based on three observations:
  - Respirations
  - Circulation
  - Mental status

This triage method assures rapid initial assessment of all patients as the basis for assignment to treatment and as the first medical assessment of the incident.

So how does it work?

- Begin where you are.
- Relocate green (minor) tag patients.
- Move in an orderly pattern, tagging patients as you go.
- Maintain count (how many red, yellow, black, and green tags).
- Provide minimal treatment.

START permits rescuers to quickly and accurately categorize patients into four treatment groups:

- *Red*—Immediate (highest priority). Typical problems are:
  1. R = Respirations/airway
  2. P = Perfusion/pulse
  3. M = Mental status
- *Yellow*—Delayed (second priority). Typical problems are:
  1. Burn patients without airway problems
  2. Major or multiple bone or joint injuries
  3. Back and spine injuries
- *Green*—Minor (third priority). Typical problems are:
  1. "Walking wounded" (The ability to "walk" does not necessarily mean that this is a "minor" patient. Minor cuts and bruises are acceptable criteria for this type of patient.)
  2. Minor painful swollen deformities
  3. Minor soft tissue injuries
- *Black*—Dead/nonsalvageable (lowest priority) (These are nonbreathing patients whose resuscitation would normally be attempted but who are not salvageable given the resources available early in an MCI response.)

The START Process

1. Begin where you stand.
2. Identify those injured who can walk. Make a clear announcement that those who can walk should get up and do so to an easily recognized point.

Relocate Green Patients

1. Relocate to a designated area (away from immediate danger and outside the initial triage area).
2. Tag each of these as a green patient.

Triage Patients in an Orderly Pattern

1. Move through the patients in an orderly pattern.
2. Assess each casualty and mark the category using triage ribbons or triage tags.

Maintain a Patient Count

1. Maintain a count of the casualties.
2. Mark on 2 to 3 in tape on thigh.
3. Save a small piece of triage ribbon and place in your pocket.

Steps in START Assessment (Fig. 42-4)

- *Step 1—Move green tag patients.*
- *Step 2—Respiration.* Check for respiratory compromise.
  - If airway is closed, open the airway.
  - *None—black* tag (dead).
  - More than 30 breaths per minute—*red* tag (immediate).
  - Less than 30 breaths per minute—*further evaluation required*—go to Step 3 (perfusion).
- *Step 3—Perfusion.* Radial pulse check.
  - Not palpable—*red* tag (immediate).
  - Control severe bleeding—bystanders use direct pressure, raise legs.
  - Palpable—*further evaluation required*—go to Step 4 (mental status).
- *Step 4—Mental status.* Check for compromise of mental status.
  - Altered mental status—*red* tag (immediate).
  - Mental status appropriate—*yellow* tag (delayed) or green (minor) according to other findings (obvious injuries or illnesses).

Secondary Triage

Secondary triage and tagging can be done:

- On a stretcher on the way to a treatment area
- In the treatment area
- In the ambulance on the way to the hospital
  - Secondary triage is an in-depth reassessment based on clinical experience and judgment.
  - Triage is an on-going process and should be done continuously.

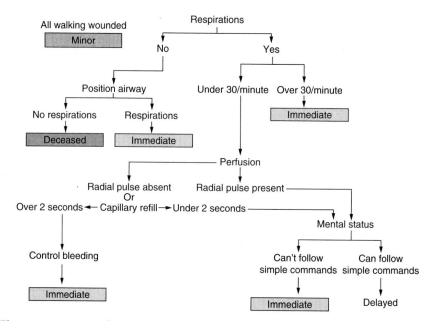

Figure 42-4 START flowchart. *(From http://www.citmt.org/start/flowchart.htm. Reprinted with permission from the Critical Illness and Trauma Foundation.)*

? CHAPTER QUESTIONS

1. The first phase of an incident is called:

   a. stabilization
   b. initial notification
   c. operations
   d. de-escalation

2. You are completing the START triage evaluation on a 27-year-old man who is complaining of difficulty breathing secondary to being involved in a building explosion. There are 53 patients that need to be triaged; all green tag patients have already been removed. The patient presents with the following during triage:

   • respiratory rate of 28
   • radial pulses are present and capillary refill is less than 2 seconds
   • follows simple commands

   What color triage tag should this patient receive?
   a. red
   b. yellow
   c. green
   d. black

3. START stands for:

a. Slow Triage and Ridiculous Treatment

b. Simple Teaching and Rapid Transport

c. Simple Triage and Rapid Treatment

d. Simple Triage and Rapid Transport

Reference

US Department of Transportation, National Highway Traffic Safety Administration. *EMT-Basic National Standard Curriculum*. Washington, DC: US Department of Transportation, National Highway Traffic Safety Administration; 1994.

Chapter 43

Response to Weapons of Mass Destruction Incidents

It is a particularly busy day for the local emergency medical services (EMS) units, humidity is at 75% and it feels like it is 100°F, and you are working on your tenth assignment for the shift. A known terrorist group has successfully detonated an explosive device in a tanker truck that was transporting liquefied chlorine across a well-known bridge in your response area. Multiple calls are coming into the 911 system regarding this assignment.

Moments later, your unit is dispatched to the staging area of this scene. Due to the close proximity of this assignment, you and your partner will be the first arriving EMS unit.

What type of scene size-up should you perform, and should you enter the scene?

TERRORISM

"The unlawful use of or threatened use of force or violence against individuals or property to coerce or intimidate governments or societies, often to achieve political, religious, or ideological objectives."—U.S. Department of Defense

Throughout history, terrorism has been a global threat from which no community is free. Terrorism surpasses all geographic and demographic boundaries; suburban, urban, and rural neighborhoods are at risk.

Terrorists have demonstrated the ability to strike anywhere in the world.

- International terrorists continue to pose a threat to the interests of the United States (Fig. 43-1). Many terrorist groups and loosely affiliated extremists view the United States as an enemy.
- Increasingly, emergency responders must deal with incidents arising from domestic sources. According to the Federal Bureau of Investigation (FBI), domestic groups or individuals are more likely to be the source of an incident involving weapons of mass destruction (WMD) than are international organizations.

THE THREAT OF TERRORISM

Terrorists have the knowledge, capability, and patience to strike anywhere, and at any time. In the past, we have seen that when properly motivated they will perform any task to achieve their goals. All communities, especially those of free societies, are vulnerable to terrorism. Any community in the United States has some form of high-profile target.

Figure 43-1   World Trade Center, September 11, 2001. *(Used with permission from Peter DiPrima.)*

Examples of critical infrastructures that become targets for criminal terrorist activity include:

- Places of public assembly
- Public buildings (ie, schools)
- Mass transit systems
- Places of high economic impact
- Telecommunications centers
- Information and communications
- Banking and finance
- Water supplies
- Electrical power, oil, and gas production and storage
- Places of historical or symbolic significance
- Apartment buildings
- Medical clinics (abortion clinics)
- Research facilities
- Transportation hubs
- Emergency services

WHY WMD: *TERRORISM?*

- Chemical and biological agents are relatively easy to manufacture. Most agents can be produced by knowledge gained in college. Weapons of mass destruction are readily available and are cheap to produce. Libraries contain the "recipes" required. Chemicals are readily available in school laboratories. Biological pathogens can be obtained from nature, hospital labs, and university research facilities. Radiological materials are found in industry and in research labs.

- WMD terrorism is spread relatively easy by air. A clever person can easily devise methods to disseminate a chemical, biological, or radiological weapon that results in little, if any, signature. For example, the first indication of a chemical attack may be when people begin to collapse as in the Tokyo incident. The first indication of a biological attack may be an influx of people beginning to develop symptoms of disease hours to days after infection. And last, there may never be any obvious indication of a radiological attack. Regardless of what type of agent is used, decontamination is required. Terrorist attacks cause a psychological impact that will extend far beyond their actual effects. Psychological effects of terrorism cause people to live in fear. A few examples of this were:
  - During the Gulf War, when Israeli citizens boarded up their homes fearful of Iraqi chemical attacks.
  - Post September 11, 2001, when after strong media coverage, many people feared planes flying overhead, traveling on mass transit, and being in large crowded areas.

Limitations of WMD

- Chemical weapons need large quantities in open areas.
- Delayed effects can detract from impact.
- Potentially hazardous to the terrorists.
- Development and use require skill.

INDICATORS OF WMD ATTACK

Primary Indicators May Include

- Similar symptoms of victims
- Mass casualties
- Casualty patterns
- Finding a dissemination device, and observing it functioning
- Detectors
- Warning given or credit taken

Secondary Indicators May Include

- Dead animals or birds
- Statements of victims
- Unexplained liquids or strange smells
- Test results confirmed

POTENTIAL OUTCOMES OF TERRORIST WMD EVENT

- Mass casualties
- The overwhelming of emergency response systems
- Disruption of normal routine
- Shutdown and decontamination of contaminated facilities
- Panic and confusion

- Loss of faith in government
- Loss of faith in emergency services

WEAPONS OF MASS DESTRUCTION: CHEMICAL AGENTS

Classes of Chemical Agents

- Choking agents
  - *Choking agents (lung-damaging agents)* include phosgene (CG), diphosgene (DP), chlorine, and chloropicrin (PS). These agents produce injury to the lungs and irritation of the eyes and respiratory tract. They may cause intractable pulmonary edema and predispose to secondary pneumonia
- Blister agents
  - *Blister agents (vesicants)* include sulfur mustard (H/HD), nitrogen mustard (HN), arsenicals (Lewisite [L]), and phosgene oxime (CX). Blister agents produce pain and injury to the eyes, reddening and blistering of the skin, and when inhaled, damage to the mucous membranes and respiratory tract. Mustard may produce major destruction of the epidermal layer of the skin
- Blood agents
  - *Blood agents (cyanogens)* include hydrogen cyanide (AC) and cyanogen chloride (CK). These agents are transported by the blood to all body tissues where the agent blocks the oxidative processes, preventing tissue cells from utilizing oxygen. The CNS is especially affected and leads to cessation of respiration followed by cardiovascular collapse.
- Nerve agents
  - *Nerve agents (anticholinesterase)* include tabun (GA), sarin (GB), soman (GD), GF, and V-Agent (VX). They inhibit cholinesterase enzymes. The cholinesterase enzymes are responsible for the hydrolysis of acetylcholine (ACh), a chemical neurotransmitter. The inhibition creates accumulation of ACh at the cholinergic synapses that disrupts the normal transmission of nerve impulses. Cholinergic synapses are located in the CNS, neuromuscular end plates of the peripheral voluntary nervous system, parasympathetic endings, and sympathetic presynaptic ganglia of the autonomic nervous system (Table 43-1).

TABLE 43-1: Signs and Symptoms of Nerve Agent Exposure

	Signs/Symptoms	Vapor Exposure	Liquid Exposure
Mild	**P** Pin point pupils (miosis)	X	
	S Salivation	X	
	L Lacrimation	X	
Severe	**U** Urination	X	X
	D Defecation	X	X
	G Gastrointestinal distress pain/gas	X	X
	E Emesis	X	X
	M Muscle twitching	X	X
	C Convulsions	X	X

WEAPONS OF MASS DESTRUCTION: BIOLOGICAL AGENTS

Biological Warfare Agents

Biological warfare involves the use of several broad categories of agents. Two of these are infectious microbial pathogens—bacteria and viruses, both of which cause disease in humans, animals, and plants. The third is known as biological toxins, which are poisons extracted from biological sources previous to their use as weapons.

Characteristics of Biological Agents

- Do not penetrate unbroken skin.
- Nonvolatile.
- More toxic than chemicals by weight.
- Undetectable by senses.
- Some detection devices are available depending on the agent involved.
- Disseminate as aerosols.

Types of Biological Agents

- *Bacteria* are single-cell, free-living organisms that reproduce by division. Bacteria cause disease in humans by invading tissues and/or producing toxins; this causes the body's immune system to be overcome.
- *Viruses* cannot replicate by themselves. Viruses require a host cell in order to reproduce and are technically described as obligate intracellular parasites. Viruses cause epidemics.
- *Toxins* are poisonous substances produced as a by-product of pathogens or plants and even some animals. (Snake venom is an example of a toxin.)

Potential Biological Agents

- Anthrax (bacteria)
- Plague (bacteria)
- Q fever (rickettsia)
- Small pox (virus)
- Ebola (virus)
- Venezuelan equine encephalitis (VEE)(virus)
- Staphylococcal enterotoxin B
- Botulinum (neurotoxin)
- Ricin (cytotoxin)

WEAPONS OF MASS DESTRUCTION: RADIOLOGICAL/NUCLEAR WEAPONS

Characteristics of Nuclear Agents

- Of the three categories, chemical, biological, or nuclear, nuclear agents in the past were considered to be the least likely of the threats. However, the potential risk is increasing with current intelligence. Threats of using a "dirty bomb" with radioactive material are on a steady increase.

- In its simplest definition, radiation can be defined as either electromagnetic or particulate emission of energy.
- This energy, when impacting on or passing through material, including us, can cause some form of reaction. This radiation is referred to as *ionizing radiation*.
- When absorbed by our bodies, it can cause changes in our cells. Small amounts can be tolerated; larger amounts can be harmful.

For EMS purposes, radiation can be classified as:

- Alpha particles—Slow moving
- Beta particles—Higher in energy
- Gamma particles—Highly energized

Ionizing radiation cannot be seen, felt, or heard. Therefore, a detection device is required to measure the radiation being emitted by the radioactive source. The most commonly used is the Geiger counter. The rate of radiation is measured in roentgens per hour (R/h) or milliroentgens per hour (mR/h).

- The unit of local tissue energy deposition is called radiation absorbed dose (RAD). Roentgen equivalent in man measure (REM) provides a gauge of the likely injury to the irradiated part of the organism. Simply stated, ionizing radiation causes alterations in the body's cell, primarily the DNA. Depending upon dosage received, the changes can be in cell division, cell structure, and cellular biochemical activities.

Ways to Limit Exposure

- *Time*—Cutting down your time reduces your exposure
- *Distance*—The farther you are from the source the better
- *Shielding*—Through various materials

DISSEMINATION DEVICES

There are five types of dissemination devices:

- Direct deposit
- Breaking devices

TABLE 43-2: Dose-Effect Total Body Exposure

Radiation Absorbed Dose (RAD)	Effect
5-25	asymptomatic, normal blood studies
50-75	asymptomatic, minor depression in WBC
75-125	anorexia, nausea, vomiting, fatigue within 2 days
125-200	nausea, vomiting, diarrhea, anxiety, tachycardia
200-600	nausea, vomiting, diarrhea within several hours, 50% fatal within 6 weeks, untreated
600-1000	severe nausea, vomiting, diarrhea within several hours, fatal 100% within 2 weeks, untreated
1000+	burning sensation within minutes, nausea and vomiting, confusion, ataxia, and prostration within 1 hour

Fatal 100% within short time without prompt treatment!

- Bursting/exploding devices
- Spraying devices
- Vectors

Direct Deposit

- Mechanical
- Point source
- No collateral damage
- Easily controlled
- Fitted into cans, umbrellas, pens, and the like

Breaking Devices

- Mechanical.
- Point source.
- Breaking devices are those mechanical weapons which encapsulate the agent and release it when broken (small drilled hole in the base, agent inserted, and hole sealed).

Bursting/Exploding Devices

Bursting or exploding devices are those which employ an explosive to break the agent container and disseminate the agent.

Spraying Devices

Mechanical spraying devices also contain an agent reservoir, but rather than an explosive charge, they employ pressure to disseminate the agent.

Vectors

Usually disseminate living biological agents. A vector is a carrier of the bacteria, and may be an insect or a contaminated item such as clothing, food, or water.

PERSONAL PROTECTION

- As stated earlier, personal safety takes precedence. If we become incapacitated, injured, or even die responding to an incident, we will be unable to provide the services needed to control the scene. Becoming a victim at an incident endangers your partners and other rescuers involved.
- We must understand that nuclear, biological, and chemical agents were deliberately developed to cause injury or death to individuals. They are all very toxic to humans and animals; however, they are not the end of the world. The majority of agents can be detected, protected against, and can be treated and decontaminated.

Regulations Involving Personal Protective Equipment (PPE)

OSHA standards mandate specific training. OSHA's final rule (March 6, 1989, 29 CFR [1910.120]) as it applies to Emergency Medical Personnel: training shall be based on the duties and functions to be performed by each responder of an emergency response organization. No single combination of protective equipment and clothing is capable of protecting against all hazards. PPE should be used in conjunction with other protective measures. So training is essential before any individual attempts to use PPE.

Protecting Yourself against Chemical Agents

- Self-contained breathing apparatus (SCBA)
- Protective clothing

Protecting Yourself against Biological Agents

- Mask (high-efficiency particulate air [HEPA] filters or SCBA)*
- Clothing
- Sanitation measures
- Decontamination
- Medical treatment
- Bloodborne pathogen universal precautions

If you know you are responding to a potential biological agent incident:

- *SCBA or protective mask combined with your clothing and unbroken skin are your first line of defense.*
- *Use good sanitation measures, which include not eating or drinking in the immediate area. Wash your hands with soap and water if you touch something.*
- *Decontaminate with 0.5% Hypochlorite solution.*
- *Don't ignore early flu-like symptoms, seek medical attention immediately.*

Levels of Protection

(See also Fig. 41-4)

The Environmental Protection Agency (EPA) designated four levels of respiratory protection and protective clothing.

- Level A protection should be worn when the highest level of respiratory, skin, eye, and mucous membrane protection is needed. It consists of a fully encapsulated, vapor-tight, chemical-resistant suit, chemical-resistant boots, chemical-resistant inner/outer gloves, coveralls, hard hat, and SCBA.
- Level B protection should be worn when the highest level of respiratory protection is needed and a lesser degree of skin and eye protection. It differs from a Level A suit in that it provides splash protection through the use of chemical-resistant clothing (two-piece chemical splash suit, or fully encapsulated nonvapor tight suit and SCBA).
- Level C protection should be selected when the type of airborne substances is *known*, concentration measured, and all criteria for air purifying systems are met, and skin and eye exposures are unlikely.
- Level D is a primary work uniform.

Protecting Yourself against Nuclear Agents

- Time
  - Cutting down your time reduces your exposure.

> **▶Note:**
>
> *Clothing contaminated with nerve agents can "OFF-GAS," creating a problem for individuals around undecontaminated clothing and who are unprotected.*

---

*Depends on biological agent involved.

▶Note:

Because of the ease of protecting from alpha and beta radiation, our main concern from these substances are inhalation and ingestion of actual radioactive material in the form of dust or contaminated food or water. Gamma is more difficult to protect against, so time, distance, and shielding are vital.

- Distance
  - *Distance*—Referring back to forms of radiation, alpha particles only travel a little over an inch in air. Beta particles will not travel for more than a few yards in air. However, gamma particles will travel extensive distances and this is the radiation we are the most concerned with. The farther you are from the source the better
- Shielding
  - Radiation can also be blocked or partially blocked by various materials. A sheet of paper stops alpha particles; beta particles are stopped by aluminum foil or clothing; and gamma rays are only reduced by dense materials such as lead or earth

? CHAPTER QUESTIONS

1. The unlawful use of force to intimidate or coerce a segment of a population for political or social reasons is:

   a. terrorism

   b. conflict

   c. warfare

   d. negotiation

2. Biological weapons target all but:

   a. utilities

   b. animals

   c. people

   d. agriculture

3. Explosives are the terrorist's weapon of choice.

   a. True

   b. False

4. Which weapons material is easiest to obtain?

   a. biological

   b. chemical

   c. nuclear

   d. incendiary

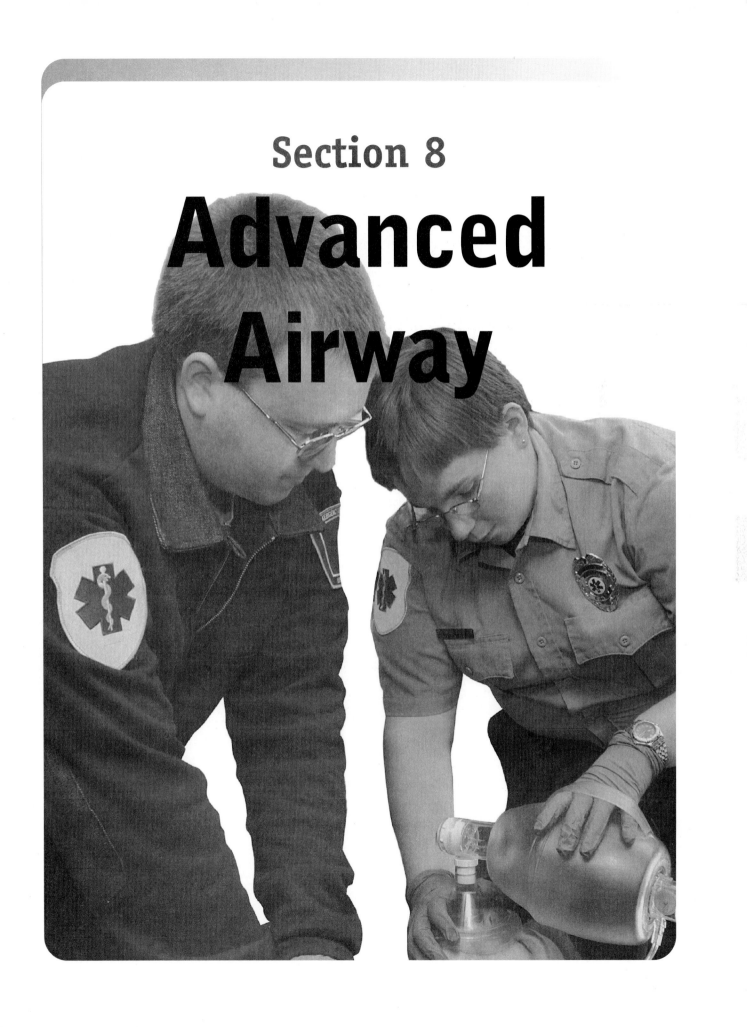

Section 8
Advanced
Airway

Chapter 44
Advanced Airway Management

After you witness the endotracheal (ET) tube pass the vocal cords of an unconscious respiratory arrest patient, you hear lung sounds only on the right side of the chest.

What are some of the causes of this to occur, and how can you correct them?

REVIEW OF THE BODY'S NEED FOR OXYGEN

- Brain death occurs within 6 to 10 minutes.
- Our body requires proper ventilation to sustain life.
- This includes the removal of wastes (CO_2) and the introduction of oxygen.

Primary objective in advanced airway management includes:

- Ensuring optimal ventilation
- Delivery of high-concentration oxygen
- Elimination of CO_2

ANATOMY AND PHYSIOLOGY OF THE RESPIRATORY SYSTEM

Primary function of the upper airway is to:

- Warm
- Filter
- Humidify

Pharynx

- Nasopharynx is formed by the union of facial bones.
- Orientation of nasal floor is toward the ear, not the eye.
- Separated by septum which is lined with mucous membranes, cilia.

Turbinate

- Parallel to nasal floor
- Provide increased surface area for air
- Filtration

- Humidifying
- Warming

Sinuses

- Cavities formed by cranial bones
- Appear to further trap bacteria and act as tributaries for fluid to and from eustachian tubes and tear ducts
- Commonly become infected
- Fracture of certain sinus bones may cause cerebral-spinal fluid (CSF) leak

Tissues are extremely delicate and vascular. Improper or overly aggressive placement of tubes or airways will cause significant bleeding which may not be controlled by direct pressure.

ANATOMY OF THE OROPHARYNX

Teeth

- 32 in an adult
- Requires significant force to dislodge
- May fracture or avulse causing obstruction

Tongue

- Large muscle attached at the mandible and hyoid bones
- Most common airway obstruction

Palate

- Roof of mouth separates oro/nasopharynx.
- Anterior is hard palate.
- Posterior (beyond the teeth) is soft palate.

Adenoids

- Lymph tissue located in the mouth and nose that filters bacteria
- Frequently infected and swollen

Epiglottis

Vallecula

- "Pocket" formed by the base of the tongue and epiglottis
- Important landmark for ET intubation

ANATOMY OF THE LARYNX

Larynx

- Attached to hyoid bone
- Supports trachea
- Made of cartilage

Thyroid Cartilage

- First tracheal cartilage
- "Shield shaped"
- Cartilage anterior
- Smooth muscle posterior

Laryngeal Prominence

- "Adam's Apple," anterior prominence of thyroid cartilage
- Glottic opening directly behind

Glottic Opening

- Narrowest part of adult trachea
- Patency heavily dependent on muscle tone
- Contains vocal bands
- White bands of cartilage
- Produces voice

Arytenoid Cartilage

- "Pyramid-like" posterior attachment of vocal bands
- Important landmark for ET intubation

Pyriform Fossae

- "Hollow pockets" along the lateral borders of the larynx

Cricoid Ring

- First tracheal ring
- Completely cartilaginous
- Compression occludes esophagus (Sellick maneuver)

Cricothyroid Membrane

- Fibrous membrane between cricoid and thyroid cartilage
- Site for surgical and alternative airway placement

ASSOCIATED STRUCTURES

Thyroid Gland

- Located below cricoid cartilage
- Lies across trachea and up both sides

Carotid Arteries

- Branches cross and lie closely alongside trachea

Jugular Veins

- Branch across and lie close to trachea

ANATOMY OF LOWER AIRWAY

Function of the lower airway includes:

- Exchange of O_2 and CO_2
- Location of the lower airway
  - From fourth cervical vertebrae to xyphoid process
  - From glottic opening to pulmonary capillary membrane

Structures of the Lower Airway

- Trachea
- Trachea bifurcates at carina into the right and left mainstem bronchi
- Right mainstem has lesser angle
  - Foreign bodies, ET tubes commonly displace here
  - Lined with mucous cells
  - Beta$_2$ receptors—Dilate bronchioles (ie, albuterol sulfate)

Bronchi

- Mainstem bronchi enter lungs at the hilum
- Branch into narrowing secondary and tertiary bronchi which branch into bronchioles

Bronchioles

- Branch into alveolar ducts which end at alveolar sacs

Alveoli

- "Balloon-like" clusters.
- Site of gas exchange.
- Lined with surfactant.
- Decreases surface tension of alveoli which facilitates ease of expansion.
- Alveoli become thinner as they expand which makes diffusion of oxygen and carbon dioxide easier.
- If surfactant is decreased or alveoli are not inflated, alveoli collapse (atelectasis).

Lungs

- Right lung
  - Three lobes
- Left lung
  - Two lobes
- Lobes made of parenchymal tissue
- Membranous outer lining called pleura

DIFFERENCES IN THE PEDIATRIC AIRWAY

Pharynx

- A proportionately smaller jaw causes the tongue to encroach upon the airway.
- Omega shaped, floppy epiglottis.
- Absent or very delicate dentition.

Trachea

- Airway is smaller and narrower at all levels.
- Larynx lies more superior.
- Larynx is "funnel shaped" due to narrow, undeveloped cricoid cartilage.
- Narrowest point is at cricoid ring before 10 years of age.
- Further narrowing of the airway by tissue swelling of foreign body results in major increase in airway resistance.

Chest Wall

- Ribs and cartilage are softer.
- Cannot optimally contribute to lung expansion.
- Infants and children tend to depend more heavily on the diaphragm for breathing.

LUNG/RESPIRATORY VOLUMES

- Adult male approximately 6 liters.
- Not all inspired air enters alveoli.
- Minor diffusion of oxygen takes place in alveolar ducts and terminal bronchioles.
- *Tidal volume*—Volume of gas inhaled or exhaled during a single respiratory cycle:
  - 5-7cc/kg (500 cc normally)
- *Dead space air*—Air remaining in air passageways, unavailable for gas exchange (approximately 150 cc).
- *Physiologic dead space*—Dead space formed by factors like disease or obstruction, such as:
  - Chronic obstructive pulmonary disease (COPD)
  - Atelectasis
- *Minute volume*—The amount of gas moved in and out of the respiratory tract per minute and determined by tidal volume—dead space volume multiplied by the respiratory rate.
- *Functional reserve capacity* (after optimal inspiration)—Optimum amount of air that can be forced from the lungs in a single forced exhalation.
- *Residual volume*—Volume of air remaining in lungs at the end of maximal expiration.
- *Alveolar*—Air reaching the alveoli for gas exchange (alveolar volume) is approximately 350 cc.
- *Inspiratory reserve*—Amount of gas that can be inspired in addition to tidal volume.
- *Expiratory reserve*—Amount of gas that can be expired after a passive (relaxed) expiration.
- *FiO_2*—Percentage of oxygen in inspired air (increases with supplemental oxygen):
  - Commonly documented as a decimal (eg, FiO_2 = .85)
- *Respiration*—Exchange of gases between a living organism and its environment. The major gases of respiration are oxygen and carbon dioxide.
  - External respiration—Exchange of gases between the lungs and the blood cells
  - Internal respiration—Exchange of gases between the blood cells and tissues

THE TRANSPORTATION OF OXYGEN AND CARBON DIOXIDE IN THE HUMAN BODY

Diffusion—Passage of solution from area of higher concentration to lower concentration

- Oxygen and carbon dioxide dissolve in water and pass through alveolar membrane by diffusion.

Oxygen Content of Blood

- Dissolved oxygen crosses pulmonary capillary membrane and binds to hemoglobin (Hgb) of red blood cell. Oxygen is carried bound to Hgb and is dissolved in plasma. Approximately 97% of total oxygen is bound to hemoglobin.
- Oxygen saturation is the percent of hemoglobin saturated and usually is greater than 98%.

Carbon Dioxide Content of the Blood

- Carbon dioxide is a byproduct of cellular work (cellular respiration).
- Carbon dioxide is transported in blood as bicarbonate ion.
- About 33% is bound to hemoglobin.
- As oxygen crosses into blood, carbon dioxide diffuses into alveoli.
- Carbon dioxide in the blood ($PaCO_2$).

Cause of Increasing Carbon Dioxide in Blood

Hypoventilation

The Measurement of Gases

The combined pressure of all atmospheric gases

- 100% or 760 torr at sea level

PATHOPHYSIOLOGY OF AN OBSTRUCTION

The tongue is the most common airway obstruction and is the cause of snoring respirations. These obstructions are corrected with positioning of the patient's head.

Foreign Body

- May cause partial or full obstruction
- Symptoms include:
  - Choking
  - Gagging
  - Stridor
  - Dyspnea
  - Aphasia (unable to speak)
  - Dysphasia (difficulty speaking)

Laryngeal Spasm and Edema

Spasm

- Spasmodic closure of vocal cords

Edema

- Glottic opening becomes extremely narrow or totally obstructed
- Most frequently caused by:
  - Epiglottitis (a bacterial infection of the epiglottis)
  - Anaphylaxis (severe allergic reaction)
- Aggressive ventilation
- Forceful upward pull of the jaw
- Muscle relaxants

Aspiration

- Significantly increases mortality
- Obstructs airway
- Destroys delicate bronchiolar tissue
- Introduces pathogens
- Decreases ability to ventilate

ENDOTRACHEAL TUBE

- Tube passed into the trachea in order to provide externally controlled breathing through a BVM or ventilator.
- ET intubation is the preferred method in controlling the airway in patients who are unable to maintain an open airway.

Sizes

- About 2.5 to 9.0 mm inside diameter (id)
- Length 12 to 32 cm

Types of Endotracheal Tubes

Cuffed 5.0 to 9.0

- Proximal-end 15 mm adapter
- Proximal-end inflation port with pilot balloon
- Centimeter markings along length
- Distal-end beveled tip
- Distal-end balloon cuff

Uncuffed 2.5 to 4.5

- Proximal-end 15 mm adapter
- Distal-end bevel tip
- Distal-end depth markings
- No balloon cuff or pilot balloon

Indications for Endotracheal Intubation

- Present or impending respiratory failure
- Apnea
- Failure to protect own airway

Contraindications

- None

Advantages

- Provides a secure airway
- Protects against aspiration
- Route for medication

Disadvantages

- Special equipment needed
- Bypasses physiologic function of upper airway (warming, filtering, moisture)

Complications

- Bleeding
- Laryngeal swelling
- Laryngospasm
- Vocal cord damage
- Mucosal necrosis
- Barotrauma

OROTRACHEAL INTUBATION

Orotracheal intubation by direct laryngoscopy means directly visualizing the passage of an ET tube into the trachea.

Indications

- Apnea
- Hypoxia
- Poor respiratory effort
- Suppression or absence of gag reflex

Contraindications

- Caution in unsuppressed gag reflex

Advantages

- Direct visualization of anatomy and tube placement
- Ideal method for confirming placement
- May be performed in breathing and apneic patients

Disadvantages

- Requires special equipment

Complications

- Dental trauma
- Laryngeal trauma
- Misplacement
- Right mainstem
- Esophageal

Equipment Needed

- Laryngoscope
- Device used to visualize glottis during ET intubation
- Battery pack/handle with interchangeable blades
- Blade types
    ◦ Straight (Miller) lifts epiglottis
    ◦ Curved (Macintosh) lifts epiglottis by fitting into vallecula
- 10 cc syringe to inflate/deflate balloon cuff
- Water-soluble lubricant to lubricate ET tube, promote ease of passage, and decrease trauma
- Stylet—Semirigid wire for molding and maintaining tube shape
- Securing device
    ◦ Tape
    ◦ Commercially available ET tube holder
- Suction
- Body substance precautions
    ◦ Gloves
    ◦ Mask
    ◦ Eyewear or face shield

Method

- Sniffing position is the position used when the potential for c-spine injury does not exist.
- Optimal hyperextension of head with elevation of occiput.
- Brings the axis of the mouth, the pharynx, and the trachea into alignment.

When potential for c-spine injury exists, head is held firmly in neutral position during intubation.

- Ensure optimal oxygenation and ventilation with 100% O_2.
- Ensure all equipment is prepared.
- Lubricated tube with stylet in place.
- Best position is "hockey stick."
- Bend directly behind balloon cuff.

Working Laryngoscope

- Blade locks securely in place.
- Light is bright and steady (unpleasant to look at).
- Test cuff by inflating and then deflating.
- Ideally, hyperoxygenate patient for 30 seconds to 1 minute.
- Insert laryngoscope blade.

- Gently insert to hypopharynx.
- Lift tongue and jaw with firm, steady pressure.
- Avoid fulcrum against teeth.
- Identify vocal cords.
- Gently pass ET tube until passage of balloon cuff past cords is observed.
- Remove stylet.
- Inflate balloon cuff.
- Ventilate patient.
- Confirm placement with multiple methods.
- Reconfirm placement with major patient movement or head movement.

Methods in Confirming Placement

- Direct revisualization (revisualize the glottis)
- Note tube depth:
  - Average tube depth in males is 22 cm at the teeth.
  - Average tube depth in females is 21 cm at the teeth.
- Note condensation in the tube
- Auscultation
  - Epigastric area
    — Air entry into stomach indicates esophageal placement.
  - Bilateral bases
    — Equal volume and expansion
  - Apices
    — Equal volume
- Palpation of balloon cuff at sternal notch by compressing pilot balloon
- Pulse oximetry
- End-tidal CO_2 detector—Measures presence of CO_2 in expired air
  - Colormetric
  - Digital
  - Digital/waveform

Unequal or absent breath sounds indicate:

- Esophageal placement
- Right mainstem placement
- Pneumothorax
- Bronchial obstruction

Increased resistance to bag-valve-mask (BVM) compliance may indicate:

- Gastric distension
- Esophageal placement
- Tension pneumothorax
  - Evidence of a misplaced tube regardless of when it was last checked must be reconfirmed.
  - Confirmation must be performed.
    — By multiple methods
    — Immediately after tube placement
    — After any major move
    — After manipulation of neck (manipulation of neck may displace tube up to 5 cm)

Corrective Measures

- Esophageal placement.
- Ready to vigorously suction as needed.
- Likelihood of emesis is increased especially if gastric distension is present.
- Ideally, preoxygenate prior to reintubation.
- Misplaced tube may be removed after proper tracheal placement is confirmed, or it may be removed beforehand provided diligent and vigorous airway suctioning is ready.
- Right mainstem placement.
- Loosen or remove securing device.
- Deflate balloon cuff.
- While ventilation continues, *slowly* retract tube while simultaneously listening for breath sounds over left chest.
- *Stop* as soon as breath sounds are heard in left chest.
- Note tube depth.
- Reinflate balloon cuff.
- Secure tube.
  - Securing the tube is as critical as the intubation itself.
  - Multiple methods and products are available.
  - Adjuncts include:
    — Securing to maxilla rather than mandible
    — Tincture of benzoin to facilitate tape adhesion

FIELD EXTUBATION

- Generally, the only reason to field extubate is the patient is unreasonably intolerant of the tube.
- Awake patients are at high risk of laryngospasm immediately following extubation. There may be a problem reinducting and reintubating a laryngospastic patient.

Indications

- Able to protect and maintain airway
- Risks for need to reintubate significantly reduced
- Must not be sedated

Contraindication

- Any risk of recurrence of respiratory failure

Complications

- Highest risk of recurrence of laryngospasm is immediately postextubation.
- Respiratory distress or failure may return necessitating reintubation.

Method of Extubating a Patient

- Ensure oxygenation.
- Intubation equipment and suction immediately available.
- Confirm patient responsiveness.
- Suction oropharynx.

- Deflate cuff.
- Remove upon cough or expiration.

Special Considerations

- Need for field extubation is extremely rare.
- Intolerance of ET tube evidenced by gag reflex should be addressed by increasing sedation rather than removing tube.

Pediatric Endotracheal Intubation

- Laryngoscope and size-appropriate blades for the pediatric patient
  - Straight (Miller) blades are preferred.
- Premature infant—0 straight
- Full-term infant to 1 year of age—1 straight
- Two years of age to adolescent—2 straight
- Adolescent and above—3 straight or curved
- Using the appropriate size ET tube:
  - Formula = (16 + age in years) ÷ 4
  - Use of a Broselow tape

General Endotracheal Tube Size Guidelines

- Premature infant—2.5 to 3.0 uncuffed
- Full-term infant—3.0 to 3.5 uncuffed
- Infant to 1 year of age—3.5 to 4.0 uncuffed
- Toddler—4.0 to 5.0 uncuffed
- Preschool—5.0 to 5.5 uncuffed
- School age—5.5 to 6.5 uncuffed
- Adolescent—7.0 to 8.0 cuffed

Depth of Insertion

- About 2 to 3 cm below the vocal cords.
  - Uncuffed—Place the black glottic marker of the tube at the level of the vocal cords.
  - Cuffed—Insert until the cuff is just below the vocal cords.
- Formula = (3 × inside diameter − 1)
- General guidelines:
  - Premature infant—8 cm
  - Full-term infant—8 to 9.5 cm
  - Infant to 1 year of age—9.5 to 11 cm
  - Toddler—11 to 12.5 cm
  - Preschool—12.5 to 14 cm
  - School age—14 to 20 cm
  - Adolescent—20 to 23 cm
- Appropriate-sized ET tube stylet
- Endotracheal tube securing device
  - Tape
  - Commercial device

Technique

- Separate parent/guardian and patient.
- Manually open airway.
- Insert appropriate airway adjunct if needed.
- Ventilate patient with 100% oxygen via age-appropriate sized bag.
- Place the patient's head in the sniffing position.
- Preoxygenate the patient with 100% oxygen a minimum of 30 seconds.
- Prepare all equipment.
- Lubricate ET tube with sterile water/saline or water-soluble gel.
- Lubricate stylet if utilized.
- Insert the laryngoscope to the right side of the mouth and sweep the tongue to the left side.
- Lift tongue with firm, steady pressure.
- Avoid fulcrum against teeth or gums.
- Use the tip of the blade to lift epiglottis.
- Identify the vocal cords.
- Introduce the ET tube to the right side of the mouth.
- Pass the tube through the vocal cords to about 2 to 3 cm below the vocal cords.
- Confirm proper tube placement.
- Observe for symmetrical chest expansion.
- Auscultate for equal breath sounds over each lateral chest wall high in the axillae.
- Absence of breath sounds over the abdomen.
- Improved heart rate and color.
- If available, end-tidal carbon dioxide detector.
- Secure tube, noting placement of distance marker at teeth/gums.
- Reconfirm tube placement.

MULTILUMEN AIRWAYS

- Pharyngotracheal lumen airway (PTL).
- An ET tube encased in a large pharyngeal tube.
- Designed to be passed blindly.
- Dual ventilation ports provide means to ventilate regardless of whether the ET tube is placed in the esophagus or the trachea.

Indication

Alternative airway control when conventional intubation procedures are not available or successful.

Advantages

- Can ventilate with tracheal or esophageal placement
- No facemask to seal
- No special equipment
- Does not require sniffing position

Disadvantages

- Cannot be used in awake patients.
- Adults only.

- Pharyngeal balloon mitigates but does not eliminate aspiration risk.
- Can only be passed orally.
- Extremely difficult to intubate around.

Method

- Head neutral.
- Preintubation precautions.
- Insert at the midline using jaw-lift.
- Ventilate through pharyngeal tube (green) first.
- Chest rise indicates ET tube is in esophagus.
- Inflate pharyngeal balloon and ventilate.
- No chest rise indicates ET tube in trachea.
- Inflate ET tube balloon cuff.
- Ventilate through ET tube.

Complications

- Pharyngeal or esophageal trauma from poor technique
- Unrecognized displacement of ET tube into esophagus
- Displacement of pharyngeal balloon

Special Considerations

- Good assessment skills are essential to properly confirm placement.
- Misidentification of placement has been reported.
- Reinforce multiple confirmations of placement techniques.

COMBITUBE

Pharyngeal and ET tube molded into a single unit

Indication

Alternative airway control when conventional intubation measures are unsuccessful or unavailable

Contraindications

- Children too small for the tube
- Esophageal trauma or disease
- Caustic ingestion

Advantages

- Rapid insertion
- No special equipment is required
- Does not require sniffing position

Disadvantages

- Impossible to suction trachea when tube is in esophagus
- Adults only

- Unconscious only
- Very difficult to intubate around

Method

- Head—Neutral position.
- Preintubation precautions.
- Insert with jaw-lift at midline.
- Inflate pharyngeal cuff with 100 cc of air.
- Inflate distal cuff with 10 to 15 cc of air.
- Ventilate through longest tube first (pharyngeal).
- Chest rise indicates esophageal placement of distal tip.
- No chest rise indicates tracheal placement; switch ports and ventilate.

Special Considerations

- Good assessment skills are essential to confirm proper placement.
- Misidentification of placement has been reported.
- Reinforce multiple confirmation techniques.

Special Patient Considerations

- Patients with laryngectomies (stomas).
- Mucous plug.
- Laryngectomies possess less efficient cough.
- Mucous commonly obstructs tubes.
- Tube may be removed/cleaned and replaced.
- Stenosis:
  - Stoma spontaneously narrows:
    — Potentially life threatening
    — Soft tissue swelling decreases stoma diameter
  - Tracheal tube is difficult or impossible to replace.
  - ET tube must be placed before total obstruction.

Suctioning

Suctioning must be done with extreme caution if laryngeal edema is suspected.

- Preoxygenate.
- Inject 3 cc sterile saline down trachea.
- Instruct patient to exhale.
- Insert suction catheter until resistance detected.
- Instruct patient to cough or exhale.
- Suction during withdrawal.

Tube Replacement

- Lubricate appropriately sized tracheotomy tube or ET tube (5.0 or greater).
- Instruct patient to exhale.
- Gently insert tube about 1 to 2 cm beyond balloon cuff.
- Inflate balloon cuff.
- Confirm comfort, patency, and proper placement.
- Ensure false lumen was not created.

Dental Appliances

- Dentures, partials, and so on.
- Best removed prior to intubation if they are loose.

AIRWAY MANAGEMENT CONSIDERATIONS FOR PATIENTS WITH FACIAL INJURIES

- Facial injuries lend to a high suspicion of cervical spine injury.
- In-line stabilization is required.
- Foreign body/blood in oropharynx:
  - Suction airway
- Inability to ventilate/intubate orally:
  - Requires surgical intervention

? CHAPTER QUESTIONS

1. The Sellick maneuver is performed by:

   a. lifting up on the back of the patient's neck

   b. lifting the patient's mandible

   c. exerting direct pressure on the patient's cricoids cartilage

   d. exerting direct pressure on the patient's sternum

2. The straight laryngoscope blade used during orotracheal intubation:

   a. fits into the vallecula

   b. is placed past the larynx

   c. directly lifts the epiglottis

   d. rests on the teeth

3. When performing orotracheal intubation on a 2-year-old man, you should use a/an:

   a. 8.0 to 8.5 mm tube

   b. 7.0 to 7.5 mm tube

   c. 6.0 to 6.5 mm uncuffed tube

   d. 4.0 to 5.0 mm uncuffed tube

4. When performing orotracheal intubation, it is necessary to visualize the:

   a. right mainstem bronchus

   b. epiglottis

   c. vallecula

   d. vocal cords

Reference

US Department of Transportation, National Highway Traffic Safety Administration. *EMT-Basic National Standard Curriculum*. Washington, DC: US Department of Transportation, National Highway Traffic Safety Administration; 1994.

Answers to Chapter Questions

Chapter 1   Introduction to Emergency Care

1. **The correct answer is d.** A patient advocate is one who speaks on behalf of the patient, protects the patient, and assures the rights of the patient are not violated.

2. **The correct answer is a.** The EMT-Basic is a physician extender of the system's medical director.

3. **The correct answer is b.** The mission of the NHTSA is to reduce death and disability by providing leadership and coordination to the EMS community in assessing, planning, developing, and promoting comprehensive, evidence-based, emergency medical services and 911 systems.

4. **The correct answer is b.**

Chapter 2   Well-Being of the EMT

1. **The correct answer is b.** The five stages of death and dying are *Denial* ("Not me.") Defense mechanism creating a buffer between shock of dying and dealing with the illness/injury. *Anger* ("Why me.") EMTs may be the target of the anger. Don't take anger or insults personally, be tolerant, and do not become defensive. Employ good listening and communication skills. Be empathetic. *Bargaining* ("OK, but first let me. . .") Agreement that, in the patient's mind, will postpone the death for a short time. *Depression* ("OK, but I haven't. . .") Characterized by sadness and despair. The patient is usually silent and retreats into his own world. *Acceptance* ("OK, I am not afraid.") Does not mean the patient will be happy about dying. The family will usually require more support during this stage than the patient.

2. **The correct answer is d.** Body substance isolation equipment includes gloves, goggles, respiratory mask, and gown.

3. **The correct answer is a.** *Depression* ("OK, but I haven't. . ."), characterized by sadness and despair. The patient is usually silent and retreats into his own world.

4. **The correct answer is a.**

Chapter 3   Medical, Legal, and Ethical Issues

1. **The correct answer is a.**

2. **The correct answer is d.** To prove negligence, the following three elements need to be established: (1) The EMT's action or lack of action incurs injury to the patient. (2) The EMT has violated the standard of care. (3) There was a duty to act.

3. **The correct answer is d.** The EMT can act under implied consent. This means the EMT can assume the patient would want emergency treatment while unconscious or unable to express verbal consent.

4. **The correct answer is c.** Abandonment refers to leaving a patient without transition of care within a hospital or medical facility, or handing over care to a lesser level of care (handing care over to a first responder).

5. **The correct answer is a.** Release of confidential information should never be made to anyone in the press. Information can be released if the EMT is subpoenaed to testify, another health-care provider needs information for the continuity of care, or for billing purposes.

Chapter 4   The Human Body

1. **The correct answer is a.** Physiology refers to the study of the functioning of living organisms.

2. **The correct answer is a.** *Lateral* means away from the midline, *posterior* means located in the rear, and *anterior* means located on the front.

3. **The correct answer is a.** The trachea carries oxygenated air to the lungs and expired air containing carbon dioxide back outside the body.

4. **The correct answer is d.** The left ventricle is responsible for pumping oxygenated blood to all the tissues of the body via the aorta.

5. **The correct answer is d.** The dorsalis pedis is located on the anterior portion of the foot.

Chapter 5   Baseline Vital Signs and History Taking

1. **The correct answer is b.** The top number of the blood pressure refers to the systolic blood pressure.

2. **The correct answer is d.** SAMPLE refers to signs/symptoms, allergies, medications, past/present medical history, last oral intake, events leading to what happened.

3. **The correct answer is c.**

4. **The correct answer is b.** The blue/gray appearance occurs from inadequate tissue perfusion.

Chapter 6   Preparing to Lift and Move Patients

1. **The correct answer is a.** Avoiding using your back in lifting will reduce back injuries.

2. **The correct answer is d.**

3. **The correct answer is a.**

4. **The correct answer is b.**

Chapter 7   Airway Management, Ventilation, and Oxygen Therapy

1. **The correct answer is d.**

2. **The correct answer is a.** The number-one cause of airway compromise in an unconscious patient is airway obstruction from the tongue.

3. **The correct answer is d.**

4. **The correct answer is b.**

5. **The correct answer is b.**

6. **The correct answer is c.**

7. **The correct answer is c.**

8. **The correct answer is d.**

9. **The correct answer is c.**

10. **The correct answer is d.**

Chapter 8   Scene Size-Up/Safety

1. **The correct answer is d.** Scene size-up should be performed on every call.

2. **The correct answer is b.**

3. **The correct answer is c.**

4. **The correct answer is b.**

5. **The correct answer is c.** Every EMS response has the possibility of being dangerous to operate at.

Chapter 9   Patient Assessment

1. **The correct answer is b.** Mechanism of injury refers to what caused the injury or how the patient was injured.

2. **The correct answer is e.**

3. **The correct answer is d.**

4. **The correct answer is a.**

5. **The correct answer is e.**

6. **The correct answer is a.**

7. **The correct answer is c.**

8. **The correct answer is c.**

9. **The correct answer is d.**

10. **The correct answer is c.**

11. **The correct answer is b.**

12. **The correct answer is c.**

13. **The correct answer is b.**

14. **The correct answer is c.**

15. **The correct answer is d.**

Chapter 10   Assessment of the Geriatric Patient

1. **The correct answer is a.**

2. **The correct answer is a.**

3. **The correct answer is c.**

4. **The correct answer is c.**

5. **The correct answer is d.**

6. **The correct answer is d.**

7. **The correct answer is d.**

Chapter 11   Communications

1. **The correct answer is d.**

2. **The correct answer is d.**

3. **The correct answer is a.**

4. **The correct answer is c.**

5. **The correct answer is b.**

6. **The correct answer is b.**

7. **The correct answer is c.**

8. **The correct answer is d.**

Chapter 12   Documentation

1. **The correct answer is d.**

2. **The correct answer is c.**

3. **The correct answer is c.**

4. **The correct answer is b.**

5. **The correct answer is b.**

Chapter 13   General Pharmacology

1. **The correct answer is c.** Penicillin can only be prescribed by a physician. There are no prehospital emergency uses for penicillin.
2. **The correct answer is c.** The medication that EMTs can assist in administration that can be given this route is nitroglycerin.
3. **The correct answer is c.**
4. **The correct answer is d.** The universal medication administered by all EMS personnel is oxygen.
5. **The correct answer is b.**
6. **The correct answer is d.**
7. **The correct answer is b.**

Chapter 14   Respiratory Emergencies

1. **The correct answer is d.**
2. **The correct answer is a.**
3. **The correct answer is c.**
4. **The correct answer is b.**

Chapter 15   Cardiovascular Emergencies

1. **The correct answer is b.** High-concentration oxygen should always be administered to any patient experiencing cardiac compromise.
2. **The correct answer is d.**
3. **The correct answer is a.**
4. **The correct answer is d.**
5. **The correct answer is a.**
6. **The correct answer is a.**
7. **The correct answer is c.**
8. **The correct answer is a.**
9. **The correct answer is c.** Always check medicine for the expiration date. If it is expired, do not use it.
10. **The correct answer is c.** Nitroglycerin is a vasodilator and may cause hypotension.
11. **The correct answer is a.**

Chapter 16   Automated External Defibrillation

1. **The correct answer is c.**
2. **The correct answer is c.**
3. **The correct answer is c.**
4. **The correct answer is d.**

Chapter 17   Altered Mental Status and Diabetic Emergencies

1. **The correct answer is d.** Any insult to the central nervous system may cause a change in mental status.
2. **The correct answer is b.** A common finding when evaluating a seizure patient is lacerations on the tongue from the patient biting down during seizure activity.
3. **The correct answer is a.** The inability of insulin to take glucose into the cells causes an increase in blood sugar.
4. **The correct answer is d.** It is imperative that the patient has an intact gag reflex. A patient with a compromised gag reflex increases the risk of aspiration.

Chapter 18   Acute Stroke

1. **The correct answer is c.**

2. **The correct answer is d.**

3. **The correct answer is b.**

4. **The correct answer is c.**

Chapter 19   Seizures and Syncope

1. **The correct answer is c.** Seizures lasting greater than 10 minutes or seizures occurring without a lucid interval are considered a "true emergency."

2. **The correct answer is d.** This is a commonly prescribed antiseizure medicine.

3. **The correct answer is b.** Seizures lasting for long periods do not allow the patient to breathe properly. This causes hypoxia, in turn causing further complications.

4. **The correct answer is a.**

Chapter 20   Allergic Reactions

1. **The correct answer is b.** Massive vasodilation causes hypotension, tachycardia, and altered mental status.

2. **The correct answer is d.**

3. **The correct answer is c.** Edematous tissue is a common finding from allergic reactions. Edema is caused by fluid leaking from the tissues.

4. **The correct answer is d.** After any medication administration, the EMT-Basic should reassess the patient.

5. **The correct answer is b.** Epinephrine is an adrenergic medicine that causes bronchodilation and peripheral venous constriction.

6. **The correct answer is c.**

Chapter 21   Poisoning and Overdose Emergencies

1. **The correct answer is a.** As with any patient with inadequate ventilation, positive-pressure ventilation is the priority treatment.

Chapter 22   Drug and Alcohol Emergencies

1. **The correct answer is a.**

2. **The correct answer is c.**

Chapter 23   Acute Abdominal Pain

1. **The correct answer is b.**

2. **The correct answer is c.**

Chapter 24   Environmental Emergencies

1. **The correct answer is a.**

2. **The correct answer is d.**

3. **The correct answer is d.**

Chapter 25   Submersion, Drowning, and Diving Emergencies

1. **The correct answer is b.**

2. **The correct answer is c.**

Chapter 26   Behavioral Emergencies

1. **The correct answer is d.**

2. **The correct answer is c.**

Chapter 27   Obstetric and Gynecological Emergencies

1. **The correct answer is a.** Swelling is an indication of toxemia.

2. **The correct answer is a.** Never insert anything into the vaginal opening.

3. **The correct answer is d.**

4. **The correct answer is c.**

5. **The correct answer is c.**

6. **The correct answer is c.**

7. **The correct answer is b.**

8. **The correct answer is a.** This usually means the infant is in distress. It is an ominous sign and ALS should be requested.

9. **The correct answer is c.**

10. **The correct answer is b.**

11. **The correct answer is c.**

12. **The correct answer is c.**

13. **The correct answer is a.** Ectopic pregnancy can cause severe hemorrhage and death.

14. **The correct answer is d.**

15. **The correct answer is a.**

16. **The correct answer is c.**

17. **The correct answer is d.**

18. **The correct answer is b.**

19. **The correct answer is c.**

20. **The correct answer is d.**

Chapter 28   Mechanism of Injury, Kinematics of Trauma

1. **The correct answer is a.**

2. **The correct answer is a.**

Chapter 29   Bleeding and Shock

1. **The correct answer is a.** Hypovolemic shock is the loss of bodily fluid (blood or plasma from injury).

2. **The correct answer is b.**

3. **The correct answer is b.** Myocardial infarction causes death of cardiac muscle tissue; this results in the inability of the heart's "pump" to pump blood effectively.

Chapter 30   Soft Tissue Injuries

1. **The correct answer is d.**

2. **The correct answer is b.** Body substance isolation should be used on every EMS assignment.

3. **The correct answer is c.**

4. **The correct answer is b.**

5. **The correct answer is c.**

6. **The correct answer is b.** Puncture and penetrating wounds tend to have little or no external bleeding.

7. **The correct answer is d.** Controlling bleeding and ensuring air does not enter the wound is vital.

Chapter 31   Burn Emergencies

1. **The correct answer is a.**

2. **The correct answer is b.**

3. **The correct answer is c.**

4. **The correct answer is d.** The abdomen is equal to 9% and the anterior surface of each leg is 9% each.

5. **The correct answer is c.** Because of the increase in body surface area, the pediatric patient has a higher percentage for the head and neck.

Chapter 32   Musculoskeletal Injuries

1. **The correct answer is a.**
2. **The correct answer is a.** A strain is damage or tearing to the tendons. A sprain is overextending or stretching of the ligaments.
3. **The correct answer is d.**
4. **The correct answer is a.**
5. **The correct answer is a.**
6. **The correct answer is b.**

Chapter 33   Head Injuries

1. **The correct answer is a.**
2. **The correct answer is a.** This discoloration is indicative of a significant injury (basal skull fracture).
3. **The correct answer is a.** As intracranial pressure increases, the blood pressure increases, and the pulse decreases. This is known as Cushing reflex.
4. **The correct answer is b.**

Chapter 34   Injuries to the Spine

1. **The correct answer is d.** The cervical spine has 7 vertebrae, thoracic 12, lumbar 5, sacral 5, and the coccyx 4.
2. **The correct answer is a.**
3. **The correct answer is a.**
4. **The correct answer is a.**

Chapter 35   Injuries to the Eyes, Face, and Neck

1. **The correct answer is d.** You should always have a high index of suspicion when treating a patient with a traumatic injury to the face.
2. **The correct answer is b.**

Chapter 36   Chest, Abdomen, and Genitalia Injuries

1. **The correct answer is d.**
2. **The correct answer is c.**

Chapter 37   Agricultural and Industrial Accidents

1. **The correct answer is b.**
2. **The correct answer is c.**
3. **The correct answer is e.**
4. **The correct answer is d.**
5. **The correct answer is a.**

Chapter 38   Infants and Children

1. **The correct answer is a.** Adolescents usually think they are invincible.
2. **The correct answer is b.**
3. **The correct answer is b.**
4. **The correct answer is d.**
5. **The correct answer is b.**
6. **The correct answer is d.**
7. **The correct answer is a.** A partial airway obstruction in a pediatric patient will cause upper airway sounds such as crowing and/or stridor.

8. **The correct answer is d.**

9. **The correct answer is c.** Obtaining a blood pressure on a 2-year-old would be difficult. The best indication of adequate circulation is to evaluate mental status, skin color, moisture, and temperature.

Chapter 39   Ambulance Operations
1. **The correct answer is b.**
2. **The correct answer is b.**
3. **The correct answer is b.**

Chapter 40   Gaining Access and Extrication
1. **The correct answer is d.**
2. **The correct answer is a.**

Chapter 41   Response to Hazardous Materials
1. **The correct answer is c.**
2. **The correct answer is a.**
3. **The correct answer is b.**
4. **The correct answer is d.**
5. **The correct answer is e.**
6. **The correct answer is b.**

Chapter 42   Response to Mass Casualty Incidents/National Incident Management System
1. **The correct answer is b.**
2. **The correct answer is b.**
3. **The correct answer is c.**

Chapter 43   Response to Weapons of Mass Destruction Incidents
1. **The correct answer is a.**
2. **The correct answer is a.**
3. **The correct answer is a.**
4. **The correct answer is d.**

Chapter 44   Advanced Airway Management
1. **The correct answer is c.**
2. **The correct answer is c.**
3. **The correct answer is a.**
4. **The correct answer is d.**

ANSWERS TO CHAPTER CROSSWORDS

Chapter 6   Crossword (Preparatory Review)
Across

1. Auscultation	4. Distal
5. CISD	8. Body
10. Dermis	12. Emergency

Down

1. Anger
2. Systolic
3. Implied consent
6. Power grip
7. Medial
9. Advocate
11. Wet

Chapter 7   Crossword (Airway Review)

Across

1. Bag-valve-mask
4. Bronchi
5. Jaw thrust
10. Tidal
12. Diaphragm
13. Oxygen

Down

2. Airway
3. Suction
6. Tonsil tip
7. Rales
8. Diminished
9. Oropharynx
11. Stoma

Chapter 12   Crossword (Patient Assessment Review)

Across

1. Mechanism
5. Examination
8. CSIC
10. Assessment
13. Age
14. Pulse
15. Pelvis
16. Trauma
20. Repeater
21. Apnea
22. Burns

Down

1. MOI
2. Chief
3. NOI
4. Scene size-up
6. Flail segment
7. Alzheimer
9. GCS
11. SAMPLE
12. Tilt
17. AVPU
18. PCR
19. Skin

Chapter 27   Crossword (Medical Emergencies Review)

Across

1. Auscultation
4. Past
5. Cartoid
8. Facial
11. Stroke
12. Stone
13. Last
14. Oxygen
15. Chambers

Down

2. Contraindication
3. Nitroglycerin
5. COPD
6. Dose
7. Kyphosis
9. AED
10. Insulin

Chapter 37   Crossword (Trauma Review)

Across

1. Kinematics
10. Nines
13. Blood
15. Hypovolemic

8. Sepsis
12. Burn
14. Flail

Down

2. Impaled
4. Cardiac output
6. Cushing
9. Puncture
14. Full

3. MOI
5. Hypoperfusion
7. TBI
11. Dura

Practice Exam

1. You respond to a 25-year-old man who has a large laceration from a suicide attempt. He has blood that is bright red and spurting from the wound. This type of wound indicates what type of bleeding?
   a. venule bleeding
   b. capillary bleeding
   c. arterial bleeding
   d. venous bleeding

2. Serious bleeding is controlled during what part of patient assessment?
   a. detailed physical examination
   b. ongoing assessment
   c. focused history and physical examination
   d. initial assessment

3. The first method of bleeding control used by the EMT is:
   a. direct pressure
   b. tourniquet
   c. elevation
   d. pressure point

4. A major hemorrhage is discovered during the initial assessment of a patient. The EMT should initially:
   a. Hold the injury above the level of the heart and compress the appropriate pressure point.
   b. Apply and inflate a B/P cuff above the wound site until bleeding stops.
   c. Apply direct pressure to the site with a gloved hand.
   d. Finish the initial assessment, then control the bleeding with a pressure bandage.

5. Which of the following steps for bleeding control is in the correct order of preference:
   a. direct pressure, pressure points, tourniquet
   b. pressure points, direct pressure, elevation
   c. elevation, pressure points, direct pressure
   d. direct pressure, elevation, pressure points

6. Tourniquets:
   a. must be loosened every 10 minutes to maintain perfusion
   b. consist of a narrow band such as a belt or cord
   c. are used only to control bleeding of an amputated extremity
   d. aid in the immobilization of an extremity when placed over a joint

7. If you suspect internal bleeding in your patient, remember:
   a. Head injury is more likely to cause unexplained shock than internal bleeding.
   b. Internal bleeding is very obvious and should be identified quickly.
   c. Your suspicion of internal bleeding may be based solely on the mechanism of injury.
   d. The two most common causes of internal bleeding are ruptured aortic aneurysm and ulcers.

8. Signs and symptoms of internal bleeding in an adult patient include:
   a. constricted pupils that are sluggish to respond
   b. capillary refill greater than 2 seconds
   c. slow, deep respirations
   d. dropping blood pressure as a late sign

9. Emergency care for internal bleeding includes:
   a. applying direct manual pressure to affected areas
   b. transporting the patient with head and torso elevated to maintain perfusion to the brain
   c. applying supplemental oxygen via nasal cannula only to prevent cardiac overload
   d. immediate transport for patients with signs and symptoms of shock

10. Important fact(s) about hypoperfusion (shock) that the EMT must remember include:
    a. Tachycardia and tachypnea are late signs of shock.
    b. Restlessness, anxiety, and AMS are usually not associated with shock.
    c. Pediatric patients can compensate and maintain their blood pressure until their blood volume is depleted by almost one-third.
    d. Mechanism of injury is not helpful in determining if the patient is in shock.

11. Which of the following is true regarding hypoperfusion and the body's response?
    a. Death is due to the brain losing control of the body's systems.
    b. Blood is shunted to organs located in the head and trunk of the body.
    c. Most forms of shock can be adequately treated in the field and while en route to the ER.
    d. Peripheral and skin perfusion are generally increased.

12. Which of the following is *true* regarding the causes of shock?
    a. Shock caused by hypoxia is caused by decreased oxygen in the blood, causing the blood vessels to leak.
    b. The brain releases hormones that cause the heart to beat slower, but stronger and the blood vessels to dilate.
    c. Spinal cord damage can cause shock due to systemic vasodilatation.
    d. Heart attack may cause shock due to the constriction of blood vessels, reducing blood flow to the cells.

13. There are several types of shock, but signs and symptoms are generally the same. Medical causes of shock include:
    a. hypovolemic shock from dehydration due to excessive vomiting, diarrhea, and urination
    b. vasogenic shock caused by toxins producing a severe infection, causing vasodilation

   c. anaphylactic shock, caused by an allergic reaction causing blood to leak
      from their vessels

   d. cardiogenic shock, caused by profuse swelling during an illness

14. Blood is shunted away from less vital organs and redirected to the brain,
    heart, and lungs during which stage of shock?

   a. compensated shock

   b. irreversible shock

   c. late-stage shock

   d. progressive or decompensated shock

15. The stage of shock known as compensated shock, shows signs and symptoms
    including:

   a. mutlisystem organ damage

   b. redirection of blood to the vital organs

   c. increased heart rate and vasoconstriction

   d. the need for outside intervention to correct this condition

16. Which of the following is correct regarding irreversible shock?

   a. Even with treatment, if shock has reached this stage, death will result.

   b. The body is able to use its normal defense mechanisms to maintain perfu-
      sion and function without noticeable signs or symptoms.

   c. The need for outside intervention is required for the body to correct itself.

   d. If the blood loss is stopped, the body may replenish the lost volume within
      24 hours.

17. A wound under the skin that involves a blood vessel, characterized by a large
    lump with bluish discoloration is called a(n):

   a. crush injury

   b. concussion

   c. hematoma

   d. contusion

18. When performing the initial assessment and focused history and physical
    examination on a trauma patient, keep in mind that:

   a. Severe bleeding should be treated as soon as your initial assessment is
      completed.

   b. BSI precautions should be taken if there is any external bleeding.

   c. Check for DCAP-BTLS during your rapid trauma assessment.

   d. Obtain a SAMPLE history prior to your physical examination.

19. All types of open wounds have one thing in common, that is:

   a. They all involve underlying soft tissue that is torn loose or pulled com-
      pletely off.

   b. The patient is at risk for contamination with dirt, bacteria, and infection.

   c. They are all more serious internally than they appear externally.

   d. The wounds are all linear.

20. Scraping, rubbing, or shearing away of the outermost layer of the skin is
    called a(n):

   a. contusion

   b. laceration

   c. abrasion

   d. avulsion

21. Which of the following statements is true regarding punctures and penetrations?
    a. Powder burns around a gunshot wound are indicative of a small caliber bullet.
    b. They are often more serious internally than they appear externally.
    c. The entrance wound of a gunshot is larger than the exit wound when shot at close range.
    d. Stab wounds are always easily detected due to the external bleeding.

22. When caring for a patient with a large, open neck injury, remember:
    a. Dark, oozing blood indicates the carotid artery has been damaged.
    b. Apply a pressure dressing circumferentially around the neck to control bleeding.
    c. Cover the wound with an occlusive dressing, taped on three sides.
    d. Immediately place a gloved hand over the wound to prevent air embolism.

23. The layers of skin are:
    a. the epidermis, dermis, and subcutaneous layer
    b. the superficial layer, the partial thickness layer, and the full thickness layer
    c. the primary dermis, secondary dermis, and adjunct dermis
    d. the superior layer, medial layer, and inferior layer

24. Which of the following statements concerning degrees of burn is true?
    a. A first-degree burn is the most serious, and is the most deepest.
    b. A full-thickness burn is also known as a third-degree burn.
    c. A second-degree burn is characterized by red, dry skin.
    d. A superficial burn is also called a second-degree burn.

25. According to the Rule of Nines, which of the following is equal to 9% of an adult's BSA?
    a. external genitalia
    b. the anterior trunk
    c. the head and neck
    d. each lower extremity

26. A patient has sustained hot-liquid burns to the abdomen and anterior portion of each leg. What percentage of BSA has been burned, according to the Rule of Nines?
    a. 45%
    b. 27%
    c. 18%
    d. 36%

27. The difference in the Rule of Nines for a child as opposed to an adult is:
    a. Each lower extremity of the child is 9%.
    b. Each upper extremity of a child is 4.5%.
    c. The head and neck of a child is 18%.
    d. The entire back of a child is 9%.

28. The three kinds of muscles found in the body, each with a specific function, are called:
    a. voluntary, involuntary, and cardiac muscles
    b. controlled, autonomic, and contracting muscles

    c. long, flat, and specialized muscles

    d. flat, striated, and walled muscles

29. Injuries to the musculoskeletal system include:

    a. a dislocation, which is the displacement of a bone

    b. a strain, which is damage to, or tearing of, ligaments

    c. a sprain, which is the overextending or stretching of a muscle and/or tendon

    d. a comminuted injury, which is the detachment of a muscle from a bone

30. Bone and joint injuries may exhibit crepitus, which is:

    a. deformity or angulations of the injured extremity

    b. swelling of the injury site

    c. the discoloration of the skin at and around the injury site

    d. the sound or feeling of broken bone fragments grinding against each other

31. Emergency medical care of bone and joint injuries should include:

    a. splinting any painful extremity

    b. applying a heat pack to the injury to alleviate pain

    c. determining the nature of the injury, such as a fracture, dislocation, etc

    d. realigning deformed extremities prior to splinting

32. The basic reasons for splinting a bone or joint injury include:

    a. preventing further movement to reduce the chance of further injury

    b. replacing exposed bone ends back into the extremity

    c. setting the bone ends back into their proper position

    d. preventing swelling which might complicate the ER physician's examination

33. When caring for an extremity injury, the EMT should assess the distal pulse, motor function, and sensation:

    a. after application of a splint

    b. both before and after application of a splint

    c. prior to application of a splint

    d. every 5 minutes until arrival at the hospital

34. The outermost layer of the three meninges is called the:

    a. pia mater

    b. dura mater

    c. alma mater

    d. arachnoid

35. Signs and symptoms of a brain injury may include:

    a. discoloration noted behind the ears "battle signs"

    b. a ketone odor to the breath, which indicates the presence of CSF

    c. neck vein distention

    d. total or partial paralysis

36. Cushing reflex is a sign of severe head injury, and causes:

    a. seizure-like activity and apnea

    b. increased B/P, decreased pulse, and respiratory pattern changes

    c. decorticate posturing and abnormal breathing patterns

    d. unconsciousness, decerebrate posturing, and vomiting

37. The 12 vertebrae that comprise the upper back are the:
    a. sacral spine
    b. coccyx
    c. lumbar spine
    d. thoracic spine

38. During the initial assessment of a trauma patient:
    a. Initiate immediate manual in-line spinal stabilization based on mechanism of injury.
    b. Open the airway of the unconscious patient using the head-tilt, chin-lift method.
    c. The patient's skin may be cool, pale, and moist below the site of spinal injury, and warm and dry above the site of injury.
    d. Inadequate breathing will result from spinal cord damage involving the lumbar spine.

39. Signs and symptoms of neurogenic shock include:
    a. tachycardia, tachypnea, and hypotension
    b. hypotension, tachycardia, and cool, clammy skin
    c. hypertension, bradycardia, and abnormal breathing patterns
    d. hypotension, bradycardia, and warm, dry skin

40. The three major complications of spinal injury include which of the following?
    a. systemic vasodilation, resulting in reduced perfusion to the tissues
    b. paralysis of the respiratory muscles, occurring with injury to the lumbar spine
    c. paralysis to only one side of the body that does not resolve
    d. inadequate circulation indicated by tachycardia and cool, clammy skin

41. The steps in immobilizing a supine patient to a long backboard include:
    a. securing the patient's torso to the board prior to securing the head
    b. removing the C-collar once the patient is immobilized on the board
    c. no padding placed on the board, as it might move the spine out of alignment
    d. using the log roll, a move ideally performed by two rescuers, one at the head, the other at the hips

42. A patient that sustained a traumatic injury to the face must also be assessed for:
    a. brain injury
    b. airway obstruction
    c. spinal injury
    d. all of the above

43. Double vision, a marked decrease in vision, or a loss of sensation above the eyebrow, over the cheek, or in the upper lip may be caused by:
    a. detached retina
    b. orbital fracture
    c. cervical spine injury
    d. temporal bone fracture

44. Treatment for a patient with a chemical burn to the eye includes:
    a. transporting the patient on his side and continue irrigation throughout the transport
    b. irrigating chemicals from the eye from the corner of the eye, across the bridge of the nose

   c. flushing the eye with a chemical antidote, such as baking soda solution

   d. leaving contact lenses in, as trying to remove them may cause damage to the eye

45. Paradoxical movement is caused by:

   a. increased use of the diaphragm to breathe due to injury to the chest

   b. a flail segment moving in the opposite direction of the uninjured side of the rib cage

   c. one damaged lung not inflating as much as the undamaged lung

   d. a tension pneumothorax limiting the expansion of the injured side of the chest

46. A patient presents with a right-sided flail chest segment, difficulty breathing, diminished lung sounds, and tracheal deviation toward the left side. You suspect:

   a. a tension pneumothorax

   b. an open wound that you cannot see

   c. a hemothorax

   d. a pneumothorax

47. You should immediately seal, with a gloved hand, any open injury to the:

   a. axillary area

   b. back

   c. chest

   d. all of the above

48. Vital signs of an unstable patient should be reassessed and recorded:

   a. every 15 minutes

   b. every 10 minutes

   c. every 5 minutes

   d. whenever a new care provider assumes care

49. An EMT is permitted, with medical direction, to administer, or assist the patient in administering, all of the following *except:*

   a. nitroglycerin

   b. oxygen

   c. penicillin

   d. oral glucose

50. Medications administered sublingually are:

   a. swallowed

   b. inhaled

   c. dissolved under the tongue

   d. injected under the skin

51. EMTs can assist with administration of which of the following medications?

   a. epinephrine

   b. metered-dose inhalers

   c. nitroglycerin

   d. all of the above

52. Which of the following is true regarding medication routes-of-administration?
    a. Most medications administered by the EMT-Basic are administered by injection.
    b. All medications are administered by the oral route.
    c. The route that is chosen controls how quickly the medication is absorbed by the body.
    d. Drugs administered by the sublingual route have a relatively slow rate of absorption.

53. A drug administered by EMTs which is used for a wide range of medical and traumatic emergencies are:
    a. Tylenol
    b. glucose
    c. nitroglycerin
    d. oxygen

54. The EMT-Basic may administer which of the following medications to treat a severe allergic reaction?
    a. Glutose
    b. Adrenalin
    c. LiquiChar
    d. Alupent

55. A 26-year-old female patient has breathing difficulty, and has been prescribed a bronchodilator. Having met all the requirements to administer the medication, the steps include:
    a. placing the patient on a nasal cannula for convenience
    b. leaving the oxygen off the patient until you can assess if the medication worked
    c. having the patient inhale fully, then place her lips around the mouthpiece
    d. having the patient hold her breath as long as is comfortable after inhaling the medication

56. When administering a metered-dose inhaler, tips for the procedure include:
    a. depressing the canister just before the patient begins inhaling
    b. coaching the patient to hold his breath as long as possible after inhaling the medication
    c. having the patient breathe in and out quickly
    d. being careful not to shake the canister

57. A disease process characterized by destruction of the alveolar walls and distention of the alveolar sacs is a type of COPD called:
    a. asthma
    b. chronic bronchitis
    c. pneumonia
    d. emphysema

58. Trace, in order, the pathway the blood takes through the heart and lungs:
    a. aorta, right atrium, right ventricle, lungs, left atrium, left ventricle, pulmonary artery
    b. pulmonary vein, right atrium, right ventricle, lungs, left atrium, left ventricle, aorta

   c. vena cava, right atrium, right ventricle, pulmonary arteries, lungs, pulmonary veins, left atrium, left ventricle, aorta

   d. vena cava, left atrium, left ventricle, lungs, right atrium, right ventricle, aorta

59. Which of the following is true regarding the heart and blood vessels?

   a. The pulmonary veins carry oxygen-depleted blood from the heart to the lungs.

   b. The left ventricle pumps blood from the heart to the lungs.

   c. The right ventricle has the largest muscle mass of the heart.

   d. The pulmonary arteries carry oxygen-depleted blood from the heart to the lungs.

60. The purpose of the valves in the heart is to:

   a. push the flow of blood in the proper direction

   b. prevent the blood from leaving the heart too soon

   c. keep the oxygen-depleted blood from mixing with oxygen-rich blood

   d. prevent a backflow of blood in the system

61. Trace an electrical impulse through the conduction system of the heart, in order:

   a. SA node, bundle of His, AV node, Purkinje fibers

   b. AV node, Purkinje fibers, SA node, bundle of His

   c. SA node, AV node, bundle of His, Purkinje fibers

   d. AV node, bundle of His, SA node, Purkinje fibers

62. Which of the following statements is *true* regarding blood pressure?

   a. The diastolic pressure represents the pressure exerted against a venous wall during contraction of the left ventricle.

   b. The systolic pressure represents the pressure exerted against an arterial wall during relaxation of the left ventricle.

   c. Two distinct pressures can be obtained when using only a sphygmomanometer.

   d. The smaller the artery the greater the resistance and the higher the diastolic pressure.

63. If blood is not circulated adequately through the body's capillaries, cells become starved for oxygen and nutrients and become overloaded with carbon dioxide and waste products. This condition is known as:

   a. circulatory depression

   b. hypotension

   c. hypoperfusion

   d. cardiac compromise

64. In events that compromise cardiac function, time becomes a crucial element for patient survival. Which of the following is *true* regarding cardiac compromise?

   a. Any adult with chest pain should be treated as a cardiac emergency until proven otherwise.

   b. Immediate transport of the patient with a cardiac emergency is not necessary, as the damage has already been done.

   c. CPR should be started within 4 minutes of the event to be effective.

   d. Unfortunately, there are no medications currently used that limit damage to heart muscle during a cardiac event.

65. When treating a child 8 years of age or younger who is unresponsive and has no breathing or pulse, you should do all of the following *except:*
a. Ventilate with high-concentration oxygen.
b. Begin CPR.
c. Apply an automated external defibrillator that is equipped for pediatric defibrillation.
d. Ensure an open airway.
e. Administer high-concentration oxygen via nonrebreather mask.

66. When assessing a *responsive* adult patient with a possible cardiac compromise, you should:
a. Insert an airway adjunct.
b. Apply oxygen at 15 L/min via non-rebreather mask.
c. Ventilate with high-concentration oxygen.
d. Begin CPR.

67. The mnemonic used to obtain a description of the patient's chest pain is:
a. SAMPLE
b. AVPU
c. DCAP-BTLS
d. OPQRST

68. When asking about the quality of chest pain, you are asking:
a. if the pain is sharp, dull, burning, or squeezing
b. what the patient was doing at the time the pain began
c. for the patient to rate the pain on a scale of 1 to 10
d. if the pain travels to any other part of the body

69. When using the mnemonic OPQRST, the "P" stands for:
a. pressure
b. pallor
c. perspiration
d. provocation

70. You assess your cardiac compromise patient for peripheral edema because:
a. This condition suggests heart failure.
b. The patient might be going into shock from fluid shifting.
c. This may indicate cardiac tamponade.
d. This condition indicates hypoxia.

71. When caring for a conscious patient with cardiac compromise, you should place him in:
a. a position of most comfort to him
b. the Trendelenburg position
c. the left lateral recumbent position
d. a supine position

72. Nitroglycerin eases chest pain by:
a. constricting blood vessels and sending more blood back to the heart
b. increasing the amount of oxygen absorbed by the blood in the lungs
c. increasing the diameter of blood vessels and decreasing the workload of the heart
d. relaxing the patient and reducing anxiety

73. Which of the following is true regarding AED's?

    a. Manual defibrillators can deliver the first shock more quickly than AEDs.

    b. The AED operator must know how to recognize various heart rhythms.

    c. AEDs allow "hands-free" defibrillation which is safer for EMS personnel.

    d. AEDs require paramedics to operate them.

74. On which of the following patients would the AED *not* be applied?

    a. a traumatic cardiac arrest patient involved in a motor vehicle crash

    b. a 54-year-old female patient, pulseless, apneic, who collapsed in the kitchen

    c. a 64-year-old man, conscious and breathing, with a heart rate of 188 per minute

    d. a 6-year-old girl electrocuted with no pulse and no breathing

75. As soon as you find your adult patient is in cardiac arrest you should immediately:

    a. begin CPR for a minimum of 2 minutes and apply the AED and begin the defibrillation process

    b. obtain the patient's history from family or bystanders if possible

    c. begin ventilating the patient with high-concentration oxygen

    d. manage the airway by inserting an oropharyngeal airway

76. While transporting a patient with no pulse, remember:

    a. to arrange for an advanced life support rendezvous, if possible

    b. if the patient regains a pulse, then goes back into cardiac arrest, you may administer the maximum number of shocks allowed again

    c. no matter what the maximum number of shocks you may give per protocol, medical control can order you to make additional attempts at defibrillation

    d. all of the above

77. A change in a patient's mental status is an indication that the central nervous system has been affected in some manner. Causes may include:

    a. brain injury due to trauma

    b. alteration in the patient's blood oxygen level

    c. alteration in the patient's blood sugar level

    d. any of the above

78. Common signs and symptoms of altered mental status associated with trauma include:

    a. stiff neck

    b. abnormal respiratory pattern

    c. hot, dry, red skin

    d. pinpoint pupils

79. During your assessment of a patient with altered mental status, you note lacerations to the tongue. You should become suspicious of:

    a. a physical attack on the patient

    b. seizure activity

    c. loose dentures and possible airway compromise

    d. a suicide attempt

80. A high level of glucose in the blood is caused by:

    a. a lack of insulin to take glucose into the cells

    b. an adequate amount of insulin, but too much glucose in the blood

    c. too much glucose entering the cells of the body

    d. too much insulin leaving too much glucose in the blood

81. Contraindications to the use of glucose in a patient with altered mental status and a history of medication-controlled diabetes include:

    a. If it is unknown if the patient has taken insulin today.

    b. The patient taking insulin today, but not eating.

    c. A history of type II diabetes.

    d. The patient does not have an intact gag reflex.

82. Signs and symptoms of a neurological deficit include:

    a. chest pain

    b. cool, clammy skin

    c. paralysis or weakness

    d. deep, regular respirations

83. General signs and symptoms of stroke include:

    a. severe headache

    b. sudden weakness or paralysis of face, arm, or leg

    c. difficulty speaking or slurred speech

    d. all of the above

84. Which of the following is correct regarding stroke, or CVA?

    a. The cause is very different from that of a heart attack.

    b. Stroke may cause loss of bladder or bowel control, nausea, and vomiting.

    c. About 25% of all stroke victims die.

    d. The onset of the signs and symptoms is usually gradual, sometimes over days.

85. Which of the following statements is true regarding paralysis caused by stroke?

    a. It is common for both sides of the body to be paralyzed from stroke.

    b. It is difficult to distinguish stroke from spinal injury, as both can cause paralysis to both legs.

    c. Typically, paralysis from strokes affects only one side of the body.

    d. It is a good sign when weakness is only experienced in the extremities, as these patients will not deteriorate further.

86. Seizure patients should be classified as a priority for transport if:

    a. The patient has a history of epilepsy and has not taken antiseizure medication for more than 24 hours.

    b. The seizure lasts longer than 5 minutes.

    c. A second seizure occurs without a period of responsiveness between the seizure episodes.

    d. The patient is still in the post-ictal state upon your arrival.

87. Medications commonly used in the treatment of epilepsy include:

    a. Nitrostat

    b. Proventil

    c. epinephrine

    d. phenobarbitol

88. If a seizure patient has been seizing for over 10 minutes you should:
    a. Apply high-concentration oxygen by nonrebreather mask and transport immediately.
    b. Insert a nasopharyngeal airway and begin positive pressure ventilation.
    c. Protect the patient from injuring himself until the seizure stops.
    d. Begin CPR and transport immediately.

89. A sudden, temporary loss of consciousness due to a temporary lack of blood flow to the brain is called:
    a. syncope
    b. a seizure
    c. stroke
    d. a TIA

90. Anaphylactic shock is brought about by:
    a. fluid loss due to tissue swelling
    b. massive systemic vasodilation
    c. decreased contractility of the heart
    d. pulmonary hemorrhage

91. An allergen may enter the body through:
    a. the respiratory tract
    b. skin
    c. the GI tract
    d. any of the above

92. During your initial assessment of a patient with an allergic reaction, you may find:
    a. a slow, bounding pulse
    b. strong distal pulses in the feet
    c. edema of the face, neck, lips, hands, and feet
    d. tiny bruises from ruptured capillaries

93. Once epinephrine has been administered to a patient you should:
    a. Routinely administer a second dose after 10 minutes, if available.
    b. Administer an over-the-counter antihistamine for long-term relief.
    c. See marked improvement and allow the patient to remain home if he wants.
    d. Reassess the patient after 2 minutes.

94. Epinephrine is the drug of choice for the emergency treatment of severe allergic reactions and:
    a. Comes packaged in a vial with a separate syringe and needle.
    b. Quickly causes peripheral vasoconstriction and relaxes the smooth muscles in the lungs to improve breathing.
    c. The same dose is administered to both children and adults.
    d. Works immediately and lasts for up to 2 hours.

95. Steps included in administering epinephrine by auto-injector include:
    a. drawing up the medication into the syringe
    b. pushing the injector firmly into the patients buttocks until the needle is deployed and the medication is delivered
    c. holding the injector in place until all the medication has been injected
    d. placing the injector back into its container for reuse

96. Emergency care for inhalation poisoning includes:
    a. starting PPV with supplemental O_2 immediately if breathing is inadequate
    b. applying O_2 via nonrebreather mask for apneic patients
    c. decontaminating completely with water from head to toe
    d. transporting the patient in the Trendelenburg position to facilitate blood flow to the brain

97. Abdominal pain is considered serious and a high priority when:
    a. There is a sudden, severe onset.
    b. It's accompanied by syncope and hypotension.
    c. It has lasted for more than an hour.
    d. It's accompanied by fever and vomiting.

98. A 59 year-old man describes a sudden onset of severe, constant abdominal pain that radiates to his lower back. The pain is described as "tearing". On physical examination, you note a pulsating abdominal mass upon palpation of the area. You suspect:
    a. esophageal varices
    b. intestinal obstruction
    c. abdominal aortic aneurysm
    d. ulcer

99. Hypothermia occurs when:
    a. The body loses more heat than it produces.
    b. Cold food or drink is ingested.
    c. The body produces more heat than it loses.
    d. Specific parts of the body are exposed to cold temperatures.

100. Emergency care for local cold injuries include:
    a. packing the affected area with snow or a cold pack
    b. encouraging the patient to walk on an injured extremity to restore circulation
    c. rubbing the affected area to restore circulation as soon as possible
    d. immersing the affected area in warm (tepid) water, just above body temperature (100°F-105°F)

101. All of the following are considered heat-related emergencies, except:
    a. heat cramps
    b. heat exhaustion
    c. heat stroke
    d. heat crabs

102. The organ through which the fetus receives oxygen and nourishment from the mother is the:
    a. placenta
    b. umbilical cord
    c. amniotic sac
    d. uterus

103. The fluid-filled bag in which the infant floats is called the:
    a. placenta
    b. uterus
    c. amniotic sac
    d. vagina

104. During the first stage of labor, which of the following occurs?

    a. The placenta separates from the uterine wall.

    b. The cervix becomes fully dilated.

    c. The infant's head appears at the opening of the birth canal.

    d. All of the above.

105. Indications that delivery is imminent include:

    a. the onset of contractions

    b. bulging of the perineum

    c. the "bloody show"

    d. the breaking of the amniotic sac

106. During the third stage of labor:

    a. The infant is actually delivered.

    b. The amniotic sac ruptures.

    c. The placenta is expelled from the uterus.

    d. The head of the infant appears at the opening of the birth canal.

107. Questions that should be asked regarding due date include:

    a. How many previous pregnancies are there?

    b. How many children does the patient have?

    c. Has the patient had any prenatal care?

    d. All of the above.

108. Which of the following conditions indicate a predelivery emergency for a pregnant patient?

    a. swelling of the face and/or extremities

    b. a fever

    c. flu-like symptoms

    d. nausea

109. Vaginal bleeding is discovered during your physical examination. You should:

    a. Place a sanitary napkin over the vaginal opening.

    b. Massage the uterus to control internal bleeding.

    c. Pack the vagina with sterile gauze or a dressing.

    d. Apply direct pressure to the vaginal area until bleeding is controlled.

110. Which of the following is true regarding trauma to a pregnant woman?

    a. Keep spine boards absolutely flat to facilitate blood flow to the fetus.

    b. Even minor trauma to the abdomen can cause serious fetal injuries.

    c. Early signs of shock are very obvious in pregnant women.

    d. If a pregnant woman dies as a result of an accident, CPR may save the life of the unborn infant.

111. Expect delivery of the infant within a few minutes if:

    a. The patient's "water breaks".

    b. The patient's abdomen gets very soft.

    c. The patient has the sensation of a bowel movement.

    d. Contractions are 5 minutes apart, and last 15 to 30 seconds.

112. Emergency care of the patient in active labor for a normal delivery includes:
    a. immediately clamping and cutting the umbilical cord if wrapped around the infant's neck
    b. suctioning the infant's nose first, as newborns are obligate nose-breathers
    c. exerting gentle pressure against the infant's skull to prevent explosive delivery
    d. having the patient lay on her left side during the delivery

113. As your patient delivers the infant, your care should include:
    a. holding the infant upside down by the feet to help drain fluid
    b. cutting, then clamping, the umbilical cord
    c. massaging the uterus to decrease vaginal bleeding after delivery
    d. yanking on the umbilical cord after delivery to assist with placental expulsion

114. Pregnancy begins with a fertilized egg. Normally, the fertilized egg attaches itself to the lining of the uterus. An ectopic pregnancy means:
    a. The egg has implanted outside the uterus.
    b. A naturally aborted fetus due to any number of reasons.
    c. A pregnancy that continues past the expected due date.
    d. The fetus is developing in an abnormal position in the uterus.

Questions 115-124 Scenarios: Each of the questions or incomplete statements below is followed by suggested answers or completions. Select the one BEST answer in each case.

115. You are called to residential neighborhood at 1:00 AM where your patient has just finished eating a super-sized meal of deep fried food. The patient is now complaining of "crampy" pain in the right upper quadrant "RUQ" and has had two episodes of nausea and vomiting with green emesis. You suspect that your patient is suffering from:
    a. a peptic ulcer
    b. an intestinal obstruction
    c. cholecystitis (gall bladder attack)
    d. appendicitis

116. You are called to a private residence for an unknown emergency. Law enforcement is not on scene. You walk into the residence and find an elderly man sitting among bottles of whiskey, crying over a picture. You observe a pistol in the patient's waistband. Your first action should be to:
    a. Ask the patient why he is so sad.
    b. Determine if the patient wants to kill himself.
    c. Slowly and calmly back out of the room.
    d. Charge the patient and pin him down.

117. It is mid-summer and you have been dispatched to a local park for a man down. You arrive and observe a workman who appears to be in his 40s lying supine. He is in the full sun and is next to a ditch. A coworker informs you that the patient was digging the ditch and just passed out. The patient's eyes are closed and he does not respond to your voice or painful stimuli. His respirations are deep and rapid. His pulse is 110 per minute, regular, and strong. His skin is hot and slightly moist. The coworker further informs you that the patient had complained of a headache and nausea for at least 30 minutes prior to passing out. Which action should be taken first?
    a. Administer oxygen at 15 L/min.
    b. Apply cold packs to the patient's body.
    c. Remove the patient's clothing.
    d. Move the patient to a cooler environment.

118. The patient in the above question would be considered:
   a. a high-priority transport
   b. a medium priority transport
   c. a low-priority transport
   d. a patient not requiring transport

119. A call comes into dispatch from a local beach. The caller tells the dispatcher there has been a drowning at cedar beach. Bystanders pulled a young man from the water who is now sitting on the beach coughing up small amounts of water. He states that he does not believe he needs to go to the hospital because he only swallowed a small amount of water. What should you do?
   a. Agree with the patient because a small amount of water is not harmful.
   b. Explain to the patient that if he wants to he can go to the hospital in his friend's car.
   c. Explain to the patient the implications involved with a near-drowning and attempt to convince the patient to allow you to transport him to be evaluated in the emergency department.
   d. Have him make an appointment to see his family physician the next day after the incident.

120. You are called to the scene for a possible chlorine leak. As you pull up to the scene, you see two victims lying on the ground by a tool shed. As an EMT your immediate action(s) include:
   a. Removing the victims from the scene to prevent further injury.
   b. Immediately providing positive pressure ventilation to the victims to prevent further hypoxia.
   c. Rapidly extricate the patients from the chlorine gas.
   d. Moving to a safe environment uphill and upwind and contacting the fire department.

121. While you are transporting a patient who has overdosed on sleeping pills, the respiratory rate decreases from 20 to 8 times a minute. Your immediate next action should be to:
   a. Administer activated charcoal.
   b. Provide positive pressure ventilations with high-concentration oxygen.
   c. Administer oxygen by nonrebreather mask.
   d. Position the patient in the Trendelenburg position.

122. Your ambulance unit arrives on-scene to find a young woman outside of the residence hysterically crying. She ushers you and your partner inside where you find your patient supine on the kitchen floor. The patient's wife tells you that he just got back from running and complained of the "worst headache of my life" and fell to the ground. You suspect what type of illness?
   a. myocardial infarction
   b. hemorrhagic stroke
   c. occlusive stroke
   d. TIA

123. All suicidal or violent threats or gestures must be taken seriously. These patients should be in police custody if they pose a danger to themselves or others. If the patient poses a danger to themselves and/or others, summon police for assistance.
   a. True
   b. False

124. If chest pain is present, the patient possesses nitroglycerin prescribed by his/her physician and has a systolic blood pressure of 120 mm Hg or greater, the EMT may assist the patient in self-administration of the patient's prescribed sublingual nitroglycerin as indicated on the medicine container.
    a. True
    b. False

125. If patient has an early *or superficial* local cold injury:
    a. Remove jewelry.
    b. Cover the exposed area with dry dressings.
    c. Do not rub, massage, break blisters, apply heat, rewarm, or allow the patient to walk on the affected extremity.
    d. All of the above is correct.

126. Generalized hypothermia treatment includes the following *except*:
    a. Place the patient in a warm, draft-free environment.
    b. Gently remove wet clothing.
    c. Assess pulses for 30 to 45 seconds. If no pulse, begin CPR.
    d. Walk the patient to the ambulance.

Please refer to the following diagram for questions 127 and 128.

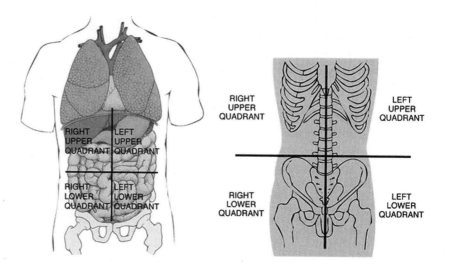

127. The main organ found in the Right Upper Quadrant is:
    a. stomach
    b. urinary bladder
    c. liver
    d. heart

128. The main organ found in the Left Upper Quadrant is:
    a. stomach
    b. urinary bladder
    c. liver
    d. heart

129. Your patient complains of chest pain. He has no known prior history of this sort of pain. Which of the following questions should you ask?
    a. "Is your pain crushing and heavy?"
    b. "Is your pain dull?"
    c. "How would you describe your pain?"
    d. All of the above.

130. Your patient is a 78-year-old man with a history of chest pain. You should find out which medications he takes during the
    a. SAMPLE history
    b. OPQRST examination
    c. ongoing assessment
    d. initial assessment

131. A 23-year-old patient just had a seizure. Following the seizure, he is awake enough to tell you he is an epileptic. Why is this history important?
    a. It provides you information to give to the hospital staff.
    b. The history helps determine what interventions you may take.
    c. The history helps determine the nature of the illness.
    d. All of the above.

132. Your 36-year-old male patient tells you he is a diabetic. What is the first step of your focused history and physical examination?
    a. Conduct a rapid physical examination.
    b. Obtain baseline vital signs.
    c. Gather a SAMPLE history.
    d. Conduct a focused physical examination.

133. A 77-year-old male patient is unresponsive but breathing. You should obtain pertinent patient information from:
    a. bystanders or family
    b. the family physician
    c. the responding advanced life support unit
    d. all of the above

134. A 10-year-old medical patient is unresponsive. The first step in the focused history and physical examination should be:
    a. a SAMPLE history from family members
    b. a rapid physical examination
    c. a history of childhood illnesses from family members
    d. physical examination of the head and chest

135. A 25-year-old female patient is unresponsive. During the rapid physical examination of her neck you should look for:
    a. jugular vein disclosure
    b. a medical identification device
    c. paradoxical respirations
    d. muscle spasms

136. A disease which affects the elderly commonly called "hardening of the arteries" is:
    a. arteriosclerosis
    b. cardiac hypertrophy
    c. kyphosis
    d. osteoporosis

137. A "mini stroke" having a similar presentation to a CVA in which signs and symptoms subside within 24 hours is called a(n):
    a. TIA
    b. ICP
    c. CHF
    d. COPD

138. Alzheimer disease is responsible for more than 100,000 deaths each year in the United States. While the disease does not directly cause death, it can result in:
    a. sudden cardiac arrest
    b. numerous infections
    c. CVA
    d. hypoglycemia

139. Epinephrine supplied in auto-injectors is a medication that is:
    a. administered sublingually
    b. sprayed into a patient's airway
    c. given by mouth
    d. administered intramuscularly

140. Oral glucose comes as what form of medication?
    a. fine powder
    b. gel
    c. sublingual spray
    d. liquid

141. A 50-year-old female patient has chronic bronchitis. The initial assessment finds her breathing rate is 6 times per minute and her skin is cool and clammy to the touch. Your next action should be to:
    a. Administer oxygen by nasal cannula at 15 L/min.
    b. Assist respirations with positive pressure ventilations and supplemental oxygen at 15 L/min.
    c. Administer oxygen by non-rebreather mask at 15 L/min.
    d. Place the patient in sitting position, and reassess breathing.

142. When using an automated external defibrillator, you should defibrillate:
    a. after analysis of rhythm and shock is indicated
    b. after hooking up oxygen
    c. after on-line approval from medical direction
    d. after hooking up oxygen and obtaining on-line medical approval

143. Hypoglycemia is a condition characterized by:
    a. low blood sugar
    b. high blood insulin level
    c. high blood sugar
    d. low blood insulin level

144. A diabetic with high blood sugar levels needs which of the following to correct the condition?

    a. Orinase

    b. Diabinese

    c. insulin

    d. Insta-glucose

145. Your diabetic patient became unresponsive after you administered oral glucose. Your next step should be to:

    a. Give a second dose of oral glucose.

    b. Use tongue depressor to inspect the airway.

    c. Ensure an open airway.

    d. Use a tongue depressor as a bite-block in case of seizures.

146. You arrive on the scene where a patient is experiencing seizure activity. A bystander has placed a spoon in the patient's mouth. You should:

    a. Restrain the patient's movements.

    b. Gently hold the spoon in place.

    c. Remove the spoon.

    d. Hold the spoon in place and grab the patient's tongue.

147. All of the following are stages of the grand mal seizure *except* the:

    a. syncopal stage

    b. aura

    c. clonic phase

    d. postical state

148. Status epilepticus is defined as a seizure which lasts longer than:

    a. 3 minutes

    b. 5 minutes

    c. 10 minutes

    d. 15 minutes

149. A 23-year-old female patient has a history of allergies to bee stings. She is complaining of breathing difficulty after being stung by a wasp. She has a prescribed epinephrine auto-injector. Your next action should be to:

    a. Administer oxygen and transport.

    b. Identify the insect that stung her.

    c. Administer oxygen and assist the patient with the auto-injector.

    d. Perform ongoing assessment and administer oxygen.

150. Carbon monoxide is a poison which may enter the body by:

    a. inhalation

    b. ingestion

    c. absorption

    d. all of the above

Practice Exam Answers

1. The correct answer is "c".

2. The correct answer is "d".

3. The correct answer is "a".

4. The correct answer is "c".

5. The correct answer is "d".

6. The correct answer is "a".

7. The correct answer is "c".

8. The correct answer is "d".

9. The correct answer is "d".

10. The correct answer is "c".

11. The correct answer is "b".

12. The correct answer is "c".

13. The correct answer is "a".

14. The correct answer is "d".

15. The correct answer is "c".

16. The correct answer is "a".

17. The correct answer is "d".

18. The correct answer is "b".

19. The correct answer is "b".

20. The correct answer is "c".

21. The correct answer is "b".

22. The correct answer is "d".

23. The correct answer is "a".

24. The correct answer is "b".

25. The correct answer is "c".

26. **The correct answer is "b".** The external genitalia is =1%, the anterior trunk =18%, each lower extremity is =18%.

27. **The correct answer is "c".**

28. **The correct answer is "a".**

29. **The correct answer is "a".** A **strain** is an injury to a muscle or tendon in which the muscle fibers tear as a result of overstretching. A sprain is an injury to ligaments that is caused by being stretched beyond their normal capacity and possibly torn.

30. **The correct answer is "d".**

31. **The correct answer is "d".**

32. **The correct answer is "a".**

33. **The correct answer is "b".**

34. **The correct answer is "b".** The middle layer is the arachnoid and the innermost layer is called the pia mater.

35. **The correct answer is "a".**

36. **The correct answer is "b".**

37. **The correct answer is "d".**

38. **The correct answer is "a".**

39. **The correct answer is "b".**

40. **The correct answer is "a".**

41. **The correct answer is "a".**

42. **The correct answer is "d".**

43. **The correct answer is "b".**

44. **The correct answer is "a".**

45. **The correct answer is "b".**

46. **The correct answer is "a".**

47. **The correct answer is "d".**

48. **The correct answer is "c".**

49. **The correct answer is "c".**

50. **The correct answer is "c".**

51. **The correct answer is "d".**

52. **The correct answer is "c".**

53. **The correct answer is "d".**

54. **The correct answer is "b".**

55. **The correct answer is "d".**

56. **The correct answer is "b".**

57. **The correct answer is "d".**

58. The correct answer is "c".

59. The correct answer is "d".

60. The correct answer is "d".

61. The correct answer is "c".

62. The correct answer is "c".

63. The correct answer is "c".

64. The correct answer is "a".

65. The correct answer is "e".

66. The correct answer is "b".

67. The correct answer is "d".

68. The correct answer is "a".

69. The correct answer is "d".

70. The correct answer is "a".

71. The correct answer is "a".

72. The correct answer is "c".

73. The correct answer is "c".

74. The correct answer is "c".

75. The correct answer is "a".

76. The correct answer is "d".

77. The correct answer is "d".

78. The correct answer is "b".

79. The correct answer is "b".

80. The correct answer is "a".

81. The correct answer is "d".

82. The correct answer is "c".

83. The correct answer is "d".

84. The correct answer is "b".

85. The correct answer is "c".

86. The correct answer is "c".

87. The correct answer is "d".

88. The correct answer is "b".

89. The correct answer is "a".

90. The correct answer is "b".

91. The correct answer is "d".

92. The correct answer is "c".

93. The correct answer is "d".

94. The correct answer is "b".

95. The correct answer is "c".

96. The correct answer is "a".

97. The correct answer is "b".

98. The correct answer is "c".

99. The correct answer is "a".

100. The correct answer is "d".

101. The correct answer is "d".

102. The correct answer is "a".

103. The correct answer is "c".

104. The correct answer is "b".

105. The correct answer is "b".

106. The correct answer is "c".

107. The correct answer is "d".

108. The correct answer is "a".

109. The correct answer is "a".

110. The correct answer is "d".

111. The correct answer is "c".

112. The correct answer is "c".

113. The correct answer is "c".

114. The correct answer is "a".

115. The correct answer is "c".

116. The correct answer is "c".

117. The correct answer is "d".

118. The correct answer is "a".

119. The correct answer is "c".

120. The correct answer is "d".

121. The correct answer is "b".

122. The correct answer is "b".

123. The correct answer is "a".

124. The correct answer is "a".

125. The correct answer is "d".

126. The correct answer is "d".

127. The correct answer is "c".

128. The correct answer is "a".

129. The correct answer is "c".

130. The correct answer is "a".

131. The correct answer is "d".

132. The correct answer is "c".

133. The correct answer is "a".

134. The correct answer is "a".

135. The correct answer is "a".

136. The correct answer is "a".

137. The correct answer is "a".

138. The correct answer is "b".

139. The correct answer is "d".

140. The correct answer is "b".

141. The correct answer is "b".

142. The correct answer is "a".

143. The correct answer is "a".

144. The correct answer is "c".

145. The correct answer is "c".

146. The correct answer is "c".

147. The correct answer is "a".

148. The correct answer is "c".

149. The correct answer is "c".

150. The correct answer is "a".

Index

Page numbers followed by *f* or *t* indicate figures or tables, respectively.